Therapeutic Arts in Pregnancy, Birth and New Parenthood

W0246442

Therapeutic Arts in Pregnancy, Birth and New Parenthood explores the use of arts in relation to infertility, pregnancy, childbirth and new parenthood. It is the first book to bring all these subjects together into one accessible volume with an international perspective.

The book looks at the role of the arts in health with respect to the pregnancy journey, from conception to new parenthood. It introduces readers to the ways in which art is being used with women who are experiencing different stages of childbearing – who may be unable to conceive and are struggling with infertility treatment, or who experience miscarriage and loss, a traumatic birth, or grief over the loss of a baby. It also elucidates how art-making offers a means for women to express and understand their changed sense of self-identity and sexuality as a result of pregnancy and motherhood.

The book has an international compass and is essential reading for arts therapy trainees and arts in health courses and will also be of interest to other health professionals and artists.

Susan Hogan is Professor of Arts and Health, University of Derby, and a Professorial Fellow, Institute of Mental Health, University of Nottingham. Her books to-date are: *Feminist Approaches to Art Therapy; Healing Arts: The History of Art Therapy; Gender Issues in Art Therapy; Conception Diary: Thinking About Pregnancy and Motherhood; Revisiting Feminist Approaches to Art Therapy; The Introductory Guide to Art Therapy; Art Therapy Theories: A Critical Introduction; Arts Therapies and Gender Issues: International Perspectives on Research; Gender and Difference in the Arts Therapies: Inscribed on the Body* and *The Maternal Tug: Ambivalence, Identity, and Agency.*

Therapeutic Arts in Pregnancy, Birth and New Parenthood

Edited by Professor Susan Hogan

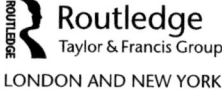

Routledge
Taylor & Francis Group

LONDON AND NEW YORK

First published 2021
by Routledge
2 Park Square, Milton Park, Abingdon, Oxon OX14 4RN

and by Routledge
52 Vanderbilt Avenue, New York, NY 10017

Routledge is an imprint of the Taylor & Francis Group, an informa business

British Library Cataloguing-in-Publication Data
A catalogue record for this book is available from the British Library

Library of Congress Cataloging-in-Publication Data
Names: Hogan, Susan, 1961- editor.

Title: Therapeutic arts in pregnancy, birth, and new parenthood/edited by Professor Susan Hogan.

Description: Abingdon, Oxon; New York, NY: Routledge, 2020. | Includes bibliographical references and index. Provided by publisher.
Identifiers: LCCN 2020014085 (print) | LCCN 2020014086 (ebook) | ISBN 9780367462246 (hardback) | ISBN 9780367462239 (paperback) | ISBN 9781003027607 (ebook)

Subjects: MESH: Pregnant Women–psychology | Art Therapy–methods | Stress, Psychological–therapy | Pregnancy Complications–psychology | Infertility–psychology | Parents–psychology

Classification: LCC RG551 (print) | LCC RG551 (ebook) | NLM WM 450.5.A8 | DDC 618.2–dc23
LC record available at: https://lccn.loc.gov/2020014085
LC ebook record available at: https://lccn.loc.gov/2020014086

ISBN: 978-0-367-46224-6 (hbk)
ISBN: 978-0-367-46223-9 (pbk)
ISBN: 978-1-003-02760-7 (ebk)

Typeset in Baskerville
by MPS Limited, Dehradun

Paperback cover image by Zoe Murdoch

In memory of Sylvia June Hogan (nee Young)

Fee Fee was my mother.

She was dismissed by her doctor as neurotic.

By the time she received a correct diagnosis her cancer was too far advanced for her to be saved.

Like many women she was compassionate and loving enough to forgive the doctor and insist that I not take legal action against him for negligence as I wished to do.

This book is in memory of *Fee* and the thousands of women like her who have been misdiagnosed, mistreated and abused by our medical and psychiatric services.

Susan Hogan

Contents

List of figures   x
List of tables   xiii
About the editor   xiv
List of contributors   xv
Foreword   xviii

1 Arts in health: pregnancy, birth and new parenthood   1
  SUSAN HOGAN

2 Metaphorically maternal: finding potential space through
  the experience of grief and loss associated with infertility   9
  SUE BULMER

3 Art Therapy and pregnancy loss: a secret grief   22
  LAURA SEFTEL

4 Overcoming severe fear in late pregnancy: the use of Art
  Therapy in maternal healthcare, in the south of Sweden   42
  HELÉN WAHLBECK

5 Lost and found: locating meaning within the landscape
  of perinatal loss   53
  CLAIRE FLAHAVAN

6 Reframing motherhood: photography as a creative
  application to re-image mother   71
  AMY LOCKHART CHILTON

 7 Representations of motherhood: normative and
    transgressive constructions   88
    MARIÁN LÓPEZ FDZ. CAO

 8 Recovery stories: transitional identities and the
    ambivalence of the maternal experience   107
    JANE HARDSTAFF

 9 Where can we make our home?: in-utero images and
    thinking in the running of a small therapeutic group
    for mothers and their young children affected by
    domestic abuse   124
    HEATHER TUFFERY

10 'Myself as a Tree': the enabling power of an Art
    Therapy intervention in clinical work with postnatally
    distressed women-mothers   138
    SOPHIA XEROS-CONSTANTINIDES

11 Obstetric violence: silenced issues   152
    DANIELA BESA TORREALBA
    TRANSLATED BY FRÉDÉRIQUE CHAMPAGNE

12 Artful trans-itions and the queering of pregnancy,
    birth and (m)othering   165
    SHERIDAN LINNELL AND ASHA ZAPPA

13 Mothering mothers: an exploration of self-referred,
    self-funded, six-week Art Therapy groups for new
    mothers   183
    ROS TAYLOR

14 Mechanisms of change within a dyadic model of Art
    Therapy for parents and their infants   196
    VICTORIA GRAY ARMSTRONG AND JOSEPHINE ROSS

15 And if the bough breaks: the use of individual Art
    Therapy within a perinatal mental health service   210
    BRIDGET GRANT

16 Cases on the border: perinatal parent–infant work
involving migrants, video analysis and art psychotherapy   228
DIANE BRUCE

17 Art Therapy for motherhood and families as a way to
support positive parenting   243
LUCIA HERVÁS HERMIDA

Index   256

Figures

2.1	Exploration of Loss 1. Sue Bulmer	12
2.2	Exploration of Loss 2. Sue Bulmer	12
2.3	Papier-mâché Vessels. Sue Bulmer	14
2.4	Dispersal. Sue Bulmer	14
3.1	Sorrow. Oil on paper, Brenda Philips	25
3.2	The Unexpected. Painting, Mary K. Flanary	26
3.3	Self-portrait (Anger). Digital art, Tammy LeMasters Gross	29
3.4	Pain Will Not Have the Last Word. Detail of scroll painting, Andrew Foster	30
3.5	Response to a Subsequent Pregnancy. Acrylic on canvas, Stephanie Paige Cole (first published in the book *Still*, 2010)	32
3.6	The Road to Motherhood. Blind contour drawing, Susan Jacobsen	33
3.7	Untitled. Oil on paper, Laura Seftel	36
4.1	The Origin of Control, 2016	47
4.2	The Room, 2016	49
4.3	The Family/Target Image, 2013	50
5.1	Adrift. Claire Flahavan	55
5.2	Unravelling. Claire Flahavan	56
5.3	Empty Nest. Claire Flahavan	57
5.4	I Can Still Feel Her Kicking. Claire Flahavan	58
5.5	Wound. Claire Flahavan	59
5.6	The Bud that Does Not Flower. Claire Flahavan	61
5.7	Vessel. Claire Flahavan	62
5.8	Willow. Claire Flahavan	65
5.9	Blooming. Claire Flahavan	68
6.1	Mind-full Mama Zen Tangle. A visual summary of some therapeutic considerations that can be experienced in matrescence, which offers an example of a Photo Art Therapy directive – combining personal photo with doodle art. Amy Lockhart Chilton, 2017	76
6.2	Mother Birth Announcement. Amy Lockhart Chilton, 2017	81
6.3	Becoming Mother Collage. Amy Lockhart Chilton, 2017	82

6.4   Matrescence photo series. Amy Lockhart Chilton, 2017   83
6.5   The Absence of I. Self-mother portrait. Amy Lockhart
      Chilton, 2015   83
7.1   Cihuateotl. Veracruz, Late Classic 600–900 CE. Xalapa
      Anthropology Museum. Photograph: Marián López Fdz. Cao   89
7.2   Cihuateotl. Veracruz, Late Classic 600–900 CE. Xalapa
      Anthropology Museum. Photograph: Marián López Fdz. Cao   90
7.3   Nativity of Mary. Oil on canvas, 101 × 142cm, Spanish,
      seventeenth century. Reproduced by kind permission:
      Wikimedia Commons, https://en.wikipedia.org/wiki/
      Nativity_of_Mary#/media/File:Nativity_of_mary.jpg   92
7.4   Virgin Suckling the Child. Hans Memling, c. 1433.
      Reproduced by kind permission: Wikimedia Commons,
      https://commons.wikimedia.org/wiki/File:Hans_Memling_-_
      Virgin_Suckling_the_Child_-_WGA14966.jpg   94
7.5   Self-Portrait on the Sixth Wedding Anniversary. Paula
      Modersohn-Becker, 1906. Reproduced by kind permission:
      Wikimedia Commons, https://commons.wikimedia.org/wiki/
      File:Paula_Moderson-Becker_-_Selbstbildnis_am_6_
      Hochzeitstag_-_1906.jpeg?uselang=fr   97
7.6   Poster distributed in Washington to defend the right to abortion.
      Barbara Kruger, 1989. Reproduced by kind permission:
      Wikimedia Commons, https://commons.wikimedia.org/wiki/
      File:Untitled_(Your_body_is_a_battleground).jpg   101
7.7   Aborto Legal Ya, Briza Maldonado, 2018. Poster for abortion
      rights in Argentina. Reproduced by kind permission of Briza
      Maldonado   102
8.1   *Wild Talents*. Digital installation, Susan Hiller, 1997. Courtesy
      of the Susan Hiller Estate   109
8.2   Unreliable Evidence. Digital prints, Jane Hardstaff, 2006   112
8.3   Motherlines. Self-portrait, acrylic, digital print, Jane
      Hardstaff, 2019   113
9.1   Salt dough work by Ahmad and Rahma   128
9.2   Untitled. Rahma's artwork   129
9.3   Untitled. Rahma's artwork   130
9.4   Fish by Ahmad and Rahma   130
10.1 My Tree is a Bush that Almost Died from Frost. Kalyca Baker   142
10.2 My Tree has Survived Fire. Nerida   143
10.3 Gum Tree. Leanne Hancock   145
10.4 Autumn Tree. Sarah-Jane Wentzki   146
11.1 Making the Woman Invisible and Abandoning Her in the Realm
      of Reproduction. Karin Carrasco, psychologist, Art Therapist
      and mother   158
11.2 Woman Object. One More Element of the Machinery. Andrea
      Gómez, nurse and mother   159

11.3   Here is the Scar and the Blood. Giorgia Pezzoli, artist and Art
       Therapist   160
11.4   Work produced by female inmate, patient of Giorgia Pezzoli   161
12.1   Self Portrait as (M)Other. Asha Zappa, digital photo, 2013   166
12.2   Dysphoria. Asha Zappa, copic marker on cardstock, 2017   171
12.3   Selfie Portraits (Series). Asha Zappa, digital photographs and
       video stills, 2018   179
13.1   Post-Natal Bliss. Pencil and coloured pencil on paper, 2017   190
13.2   Outgrown. Pen and coloured pencil on paper, 2017   191
13.3   Mothering Mothers. Pencil on paper, 2017   193
14.1   Infant engaged with painting   197
15.1   Untitled. Bridget Grant   215
15.2   A Dark 'Unbearable' Part. Nicola   218
15.3   Euphoric Moment. Nicola   219
15.4   Overlooked, Unheard and Unseen. Nicola   221
15.5   Trapped. Nicola   222
16.1   Homeland. Abi, pencil on card, 2019   234
16.2   Clay Baby. Abi, clay, tissue, glue and cardboard, 2019   235
17.1   The Tree of Life. Art Therapy in the perinatal period,
       pregnant women or recent mothers with their partners. Image
       and text by the participants of the Art Therapy workshop deve-
       loped in Calpe, Spain, 2017   243
17.2   Glow of Hope. Family Art Therapy with other members of the
       family. Image and text by the participants of the Art Therapy
       workshop developed in Aranjuez, Spain, 2015   248
17.3   Green Bowl. Family Art Therapy with a dyadic approach,
       mothers and infants participating together. Image and text by
       the participants of the Art Therapy workshop developed in
       Aranjuez, Spain, 2015   252

Tables

17.1 Principles of positive parenting (Rodrigo Lopez et al. 2010
      p. 12)   245
17.2 Mothers' issues, difficulties and needs (Hervás Hermida 2018) 246
17.3 Objectives of the intervention (Hervás Hermida 2018, p. 849)   250

About the editor

Professor Susan Hogan's books are:

Feminist Approaches to Art Therapy (as editor, 1997)

Healing Arts: The History of Art Therapy (2001)

Gender Issues in Art Therapy (as editor, 2003)

Conception Diary: Thinking About Pregnancy and Motherhood (2006)

Revisiting Feminist Approaches to Art Therapy (as editor, 2012)

The Introductory Guide to Art Therapy (with Coulter, 2014)

Art Therapy Theories: A Critical Introduction (2016)

Art Therapy Theories: A Critical Introduction in Korean translation (2017)

Arts Therapies and Gender Issues: International Perspectives on Research (commissioned by the European Consortium of Art Therapy Educators) (as editor, 2019)

Gender and Difference in the Arts Therapies: Inscribed on the Body (as editor, 2019)

The Introductory Guide to Art Therapy (with Coulter) in Korean translation (2019)

The Maternal Tug: Ambivalence, Identity, and Agency (with La-Chance Adams and Cassidy 2020)

Therapeutic Arts in Pregnancy, Birth and New Parenthood (as editor, 2020)

Art Therapy Theories: A Critical Introduction (French and Chinese translations under discussion)

Contributors

Victoria Gray Armstrong is an HCPC (UK) registered Art Therapist who co-founded Art at the Start, a project exploring the impact of the arts in the early years, based in Dundee, Scotland. This is a collaborative project between the University of Dundee and the Dundee Contemporary Arts Centre.

Diane Bruce is an HCPC (UK) registered Art Therapist and a registered VIPP-SD (Video Intervention Positive Parenting – Sensitive Discipline) intervener working for a child and adolescent mental health and perinatal parent and infant mental health service at NELFT NHS Foundation Trust.

Sue Bulmer is an HCPC (UK) registered Art Therapist working in the UK. Her professional interests include working with clients who have experienced infertility, pregnancy loss and bereavement as well as trauma. Sue graduated with a distinction from the MA Art Therapy at Derby University and was awarded the Donna Betts prize for academic achievement.

Marián López Fdz. Cao is Professor of Art Therapy and Education at Universidad Complutense of Madrid, where she was director of the Master's in Art Therapy and Artistic Education for social inclusion, 2010–2014. She was director of the Complutense Institute of Feminist Research, 2007–2011. She is an accredited Art Therapist by FEAPA and vice-chair of the European Consortium of Art Therapy Education (ECARTE).

Amy Lockhart Chilton is a Canadian Art Therapist with a Master's degree in Spirituality and Psychotherapy. Although parenthood is her current focus, she continues to research and consider the ways in which Art Therapy and photography can support matrescence.

Claire Flahavan. Prior to training as an Art Therapist, Claire worked in medicine and psychiatry across a range of mental health services for over ten years. She currently works as an Art Therapist at the National Maternity Hospital and at Children's Health Ireland – Crumlin Hospital, Dublin. Claire has particular interests in developmental trauma, loss/bereavement and psychological issues arising in the perinatal period.

Bridget Grant is an HCPC (UK) registered Art Therapist. She currently works as an Art Therapist and clinical supervisor in a perinatal mental health service in addition to running a private practice in Edinburgh, Scotland. Alongside individual work, Bridget is an experienced group and workshop facilitator and has also been a visiting lecturer on the MSc Art Therapy training at Queen Margaret University, Edinburgh.

Jane Hardstaff is currently Creative Wellbeing Coordinator at QUAD, Derby, artist in residence at the Beeches Perinatal Unit, Derby Royal Hospital, and founder of Common Threads, an arts organisation supporting mental health through creative practice. Formerly a psychotherapist, she is a freelance curator, artist and participatory arts manager.

Lucia Hervás Hermida is an artist, art therapist and Associate Professor of art therapy and education at the Autonoma University of Madrid, where she developed her PhD on Art Therapy with mothers and families as a way to support positive parenting. In recent years, she has presented her work in a number of conferences and publications. She is part of the board of the Iberoamerican Forum of Art Therapy and the Federation of Spanish Art Therapists Associations.

Sheridan Linnell is Associate Professor of Art Therapy in the School of Social Sciences at Western Sydney University, Australia, where she is Discipline Leader for Arts Therapy and Counselling. As Chief Editor of the *Australian and New Zealand Journal of Arts Therapy*, Sheridan is interested in amplifying voices from the region. She is passionate about socially just Art Therapy for a postcolonial, diverse world.

Josephine Ross is a Senior Lecturer in Psychology at University of Dundee and co-founder of the Art at the Start Project. She specialises in developmental psychology, primarily the development of children's self-awareness and its context in their relationships and interactions. She runs the university's 'Minime' lab.

Laura Seftel is an Art Therapist and Clinical Consultant with a private practice in Northampton, Massachusetts. She is the founder of the Secret Club Project and author of *Grief Unseen: Healing Pregnancy Loss through the Arts* (2006). She presents nationally on topics related to art and healing.

Ros Taylor is an HCPC (UK) registered Art Therapist based in London. Her own experience as a mother gave her the impetus to set up and run Art Therapy groups for new mothers. She currently works as an Art Therapist in a London primary school and co-facilitates a Painting Together Group for parents and babies and toddlers.

Daniela Besa Torrealba is former President of the Asociación Chilena de Arte Terapia. She is trained in psychology (Univeridad Diego Portales), Art

Therapy (Universidad Complutense de Madrid), and psychoanalytical psychotherapy (Universidad Complutense de Madrid).

Heather Tuffery is an HCPC (UK) registered Art Therapist working in Early Years service in Edinburgh, Scotland and is a visiting lecturer on the Art Therapy training course at Queen Margaret University.

Helén Wahlbeck is a registered midwife who worked in delivery and maternity healthcare for 30 years. She is based at Midwifery Clinic, Helsingborg, Sweden. She holds a behavioural science degree, and is trained in Jungian image therapy. Most recently, Helén has led a research project on the impact of Art Therapy on childbirth fear and published on this subject (*Women & Birth*, 2017; *Journal of the American Art Therapy Association*, 2020).

Sophia Xeros-Constantinides is a medical doctor and Art Therapist working in psychological medicine. She has engaged in co-conducting the PAIRS Mother-Baby Groups and the CONNECT Art Therapy Groups for distressed mothers and infants. She also works part-time offering mental health support at the University of Melbourne Health Service. Sophia has completed studio-based postgraduate studies in Fine Art, using collage and drawing to envision lived-maternity.

Asha Zappa is an Art Therapist and researcher providing expressive therapy for children who have experienced trauma in Australia. Xie is also a practising artist. Xir research focuses on Art Therapy and sex, sexuality and/or gender diverse people.

Foreword

Andrea O'Reilly

Reading this vital and vibrant collection I was reminded of a radicalising moment at the 2003 Birth: Representation and Experience conference at the Hebrew University of Jerusalem. Invited to present a keynote on the representations of birth in the fiction of Toni Morrison, I and the other feminist scholars were stunned to near speechlessness following an address by a male obstetrician. While the details of his talk are hazy, his conclusions and recommendations are anything but; with pompous and grandiose certainty he proclaimed that post-partum depression was strictly and only a biological condition and should be treated accordingly with medical intervention. I remember standing and struggling to articulate a cogent and coherent response to explain what all mothers know: our feelings post-partum cannot be simply and solely reduced to biology and that it is patriarchal culture that makes most women's transition to motherhood so arduous and perilous. Thus, what needs to be corrected is not women's minds or bodies but patriarchal motherhood. I recall explicating the crucial distinction Adrienne Rich makes between 'motherhood', the patriarchal institution of motherhood, which is male-defined and controlled and is deeply oppressive to women, and 'mothering', which is female-defined and centred and potentially empowering to women (1986, p. 13) to explain how, in Rich's words, 'motherhood as institution [throughout history] has ghettoized and degraded female potentialities' (p. 13). With this collection now on my desk, I only wish I had it at this conference; that obstetrician would certainly have received a copy.

In the introduction Hogan explains that, 'women experience often unprecedented pressures and constraints in their lives during pregnancy and after birth' (pp. 1–8). Moreover, as Hogan further elaborates, '"psychosocial risk factors" should *not* be seen as located *within* the individual woman, but rather viewed as a matrix or field of conflicting social forces which act upon women in a destabilizing manner' (emphasis in original). In other words, as Hogan emphasises, 'What women experience during pregnancy and childbirth is not merely psychological, it is social (structural)' (pp. 1–8). Post-partum depression thus cannot be simply and solely positioned, explained and treated as a biological condition; rather it must be located and understood in its cultural context, that of a patriarchal society which causes motherhood to be oppressive to women for a myriad of reasons. In her poignant and potent memoir, *Inconsolable: How I Threw My Mental Health Out with the Diapers*, Marrit Ingman replaces the word *depression* with *oppression* to describe post-partum motherhood: '[What women experience] is post-partum *oppression*: the grind of getting by in a culture that systemically devalues women and their mothering [...] and tells us we are to blame for everything we experience' (2005, p. 249, emphasis in original). Indeed, as Ingman remarks, 'when we talk about PPD we're actually describing a variety of conditions, one of which may actually be the condition of motherhood' (p. 2). Thus, as Ingman perceptively and drolly concludes, 'So maybe PPD isn't a malfunction of those mercurial female humors. Maybe it's more like a shitstorm parents endure because we are tired, frightened, isolated, confused, and apparently powerless' (p. 3).

Women's literature is replete with the anguish mothers suffer when their typical post-partum feelings are pathologised and they are blamed and shamed for 'being neurotic' and 'failing to cope'. Charlotte Perkins Gilman's classic *The Yellow Wall-Paper* is a fictionalised account of the author's own post-partum oppression following the birth of her child. Diagnosed with a nervous disorder, Perkins Gilman was prescribed Dr Weir Mitchell's infamous Rest Cure and instructed: 'To live a domestic life as possible, to have your baby with you at all times and never touch pen, brush or pencil for the reminder of your life' (Knight, 1999, p. ix). Following a nervous breakdown, Perkins Gilman garnered the resolve and courage to leave her confining marriage and began her successful career as a writer and speaker. For the unnamed narrator of *The Yellow Wall-Paper* the only liberation from her post-partum oppression is a descent into madness enacted and symbolised through the wallpaper. Tellingly, the narrative concludes with the words 'I've got out at last ... in spite of you [her husband] ... And I've pulled off most of the paper, so you can't put me back' (Perkins Gilman 1999, p. 182). More recently Lionel Shriver's award-winning novel *We Need to Talk about Kevin* details the maternal anxiety, doubt and regret of a mother who does not adjust to normative motherhood as expected as required in patriarchal culture. As Eva, the mother, remarks: 'the whole thing was going wrong from the start ... I was not following the program ... I had dismally failed us and our newborn baby. That I was, frankly, a freak' (2003, p. 83). Later Eva describes her childbirth as

> awful ... the emotion on which I fastened to push was loathing ... And yes, I even hated the baby which had brought me unwieldiness and embarrassment and a rumbling subterranean tremor quaking through the very ocean floor of who I thought I was. In the very instant of his birth, I associated Kevin with my own limitations – not only with suffering but defeat.
>
> (Shriver 2003, pp. 75–76)

For many readers of the novel Eva is a bad mother precisely because she is seen as lacking the assumed innate desire and ability to mother as well as the happiness expected of women in and through motherhood. However, and as Vivienne Muller astutely observes, what the novel details is not failed mothering but 'the mis-fit between Eva's individual experiences of motherhood and the social discourses of mothering which relentlessly seek to claim her' (2008, p. 43). Eva's ambivalence and regret, similar to the narrator's despair and madness in *The Yellow Wall-Paper* derive not from a defective psychology but from the cultural expectations and conditions of normative motherhood.

This collection is a crucial and timely contribution to the feminist project of 'de-pathologising' women's maternal subjectivities and experiences to recognise, in the words of Hogan, 'that post-natal distress [is] understandable rather than irrational or pathological' (pp. 1–8). Moreover, with its emphasis on Art Therapy, the collection delivers specific artistic and therapeutic practices to heal and empower mothers in resistance to normative motherhood. In *Inconsolable*, Ingman writes: 'This is the slippery slope of motherhood. Too many of us are falling off and we need to catch each other' (2005, p. 250). This anthology does just that: offering understanding and support to navigate the slippery slopes of motherhood.

Andrea O'Reilly is Professor at York University in the School of Women's Studies and author/editor of 25 books on motherhood, including The Routledge Companion to Motherhood.

References

Ingman, M. 2005. *Inconsolable: How I Threw My Mental Health Out with the Diapers*. New York, NY: Seal Press.

Knight, D. 1999. Introduction. In Perkins Gilman, C., *The Yellow Wall-Paper, Herland, and Selected Other Writings*, ed. D. Knight. London: Penguin, pp. ix–xxx.

Muller, V. 2008. Good and Bad Mothering: Lionel Shriver's *We Need to Talk About Kevin*. In M. Porter & J. Kelso (eds.), *Theorizing and Representing Maternal Realities*. Newcastle: *Cambridge Scholars Press*, pp. 38–53.

Perkins Gilman, C. 1999. *The Yellow Wall-Paper, Herland, and Selected Other Writings*, ed. D. Knight London: Penguin.

Rich, A. 1986. *Of Woman Born: Motherhood as Experience and Institution*. New York: Norton.

Shriver, L. 2003. *We Need to Talk About Kevin*. New York: HarperCollins.

1 Arts in health

Pregnancy, birth and new parenthood

Susan Hogan

Art making offers a means for women to express and understand their changed sense of self-identity and sexuality as a result of pregnancy and motherhood. The aim of this book is to introduce readers to the various ways in which art is being used with women who are experiencing different stages of childbearing – who may be unable to conceive and are struggling with infertility treatment, or experience miscarriage and loss, or are facing other issues of adjustment. This work can include a myriad of factors: ambivalence, pre-natal anxiety, unhappiness and disorientation, or even dread, as well as rekindled feelings of grief for lost parents, unresolved feelings towards mothers and others, feelings of abandonment where the progenitor has fled, birth trauma, or the grief of the loss of a baby. Art can also be of help in exploring and supporting family relationships with partners involved and in supporting new families, as the final chapter in this book explores.

Metaphor and symbolism are often used around contested sites of meaning, and art making can also provide the opportunity to analyse and challenge social ideas and oppressive discourses (Hogan 1997).

This book wishes to acknowledge that ideals around pregnancy and childbirth are highly contested, that this contestation, coupled with the very liminality of the event itself is challenging, if not potentially destabilising for new mothers and their partners. Or, to put it another way, women are subject to new pressures and constraints that are potentially dislocating. Having been led to expect success and joy, some women may experience conflicting feelings and memories that have no space for expression, making pregnancy or new motherhood a challenging time. Moreover, women's actual perinatal experiences (which may be very far from imagined ideals) can be disavowed by societal expectations of maternal competency and bliss (Hogan 2017).

The English political activist and law reporter Vanessa Olorenshaw (2016) has pointed out that motherhood demands interdependence and sits uncomfortably with the dominant neo-liberal ideology of 'self' and 'individualism' as the core objects of a happy selfhood. Although childbirth is a universal experience, it is also culturally mediated – it is experienced through culture. Current fashion demands women should have thin and muscular bodies. Some women can find pregnancy distressing because of the transformation of their body shape away from such an ideal, their feelings of self-esteem being undermined.

Chronic illness is often exacerbated by pregnancy. Previously fit and healthy women can develop debilitating conditions during pregnancy such as pre-eclampsia (marked by swelling and high blood pressure). There is sometimes lack of understanding about bodily processes among pregnant women and new mothers. For example, when breastfeeding a new-born baby, women can experience uterine contractions as the baby suckles (this is quite normal), but one new mother I worked with thought this reaction was "perverted" and this false belief had caused her great distress. Our bodily autonomy is challenged: as our baby cries out, we feel our breasts filling with milk at the baby's command. The sheer profound dependence of the infant is dismaying. The 'I experience that too' aspect of group work is intensely valuable for mutual support of new mothers. There are strong cultural taboos preventing women from expressing their feelings, not least the fear that their children may be taken away from them. One of the advantages of working pictorially is that the *revealing image* allows the expression and acknowledgement of denied or unrealised feelings – it enables women to show what they cannot say and learn what they feel, but find difficult to acknowledge or grasp.

What women experience during pregnancy and childbirth is not merely psychological, it is societal (structural). Structural issues are at play during the period of pregnancy: women may be subject to increased regulation, depending on their specific milieu. This might include interference in women's activities (what she may or may not do whilst pregnant), dietary intake (what she may or may not eat or drink), even what clothes are deemed appropriate to wear. Unfortunately there is *no consensus* on these issues, so women are subject to conflicting advice, sometimes a bewildering array of conflicting guidance from family members and health professionals. This can result in conflict and tensions between members of a family about what is best.

The Nigerian writer Chimamanda Ngozi Adichie gives some words of hope and encouragement on this topic:

> Be a full person. Motherhood is a glorious gift, but do not define yourself solely by motherhood. Your child will benefit from that … Everybody will have an opinion about what you should do, but what matters is what you want for yourself, and not what others want you to want … In these coming weeks of new motherhood be kind to yourself. Ask for help. Expect to be helped … Give yourself room to fail. A new mother does not necessarily know how to calm a crying baby. Don't assume you should know everything.
>
> (2016, pp. 9–11)

Different cultures treat pregnant women differently. Here in the UK, women report being touched more (their enlarging stomachs touched) and new mothers are fair game for conversations about their new babies from an selection of strangers with whom they'd not previously spoken. In this way bodily privacy and the negotiation of public space is altered for women who are pregnant or new mothers. Indeed, a new mother can find hitherto simple tasks (such as getting on a bus and then shopping) have become extremely difficult. I found it impossible to get my buggy on a bus in London, I recall, as I was simply elbowed out of the way by determined commuters in their frantic scrum! No concession was made to the fact that I was encumbered. In contrast, in many parts of France, people with babies or young children may find themselves ushered to the front of queues and given preferential boarding on forms of transport.

In many relationships in which there has been relative equality between partners, inequality starts to develop when the first baby is born. Women often lose or reduce their paid employment and become semi-dependent on their partners, possibly for the first time in their relationships. Loss of employment at this time can result in late-in-life poverty for many women who make insufficient pension contributions throughout their careers. These decisions around early parenting have lifelong consequences. *The Economist* magazine put it like this, 'Having children lowers women's lifetime earnings, an outcome known as the "child penalty"' (*The Economist* Twitter feed, 17 November 2018). Women having time out of paid employment, or reducing their employment then puts men at the forefront of the career/wage-earning stakes within the relationship. Men may have the primary power position in terms of making an economic contribution from then on (Banyard 2011). Subsequently, it is often the man's career that is prioritised, even necessitating possible geographical relocations to seize new opportunities, which can further dislocate wives and partners from their support networks, as they become 'trailing spouses'. Women who stay on at work are likely to be subject to an array of discriminatory behaviours and lack of career progression. It doesn't have to be like this, and the more we move to genuine co-patenting the better it will be for women and men alike. A European survey summarised that 'the birth of the first child constitutes a major and irreversible change in focus, priorities, and life-course. One never sees life as one did before becoming a mother' (Stevens, de Bergeyck & de Liedekerke 2011, p.11). Stunningly, in the same report, only 50 per cent of husbands are recorded as helping 'regularly' with domestic work (housework and childcare) by 4,200 women who answered this question; nevertheless, the Second European Quality of Life Survey notes increased levels of 'life satisfaction' for couples with children (Stevens et al. 2011, p. 32).

The way women give birth varies, but in many cultures there has been a strong move towards hospital births as customary. Until the 1960s the *British Medical Journal* was advocating that for normal pregnancies the best place to give birth was in the home, (The *British Medical Journal* in 1954 was still willing to 'arbitrate decisively' that 'the proper place for the confinement is the patient's own home'; *BMJ* 24 April 1954, cited Oakley 1984, p. 215). Today the overwhelming majority of births take place in hospitals, even if entirely normal. This means that women are taken into a medical environment. Once in the medical environment, women are more likely to be subject to 'routine' medical procedures that would not be, or would be less likely to be, implemented in the home. For example, so-called 'routine induction' is common, to precipitate and speed-up childbirth. It is justified to prevent 'bed blocking', an insidious dehumanising euphemism that prioritises hospital timetables over letting the labour take its natural time – women vary and so do the length of our labours.

Routine induction is presented as a normal and usual procedure and its risks and benefits are rarely properly articulated and discussed with the labouring woman. Induction is linked to the likelihood of further medical procedures and higher levels of pain. Furthermore, women can be made to feel unreasonable if they decline offered interventions. However, induction is linked to an increased rate of episiotomy and caesarean section, which is a serious and life-threatening surgical procedure. Episiotomy is the cutting of the skin between the vagina and anus with surgical shears and can cause long-term discomfort and pain and short-term agony. Rather than being used in extreme emergencies, C-sections account for a large proportion of hospital births today. A national survey carried out in Italy between 2003 and 2017 found that episiotomy had been performed 'by deceit' on 1.6 million women: 61 per cent of whom declared they *had not given informed consent*. Of these women 15 per cent considered it to be 'a form of genital mutilation' and 13 per cent regarded it as a 'betrayal of trust'. The same survey revealed that four out of ten women (41 per cent) were subjected to practices 'that violated their dignity and psychological integrity'. This survey was useful in revealing a level of obstetric intervention that was seen as being of clear concern. Indeed 21 per cent of the women in Italy considered themselves to have been subject to 'obstetric violence' whilst giving birth. The proportion of these women to be diagnosed as being depressed in new motherhood is not reported (*Bastatacere National Survey* 2017).

The World Health Organization has also reported on disrespectful and abusive treatment experienced during childbirth globally, highlighting particular situations including:

- Failure to get informed consent for procedures.
- Lack of confidentiality.
- Gross violations of privacy.
- Coercion to undergo medical procedures (including sterilisation).
- Outright physical abuse.
- Profound humiliation and verbal abuse.
- Refusal to give pain relief.
- Neglect of women during childbirth (with the consequence of women suffering life-threatening, avoidable complications).
- Refusal to admit women to health facilities.
- Detention of women and their infants after childbirth due to their inability to pay.

The World Health Organization has produced the following statement on the prevention and elimination of disrespect and abuse during facility-based childbirth: 'Every woman has the right to the highest attainable standard of health, which includes the right to dignified, respectful care' (WHO 2014). The physiological challenges involved, even for straightforward, uncomplicated pregnancies and births, should not be underestimated and the United Nations has expressed concern about preventable deaths (UN 2010). In the UK, stillbirth rates and maternal mortality is disproportionately high for black women, due to a combination of factors (Muglu et al. 2019).

To dismiss women's reactions to pregnancy, childbirth and new motherhood as merely neurotic is unacceptable and compounds abuses of power and discriminatory cultural norms. In previous work, I have explored the 'mother blaming' aspects of various psychological theories, as women are positioned as *the problem* – first, we are positioned as deficient if we don't bounce back immediately from traumatic births and destabilising circumstances, and second, we are responsible for our children's attachment anxieties should we dare to venture out without our infants. *There is no such thing as a good enough mother*; women are condemned in much of the published psychological theorising, which is fundamentally oppressive; examples of criticism even include 'too good' mothering (Hogan 2012). Mother blaming is endemic and Caplan sardonically sums it up. I paraphrase: sit too close to your child and you are smothering and invasive; sit too far away and you are narcissistic, remote and rejecting, or possibly 'castrating'. Of her clinical experience she wrote: 'We found that mothers were blamed for virtually every kind of psychological or emotional problem that ever brought any patient to see a therapist (Caplan 2007, pp. 592–593).

In a polemical outburst Olorenshaw (2016) puts it like this,

> And the children? Hoodlum? Mother was depressed. Autism? Mother consumed a glass of wine in pregnancy. Addiction? Mother was detached in infancy. Married to a violent man? Mother failed to protect you from a violent father. Fear of commitment? Mother didn't love you enough. Desperate for love, and clingy? Mother loved you too much. Angry? Mother didn't attend to your every emotional need. Got a problem? Blame mother, show your wounds, and collect your patriarchal misogynistic matraphobic prize ... "if you really want to know why this child is a mess, just look at its mother!" (Caplan p. 37) ... So the fundamental issue that women face when they become mothers is how to navigate this minefield and how to diffuse the bomb of blame ... No matter what a mother does, she is at fault.
>
> (pp. 123–124)

Women who don't experience instinctual certainty as to what to do feel deficient because of the rhetoric about 'maternal instinct' – aren't we just *supposed* to know what to do? Not all new mothers '*fly* into motherly love' and then feel defective or monstrous and ashamed (Olorenshaw 2016, p. 103, emphasis in original). US author and poet Adrienne Rich captured this eloquently in her descriptions of a blissful love she felt for her children, which engulfs her, juxtaposed with ambivalence: 'the murderous alternation between bitter resentment and raw-edged nerves, and blissful gratification and tenderness' (Rich 1997, p. 11). Rich also describes how she was 'haunted' by the stereotype of the mother whose love is unconditional and

> by the visual and literary images of motherhood as a single-minded identity. If I knew parts of myself existed that would never cohere to those images,

weren't those parts then abnormal, monstrous? And – as my eldest son, now aged twenty-one, remarked on reading the above passages: "You seemed to feel you ought to love us all the time. But there *is* no human relationship where you love the other person at every moment." Yes, I tried to explain to him, but women – above all, mothers – have been supposed to love in that way.

(Rich 1997, p. 12)

Many of the discourses around new motherhood are orientated towards characterisations of deficient and failing-to-cope women, rather than looking at the terrain of birth itself, which is both intensely ideological and contested and destabilising (Hogan 2003, 2008). I have argued that it is a *combination* of a myriad of factors that renders childbirth and new motherhood as uniquely disorientating and potentially distressing (Hogan 2017). Childbirth and childrearing are complex, and women experience often unprecedented pressures and constraints in their lives during pregnancy and after birth (Hogan 2017). Even those wishing to support new mothers often use language that unwittingly blames the mother – 'psychosocial risk factors', for example, can point the finger of blame at the individual if used as a metaphor for a problem, like a 'seed' that is located in the individual: in this analogy the 'seed' germinates when the woman is subject to stressors, to bloom into full-blown mental illness (Hogan 2019). Some women may be more at risk of psychological distress during pregnancy, or after birth, (such as those subject to emotional or physical violence throughout their pregnancies from their partners, or women who have been coerced into proceeding with an unwanted pregnancy, or who have experienced rape, for example). However, I would suggest that the 'psychosocial risk factors' should *not* be seen as located *within* the individual woman, but rather viewed as a matrix or field of conflicting social forces which act upon women in a destabilising manner; childbirth and all of the practices surrounding it are highly contested and this contestation has repercussive effects (Hogan 2008, 2017). Indeed, current classifications 'may not adequately address the range or combination of emotional distress experienced by mothers' (Coates, de Visser & Ayres 2015, p. 1). The author Angela Garbes avers that in the US 'we tend to gloss over, ignore, judge, or, even worse, pathologise difficult emotions. Intentionally or not, we shame and isolate women who don't have the joyful pregnancy and postpartum experiences our culture expects' (2018, pp. 225–226). To blandly put forward the diagnosis of post-natal depression, with no real attempt to deconstruct what this really means, runs the risk of compounding abuses of power, which are manifold (Bohren et al. 2015; Jewkes & Penn-Kekana 2015). Talwar suggests that Art Therapists must be prepared to challenge 'power hierarchies' as part of our work (2019, p. 11). In my view, this should include an explicit acknowledgement of social constraints, pressures and institutional abuses to which women are subject when experiencing pregnancy, birth and new parenthood. Furthermore, in art therapy we want to resist a 'global reductionist' stance, in terms of what birth and motherhood means to women who experience it, even if obstetric violence is becoming a global phenomenon (Huss 2015, p. 116).

Readers of my previous books will know that I do not have a prescriptive attitude, so this volume will represent a range of ways of thinking about these topics and employ a variety of theories (Hogan 2016). This book is intended to generate discussion and debate and is the first full-length British book on this topic, although with an international cast of contributors.

I have emphasised structural aspects at play in this introduction, because I am keen to see an approach develop which recognises post-natal distress as understandable rather than 'irrational' or pathological (Hogan 1997, 2003). It is admittedly hard to shake off the rhetoric of post-natal 'illness' as the existing literature illustrates (Hogan et al. 2017), but it is important that those institutional practices and norms that are illness inducing (that is to say, they are iatrogenic) are acknowledged. Iatrogenic illness is defined as having been produced by the adverse effects of medical treatments, procedures and practices (a topic I have explored in a series of films as part of *The Birth Project*, 2014–2018). I am keen to 'de-pathologise' women's experiences, while also acknowledging real distress, rather than add to a dominant rhetoric of women's instability and inadequacy. I hope this volume is a useful step in this direction.

To conclude, this book is a *cri du coeur* for more sympathetic and deeply understanding support for women (and those who are self-defined as intersex or non-binary), throughout their reproductive journey and in new parenthood.

References

Adichie, C. N. 2016. *Dear Ijeawele: A Feminist Manifesto in Fifteen Suggestions*. London: 4th Estate.

Banyard, K. 2011. *The Equality Illusion: The Truth about Women and Men Today*. London: Faber & Faber.

Bastatacere National Survey Women and Childbirth. 2017. Commissioned by the Obstetric Violence Observatory (OVO-Italia) and completed by DOXA survey agency (www.doxa.it/en). September 20, 2017.

Bohren, M. A., Vogel, J. P., Hunter, E. C., Lutsiv, O., Makh, S. K., Souza, J. P., Aguiar, C., Saraiva Coneglian, F., Diniz, A. L., Tunçalp, Ö., Javadi, D., Oladapo, O. T., Khosla, R., Hindin, M. J., & Gülmezoglu, A. M. 2015. The Mistreatment of Women during Childbirth in Health Facilities Globally: A Mixed-Methods Systematic Review. *PLoS Medicine*, 12(6): e1001847. doi:10.1371/journal.pmed.1001847.

Caplan, P. 2007. Don't Blame Mother: Then and Now. In A. O'Reilly (ed.), *Maternal Theory: Essential Readings*. Toronto: Demeter, pp. 592–601.

Coates, R., de Visser, R., & Ayres, S. 2015. Not Identifying with Postnatal Depression: A Qualitative Study of Women's Postnatal Symptoms of Distress and Need for Support. *Journal of Psychosomatic Obstetrics and Gynecology*, 36(3): 114–121.

Garbes, A. 2018. *Like a Mother: A Feminist Journey through the Science and Culture of Pregnancy*. New York, NY: Harper Wave.

Hogan, S. 1997. *Feminist Approaches to Art Therapy*. London: Routledge.

Hogan, S. 2003. *Gender Issues in Art Therapy*. London: JKP.

Hogan, S. 2008. The Beestings: Rethinking Breast-Feeding Practices, Maternity Rituals, & Maternal Attachment in Britain & Ireland. *Journal of International Women's Studies* 10(2): 141–160.

Hogan, S. 2012. Post-modernist but Not Post-feminist! A Feminist Post-modernist Approach to Working with New Mothers. In H. Burt (ed.), *Creative Healing Through a Prism: Art Therapy and Postmodernism*. London: Jessica Kingsley Publishers, pp. 70–82.

Hogan, S. 2016. *Art Therapy Theories: A Critical Introduction*. Abingdon, Oxon: Routledge.

Hogan, S. 2017. The Tyranny of Expectations of Post-Natal Delight: Gendering Happiness: The Power of Pleasure. *Journal of Gender Studies*, Special Issue: Gendering Happiness, 26(1): 45–56.

Hogan, S. 2019. Birth Shock. In S. Hogan (ed.), *Arts Therapies & Gender in International Arts Therapies Research*. Abingdon, Oxon: Routledge, pp. 90–119.

Hogan, S., Sheffield, D., & Woodward, A. 2017. The Value of Art Therapy in Antenatal and Postnatal Care: A Brief Literature Review. *International Journal of Art Therapy*, 22(4): 169–179.

Huss, E. 2015. *A Theory-based Approach to Art Therapy*. Abingdon, Oxon: Routledge.

Jewkes, R., & Penn-Kekana, L. 2015. Mistreatment of Women in Childbirth: Time for Action on This Important Dimension of Violence against Women. *PLoS Medicine*, 12(6), e1001849. doi:10.1371/journal.pmed.1001849.

Muglu, J., Rather, H., Arroyo-Manzano, D., Bhattacharya, S., Balchin, I., Khalil, A., et al. 2019. Risks of Stillbirth and Neonatal Death with Advancing Gestation at Term: A Systematic Review and Meta-Analysis of Cohort Studies of 15 Million Pregnancies. *PLoS Medicine* 16(7): e1002838. doi:10.1371/journal.pmed.1002838.

Oakley, A. 1984. *The Captured Womb: A History of the Medical Care of Pregnant Women*. Oxford: Blackwell Publisher Ltd.

Olorenshaw, V. 2016. *Liberating Motherhood: The Birth of the Bluestockings Movement*. Cork: Womencraft Publishing.

Rich, S. 1997[1976]. *Of Women Born: Motherhood as Experience and Institution*. London: Virago.

Stevens, J., de Bergeyck, J., & de Liedekerke A., eds. 2011. *A Report by World Movement of Mothers Europe (MMM Europe)*. SSH-2009-3.2.2. Report for the European Commission.

UN. 2010. *Report of the Office of the United Nations High Commissioner for Human Rights on Preventable Maternal Mortality and Morbidity and Human Rights*. Geneva: Office of the United Nations High Commissioner for Human Rights (UNFPA). Available at: www2.ohchr.org/english/bodies/hrcouncil/docs/14session/A.HRC.14.39_AEV-2.pdf (accessed January 2019).

Talwar, S., ed. 2019. *Art Therapy for Social Justice: Radical Intersections*. New York, NY: Routledge.

WHO. 2014. *The Prevention and Elimination of Disrespect and Abuse During Facility-Based Childbirth*. Available at: https://apps.who.int/iris/bitstream/handle/10665/134588/WHO_RHR_14.23_eng.pdf;jsessionid=97E281AD0089CD206EC9BFA3DFA319C0?sequence=1 (accessed January 2019).

2 Metaphorically maternal

Finding potential space through the experience of grief and loss associated with infertility

Sue Bulmer

This chapter is an abridged arts-based research exploration of the author's personal experience of grief and loss associated with infertility. Throughout the process of the research the concept of loss and grief associated with infertility is explored through the making of three-dimensional vessels using a variety of unfamiliar art materials and techniques. The chapter focuses on the themes that arose from the creative process, rather than reflecting in depth about each particular technique or material employed.

Infertility, loss and grief

The definition of infertility is a when a couple fail to achieve a pregnancy after 12 months of unprotected sex, leaving approximately one in seven couples in the UK (or 3.5 million people) struggling to conceive (National Health Service 2018). It has been described as 'one of the most distressing life experiences a couple can face' (Seftel 2006, p. 39), with loss and grief being central components (Lindsey 2013). It can leave those who experience it with profound feelings of disbelief, failure, low self-esteem, despair, stress, anxiety and depression, envy, anger, resentment, loss of control, guilt and worthlessness (Cook 1987; Williams 1997; Cousineau & Domar 2007; Hogan 2012). People can experience the grief of loss associated with infertility on many levels, but with no actual life to grieve it is often experienced as taboo, an unseen, invisible loss, not recognised or discussed by society. It has been described as 'disenfranchised grief' (Doka 1989) and a life crisis similar to bereavement (Fertility Network UK 2018). In a pro-natal, parent-centric society where motherhood is glorified, childless women can be left feeling isolated and lost (Seftel 2006). They can experience 'identity crises' pondering their role in society if they are not a mother (Day 2013).

Methodology and rationale

Heuristic inquiry is rooted in phenomenology, which is concerned with theories of experience and how the 'lived' experience of a particular phenomenon is captured (Heidegger 1962). Heuristic inquiry, however, is autobiographical in focus, with a direct personal connection or lived experience of the investigated phenomenon being essential (Kapitan 2010). This methodology is qualitative and subjective, placing human experience above numerical evaluations (Sela-Smith 2002). It focuses on the transformation of the researcher (Hiles 2002) and involves intense introspection, described as a demanding process culminating in personal learning and change (Moustakas 1990). Furthermore, the process of art making in response to loss and grief sits well within the framework of heuristic inquiry due to the emphasis on creativity (McNiff 1998b; Ashby 2017). Arts-based research is a qualitative approach where we engage with our tacit knowing, a basic concept in heuristic discovery (Moustakas 1990). It is useful because sometimes there may not be words to express our experiences of loss (Kluger-Bell 2000), but we can rely on expression through art making: 'The image is the best way of representing meanings as yet unknown or not fully grasped' (Watkins 2000, p.198).

The six phases of Heuristic Research, now outlined, are to guide the unfolding, transformational process and to provide the framework for the basic research design (Moustakas 1990). However, I now realise that the heuristic process, like the grieving process, is not linear. The dynamics relate more closely to the grief theory of Stroebe and Schut (1999) where there is a focus on 'back and forth' movement between mourning and recovery.

Initial engagement

The process begins with a question or problem the researcher wishes to answer or explore, the aim being the discovery of meaning or essence of human experience (Moustakas 1990). It was when I began to explore grief, bereavement and loss that I realised how my own reproductive losses had deeply affected me. No one had ever explained that the process I had endured following this experience was grief. This realisation and relief at being able to name and understand what I was feeling helped me immensely. I therefore felt called by my own experience to research this issue and its effects as I knew that doing so would help me gain greater understanding of myself and may also help others.

Immersion

In the initial stages of the research process it is essential to fully immerse oneself in the phenomenon being investigated (Moustakas 1990). I embraced this opportunity by rereading old diaries, looking back over medical letters and fertility treatment protocols, reviewing artwork I made around this time, reading academic texts and self-help books, gaining knowledge of others' experiences of infertility and reproductive loss through books, blogs and podcasts. I reflected on this material in my journal notes and initial art making. Much of the 'data' or artwork was produced in the immersive stage.

Incubation

This phase of heuristic inquiry is described as a retreat from the intense con-centrated focus on the investigated phenomenon (Moustakas 1990). This allowed me the time and space to focus on other areas of my studies as well as allowing for periods of self-care and rest when I could switch off totally and let thoughts and ideas percolate through to my consciousness.

Illumination

This phase is argued to occur naturally when the researcher is open and receptive to tacit knowledge and intuition (Moustakas 1990). Illumination felt like 'lightbulb moments of realisation' where I could feel my thinking change. I felt these moments gave me new insight and understanding which settled naturally into themes. Personally, I found the stages of immersion, incubation and illumination difficult to separate from each other. I experienced them more as a natural cyclical process as described by Ashby (2017), which repeated many times throughout the research.

Explication

This part of the heuristic inquiry process involves a period of clarification when the researcher analyses, examines and develops the details of the illuminated themes (Moustakas 1990). For me this involved introspection, reading, jour-naling, making response art and mind maps and focusing more on the possible meanings of my research on a personal level. I felt the pieces of the jigsaw puzzle fit together more cohesively as understanding of my experience expanded.

Creative synthesis

During this final stage the researcher has become thoroughly familiar with the data, having explicated the meanings of the details, themes and qualities of their experience, bringing it all together to synthesise a cohesive whole (Moustakas 1990). This stage is usually presented in the form of a narrative depiction, although other it can take other forms (Ashby 2017). The completion of this written critique, an exhibition and viva voce helped me to fully creatively synthesise my experience.

The creative process

During the 'Immersion' phase of my research I began to explore images and written accounts from the time following my failed fertility treatments. Reliving this period of my life through immersion in my written and visual past worlds reminded me of the long-forgotten intense need I had to express myself creatively at that time. Looking at this work, which I had not seen for over ten years, with fresh eyes also brought all of those unwanted and uncomfortable feelings flooding back. The process left me feeling raw, vulnerable and exposed, but I felt this was necessary to help me to re-engage with the feelings. I also curiously explored these emerging feelings and repetitive forms, evocative of absence and loss, appeared in my imagery (Figures 2.1 and 2.2).

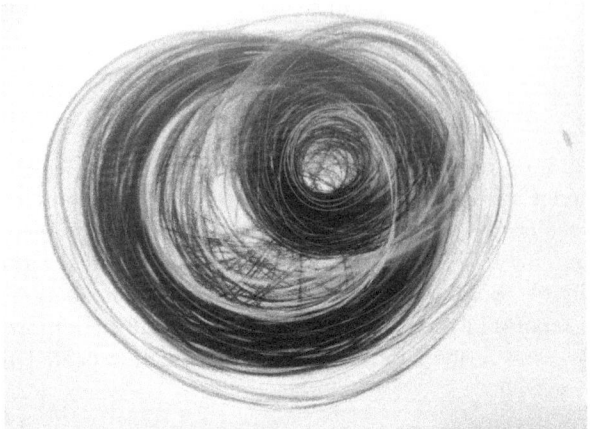

Figure 2.1 Exploration of Loss 1. Sue Bulmer.

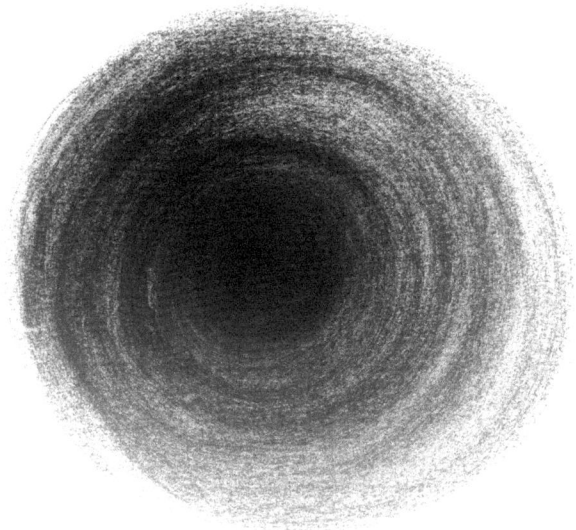

Figure 2.2 Exploration of Loss 2. Sue Bulmer.

I engaged with my tacit knowledge, opening myself up to the myriad possibilities of the art materials and entered into the unfamiliar territory of three-dimensional image-making, placing my trust in the process (McNiff 1998a). I explored ideas and themes of vessels, wombs, containers, emptiness, empty space, and the concept of inside and outside space. I wanted to portray images of empty vessels which reflected my feelings of emptiness, but also wanted to explore how vessels can be shaped by space, just as I had been shaped by the empty space of loss.

One author who explores common themes in the art of pregnancy loss and infertility is Seftel (2006) who argues that recurring motifs do appear:

- Circles – a symbol of the womb, containment, the cycle of life and death.
- Bowls, containers, teapots, vessels – which can hold or contain, be emptied and refilled.
- Empty spaces.
- Broken pieces, fragility.

Initially I worked with clay and started to make pinch pots. In the process of hollowing out the clay I immersed myself in the experience, sometimes working with my eyes closed. The formation was rhythmic and self-soothing (Berensohn 1972). I noticed that the forms I made had a corporeal quality to them, bringing to mind thoughts of my experiences of empty bellies, lost pregnancies, ugliness and deformity. Clay is a useful therapeutic tool when working with loss and can be used to create an image of the 'lost' object (Henley 2002). I wondered whether I was unconsciously making lost parts of my 'self' or whether the clay had enabled me to regress to the lost parts of my self through haptic perception and the power of touch (Elbrecht & Antcliff 2014). Manipulating clay enables a change in consciousness, allowing the emergence of powerful emotions when engaging with it (Henley 1991; Case & Dalley 2014). I noted in my reflective journal the intense feelings which arose during this period of immersion. The impact of this made me consciously aware of the need to exercise caution when introducing this medium to clients (Souter-Anderson 2010).

I next worked with plaster, my aim being to make a plaster vessel within a balloon. I tried several times to create the 'right mix' of plaster and water and noted feelings of frustration when the plaster failed to form a cohesive structure and collapsed within the balloon when it was pierced. This reminded me of the fragility of an egg as it is pierced by the needle during the IVF/ICSI procedure.

This drew parallels to my recently read diary entries – the challenges of the creative process, the struggle to create, fragility, brokenness and feelings of failure. Moon (2002) suggests that examination of our own brokenness is part of the preparatory work for being ready to nurture our clients. This helped me to recognise how far I have come in my process of recovery and how much stronger and resilient I now feel. This recognition of my increased ability to cope and accept my failures enabled me to make the decision to move on to a different media.

While working with tin foil I became tacitly aware of the strength and resilience gained from adding layers to a structure. This engagement flowed seamlessly into my first experience of working with papier-mâché. I noted initial feelings of avoidance at having to work with unfamiliar, messy media but I soon mastered the consistency and technique and made several forms using balloons as moulds.

I continued the exploration of using balloons as a supporting structure with ModRoc, another messy medium combining plaster and fabric mesh. These vessels were more solid and became transformed through the making process. I painted some of them and reflected on the inside and outside space and the

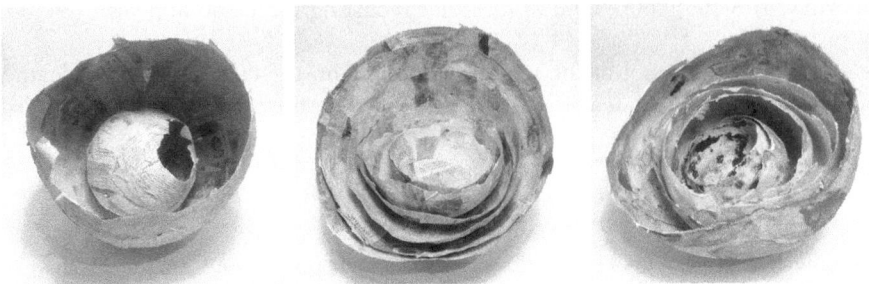

Figure 2.3 Papier-mâché Vessels. Sue Bulmer.

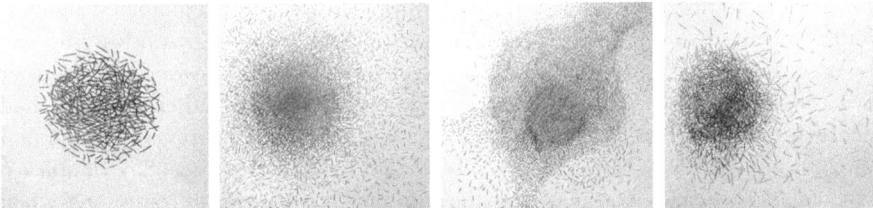

Figure 2.4 Dispersal. Sue Bulmer.

making of them around a balloon, a thin membrane which was filled and shaped by 'empty space', which then forms a structure for making something solid. At this point I felt a moment of illumination when my thoughts moved to considering the empty space as a potential space which can aid the formation of something 'other'. I began to place vessels inside one another (Figure 2.3) as I wondered at the possibilities of what this empty space could contain. My resulting images brought to mind layers of protection, feeling cocooned, being sheltered and held. It was during this period of immersion as I was creating and shaping vessels that I began to consider the extent to which I had been shaped by my lived experience of infertility. My diary entries were full of negative self-talk, failure, frustration, anger, envy, and deep sadness, themes which were echoed within previously cited literature. I wondered about the potential space created by my loss and what the exploration of this could mean for me.

My line drawings (Figure 2.4) captured my response to these thoughts. These images speak of letting go, movement from darkness into light, liberation, scattering of grief and recovery. This was explored in dry-point, a time-consuming process, causing initial frustration with the materials, the ink consistency, and the repeated effort it took to gain the image I wanted. The process reminded me of my repeated frustrating attempts to conceive and the imprint this experience has left on me. These images also speak, however, of a newfound resilience.

When I picked up the offcuts from the prints I attempted to weave them together. The discovery, when I realised that all of these separate parts could hold themselves together as a cohesive whole, was profound. This compounded and illuminated positive thoughts about internal strength, resilience and being something 'other'.

McNiff (2013) describes the unpredictable nature of arts-based research and how the process of discovery is often spontaneous. At this point I felt a complete change in direction as I unexpectedly began to explore weaving, another unfamiliar technique.

I explored the spider archetype and its links to creativity, the ancient feminine and mother complex. In Native America the spider is also seen as a keeper of the past and its connection to the future (Ronnberg & Martin 2010), a concept that resonated deeply within my work as I literally felt my past informing my present and future. Weaving and basketry also have historical connections to the transformational cycles of life, death and rebirthing, naturally integrating the concept of maternal containment (Collier 2012) which I was keen to explore.

I worked with wire, pipe-cleaners, straws and yarns, exploring uncertainty and 'not-knowing' with each new material, learning new ways of working, forming structures and vessels, and using the new knowledge I was gathering to inform what came next, tapping into my haptic perception and engaging physically in the process. While engaged in finger crochet I developed a 'double' stitch which I could neither explain nor replicate, but instinctively a vessel formed in my hands.

Reflexively stepping back to incubate and view all of the vessels together helped illuminate the fact that the vessels I had made represented multiple parts of self and my journey so far. This illumination helped me to re-engage with the physical aspects of the materials and I tacitly knew I was looking for something that reflected my current self. The wire was hard and unforgiving; the garden twine scratchy and coarse; the willow and eco fibre, while strong and solid, hurt my hands. I tried combining materials to form something new but nothing felt 'right'. I entered another period of incubation when I stepped away from the work to gain some valuable reflective time.

This facilitated further illumination and realisation that my next vessel needed to be made with something soft, forgiving and comforting. I began to explore finger crochet with wools and yarns which felt more physically pleasing to make but lacked the desired structure or form.

This led me into the final stage in my three-dimensional vessel exploration as I began to investigate the felting process, again something I had never tried before. The essential ingredient is wool, which becomes irreversibly transformed as the fibres become enmeshed into felt with the addition of friction, moisture and heat (Smith 2006). Felt can represent attributes such as protection and healing, and interestingly is the past tense of the verb 'to feel' (Collier 2012), something I was engaging with physically and emotionally through this process. The felting process was time-consuming and laborious with the repetitive rubbing motion and the resulting felt was surprisingly robust, soft but well-formed. It was the perfect representation of what I tacitly knew I needed to make and a natural final step in my three-dimensional exploration.

When we bear witness to our personal experience we step closer to experiencing its meaning (Learmonth 1994). Viewing and reflecting on the many vessels I had made led me into the explication phase of my heuristic inquiry as I began to make sense of my work. I viewed the work separately, in groups and all together, placing the vessels in different formations. A linear, chronological spiral was not a true representation of the process. All of the work was connected in ways I couldn't explain and I felt it needed to be grouped together as one; however, at this point, themes started to become apparent to me.

Discussion of themes

I fully relate to the significance of the transformational aspect of heuristic inquiry described by Moustakas (1990) especially as I felt the impact of my personal transformation on many levels. Like the fibres of my felted vessels, the threads of my themes are interlinked, enmeshed and difficult to separate, relating reflexivity, not knowing and multiplicity to identity, potential space and the therapeutic relationship.

Reflexivity, assumptions – self and potential space

> The goal is not to decide upon one option, or one truth, but to hold all the interpretations together as contributions to the whole.
>
> (Whitaker 2004, p. 8)

My initial hesitation in the two-dimensional visual response to the vessels enabled me to reflexively question my thinking about it. Resistance has been described by McNiff (2004) as a source of creative discovery. I realised that my hesitation was based on my assumption that my body of work had to be either *one thing* (three-dimensional) *or another* (two-dimensional). In this assumption I was failing to remain open and curious to the fact that it could be both, unconsciously placing boundaries on my work and thinking. McNiff (2004) stresses the importance of contemplation of our images and that we should not quickly jump to conclusions about meaning, in the act of withholding judgement we gain deeper under-standing. Case and Dalley (2014) and Moon (2002) also emphasise the importance of the Art Therapist's ability to remain open to the many levels of commu-nication of meaning that images hold.

I began to experience my work in terms of 'self' and realised the impact of my assumptions and dichotomous thinking on my identity. At the beginning of my research journey I did not consider myself as maternal. Heuristic inquiry had placed me in touch with the maternal aspects of self through the use of art materials in the search for the material that spoke to me of its 'maternal-ness'. It had helped me to see myself anew and realise things I hadn't considered before, as well as shedding new light on my own 'maternal' identity.

Contemplation of my work helped me to realise that through my client work I had been the 'good enough mother' and the metaphorical maternal presence in the therapy room. In the exploration of the empty space of loss I understood the capacity I had developed to contain and hold clients' feelings, thoughts, emotions and artworks and become the 'maternal container' (Bion 1962).

As Art Therapists, these functions are central to our work as we hold the space of 'good enough mother', accepting and containing our clients' material and returning it to them in a modified form, helping them to feel understood, aiding their transformation (Bion 1962; Edwards 2013). The space that had been created through my loss has literally been transformed through my training in Art Therapy and realised through my research. It can now be utilised in future client work as the therapeutic 'potential space' between therapist and client where play and creativity can facilitate the client's unfolding self-understanding and discovery (Winnicott 1971).

Embracing uncertainty and not-knowing

Coming from a science-based background I have found the 'not-knowing' of Art Therapy continually challenging. For this reason commencing this arts-based heuristic research felt exactly as described by Moustakas (1990, p. 13) like 'swimming into an unknown current'. Edwards (1992) talks about uncertainty and not-knowing and their centrality to the Art Therapy profession, and advocates the need to become familiar with both.

Throughout this heuristic inquiry I have intentionally embraced uncertainty through engagement with an unfamiliar research process, unknown-to-me art materials and techniques and working three-dimensionally. Repeated experience of uncertainty has enabled me to become more accustomed to it, which I believe will help me to respond more empathically to clients who undoubtedly will go through similar feelings during their therapy. Through experiencing not-knowing, I was able to transform my work and also felt the transformation within myself as explication progressed.

A willingness and ability to embrace uncertainty enables creation of (potential?) space in art therapy where possibilities for discovery of new meanings are endless and the exciting and surprising elements of our work come alive (Moon 2002). Although it may make the therapist feel uncomfortable or inadequate, being in touch with unclear or uncertain material allows valuable time to think (Lesser 2007). The pressure to know may limit the potential space. Therefore 'negative-capability' (Jemstedt 2000) or the tolerance of not-knowing by the therapist can lead to an unbounded and more authentic therapeutic space where clients are better served.

Uncertainty has also been described as a driving force of artistic transformation (McNiff 1998b). The experience of entering into the unknown with new art materials allowed me to experiment with my personal responses to them, exploring and learning more about the materials and myself in the process. Extensive knowledge of art materials is of utmost importance, enabling the therapist to help clients find the most suitable way to achieve expression of their emotions (Rubin 1999). The practical knowledge I gained from their use helped me to appreciate the expressive and tactile qualities of each, resulting in a sense of self-mastery, empowerment and confidence, equipping me with valuable skills for future client work.

Repetition and multiplicity

Using repetition of gestures, marks or forms can be indicative of an attempt on behalf of the maker to comprehend or tackle an idea or concept (Cavaliero 2016). In this heuristic study I employed the repetitive exploration of the vessel form to help me to understand my experience of infertility. While repetition may have negative connotations in terms of destruction, restriction and immobility, it has also been associated with rhythm, perseverance, knowledge assimilation, learning and communication (Cavaliero 2016). When I reviewed my body of work, the ideas around meditative growth, perseverance and resilience resonated with me. I felt my knowledge and understanding expand each time I made a new vessel. McNiff (1998a) relates the process of repetition art to the use of a familiar starting point which can generate numerous different outcomes. I think these different outcomes all related to exploring the multiple parts of self through imagery, which helped me to acknowledge my maternal-ness.

As well as repetition of form there was also repetition of movement within the making of many of the vessels I created. Whitaker (2004) explores kinaesthetics and the implications of body movement within art therapy. She links movement to art making, describing the body as a physical aspect of the personality. Therefore movement, and the images made through bodily movements, represent the personality made visible.

When we engage consciously with our movement it becomes a vehicle for understanding and transformation (Halprin 2003). Due to the repetitive movements involved with making many of the vessels I found myself becoming consciously attuned to my bodily feelings during the making process. Sheets-Johnstone (1999) explains how we come to know ourselves more deeply through the 'fundamental primacy of movement'. Maybe this engagement of kinaesthetic consciousness could explain how I was able to look more insightfully at my work and self, and acknowledge the internal strength and resilience I have developed. I believe this development of my own kinaesthetic consciousness will contribute to my overall non-verbal awareness which will help me to be more attuned to clients in my future work.

Conclusion

Through this art-based heuristic research study, I have been able to explore, in-depth, the loss and grief of infertility through engagement with art materials. This process has enabled me to explore: parts of self and identity, repetition and resilience, and the concept of 'not-knowing'. Through this journey I have also been able to appreciate my metaphorical maternal self and the potential space I have found through my loss, and have been able to consider how they can be used therapeutically with clients. I have come to realise the importance of reflexively examining my own thinking. This helped me realise that the haste to 'know', 'name' or 'label' can be limiting to self, the creative process and therapeutic work. By tolerating uncertainty and remaining open, we enhance the potential therapeutic space, leading to a richer and more authentic therapeutic relationship (Lesser 2007). Moreover, we remain open to the many layers of meaning and material clients bring. Regarding the challenges of utilising verbal language to describe visual and haptic process (McNiff 1998b), I acknowledge that I found the written translation of the creative process challenging. Through experiencing first-hand the profoundly transformational power of the creative process in the exploration of the grief and loss associated with infertility, I now believe many others could also benefit from the healing, restorative and empowering effects of art-making and art therapy. Creative synthesis is expressed in the form of a poem

Metaphorically Maternal

Unwhole, empty, not mother, other
Failure, loss, longing, lost
Envy, yearning, sadness, anger
Devoid, hollow, absence present.
What is this loss, I have to know,
I look inside it, searching for meaning.
It is part of me and I am of it.
Feeling my way through my grief,
eyes closed, memories awakened
fresh and alive in my mind,
touched by touch, touched by loss.
Circles, vessels forms emerging,
Out of the empty darkness
A whisper of light illuminates
I am more than this.
Circles, vessels, forms emerging
Informing what is next,
scattering grief, imagining potential space.
Strength, resilience and growth
I am not one or the other
But countless different things
All the colours, black and white
And many more to be

References

Ashby, E. 2017. *Surviving Creatively: An Investigation into the Impact of Working with People who have Learning Disabilities on Art Therapists Employed in the NHS.* Doctor of Philosophy, Goldsmiths College, University of London. Available at: http://research.gold.ac.uk/22953/ (accessed June 2019).

Berensohn, P. 1972. *Finding One's Way with Clay.* New York: Simon and Schuster.

Bion, W. 1962. *Second Thoughts.* London: Heinemann.

Case, C., & Dalley, T. 2014. *The Handbook of Art Therapy*, 3rd ed. London: Routledge.

Cavaliero, A. 2016. Considering the Function of Repetition in Art and Art Psychotherapy. *ATOL: Art Therapy OnLine*, 7(1). Available at: http://journals.gold.ac.uk/index.php/atol/article/view/401/pdf (accessed February 2018).

Collier, A. F. 2012. *Using Textile Arts and Handcrafts in Therapy with Women: Weaving Lives Back Together*. London: Jessica Kingsley Publishers.

Cook, E. P. 1987. Characteristics of the Biopsychosocial Crisis of Infertility. *Journal of Counselling and Development*, 65: 465–470.

Cousineau, T. A., & Domar, A. D. 2007. Psychological Impact of Infertility. *Best Practice & Research Clinical Obstetrics & Gynaecology*, 21(2): 293–308.

Day, J. 2013. *Living the Life Unexpected: Twelve Weeks to Your Plan B for a Meaningful and Fulfilling Life without Children*, 2nd ed. London: Pan Macmillan.

Doka, K. J. 1989. *Disenfranchised Grief*. Lexington and Toronto: Lexington Books.

Edwards, D. 1992. Certainty and Uncertainty in Art Therapy Practice. *International Journal of Art Therapy: Inscape*, Spring: 2–7.

Edwards, D. 2013. *Art Therapy: Creative Therapies in Practice*, 2nd ed. London: Sage.

Elbrecht, C., & Antcliff, L. R. 2014. Being Touched through Touch: Trauma Treatment through Haptic Perception at the Clay Field: A Sensorimotor Art Therapy. *International Journal of Art Therapy*, 19(1): 19–30.

Fertility Network UK. 2018. *Emotional Impact*. Available at: https://fertilitynetworkuk.org/tag/for-those-facing-the-challenges-of-childlessness (accessed November 2018).

Halprin, D. 2003. *The Expressive Body in Life, Art and Therapy*. London: Jessica Kingsley Publishers.

Heidegger, M. 1962. *Being and Time*. New York: Harper & Row.

Henley, D. 1991. Facilitating the Development of Object Relations through the Use of Clay in Art Therapy. *American Journal of Art Therapy*, 29(3): 68–77.

Henley, D. 2002. *Clayworks in Art Therapy: Plying the Sacred Circle*. London: Jessica Kingsley Publishers.

Hiles, D. 2002. *Narrative and Heuristic Approaches to Transpersonal Research and Practice*. Paper presented to CCPE, London, October. Available at: http://psy.dmu.ac.uk/drhiles/N&Hpaper.htm (accessed May 2019).

Hogan, S. 2012. A Tasty Drop of Dragon's Blood: Self-Identity, Sexuality and Motherhood. In S. Hogan (ed.), *Revisiting Feminist Approaches to Art Therapy*. New York: Berghahn Books.

Jemstedt, A. 2000. Potential Space: The Place of Encounter between Inner and Outer Reality. *International Journal of Psychoanalysis*, 9: 124–131.

Kapitan, L. 2010. *Introduction to Art Therapy Research*. London: Routledge.

Kluger-Bell, K. 2000. *Unspeakable Losses: Healing from the Miscarriage, Abortion, and Other Pregnancy Loss*. New York: Harper.

Learmonth, M. 1994. Witness and Witnessing in Art Therapy. *Inscape: Journal of the British Art Therapy Association*, 1: 19–22.

Lesser, A. 2007. Potential Space: Knowing and Not Knowing in the Treatment of Traumatised Children and Young People. *British Journal of Social Work*, 37: 23–37.

Lindsey, B. 2013. The Psychology of Infertility. *International Journal of Childbirth Education*, 28(3): 41–47.

McNiff, S. 1998a. *Trust the Process: An Artist's Guide to Letting Go*. Boston: Shambhala.

McNiff, S. 1998b. *Art-Based Research*. London: Jessica Kingsley Publishers.

McNiff, S. 2004. *Art Heals*. Boston: Shambhala.

McNiff, S., ed. 2013. *Art and Research*. Bristol: Intellect.

Moon, C. H. 2002. *Studio Art Therapy: Cultivating the Artist Identity in the Art Therapist.* London: Jessica Kingsley Publishers.

Moustakas, C. 1990. *Heuristic Research: Design, Methodology and Applications.* London: Sage.

National Health Service. 2018. *Overview: Infertility.* Available at: www.nhs.uk/conditions/ infertility (accessed November 2018).

Ronnberg, A., & Martin, K., eds. 2010. *The Book of Symbols: Reflections of Archetypal Images.* Cologne: Taschen.

Rubin, J. 1999. *Art Therapy: An Introduction.* Philadelphia: Brunner/Mazel.

Seftel, L. 2006. *Grief Unseen: Healing Pregnancy Loss through the Arts.* London: Jessica Kingsley Publishers.

Sela-Smith, S. 2002. Heuristic Research: A Review and Critique of Moustakas' Method. *Journal of Humanistic Psychology*, 42(3): 53–88.

Sheets-Johnstone, M. 1999. *The Primacy of Movement.* Amsterdam: John Benjamin's Publishing Company.

Smith, S. 2006. *Felt to Stitch.* London: Batsford.

Souter-Anderson, L. 2010. *Touching Clay, Touching What? The Use of Clay in Art Therapy.* Dorset: Archive Publishing.

Stroebe, M. S., & Schut, H. 1999. The Dual Process Model of Coping with Bereavement: Rationale and Description. *Death Studies*, 23(3): 197–224.

Watkins, M. 2000. Six Approaches to the Image in Art Therapy. In B. Sells (ed.), *Working with Mages: The Theoretical Base of Archetypal Psychology.* Woodstock: Spring.

Whitaker, P. 2004. Art Moves; Exploring the Implications of the Body and Movement within Art Therapy. *Canadian Art Therapy Association Journal*, 17(1): 3–9.

Williams, M. E. 1997. Towards Greater Understanding of the Psychological Effects of Infertility on Women. *Psychotherapy in Private Practice*, 16(3): 7–26.

Winnicott, D. W. 1971. *Playing and Reality.* London: Routledge.

3 Art Therapy and pregnancy loss

A secret grief

Laura Seftel

It's easy to guess how one becomes an expert in pregnancy loss. I had a miscarriage.

It happened 27 years ago, at a time when I didn't know this could happen to me. Writing and making art was the only path I could find through the shock and the grief. The loss of that pregnancy reverberated through my artwork for a long time – sometimes I wasn't even aware that a piece was about my miscarriage until after it was completed. I felt very alone through the grieving process, but eventually I wondered if others were using art to heal from the confusion and pain of pregnancy loss.

A few years after my miscarriage I organised an exhibit with a handful of other like-minded artists in my small Massachusetts town. That first show evolved into the Secret Club Project, a digital collection of visual art and poetry submitted by pregnancy loss survivors from around the United States and abroad (Seftel 2001). Like me, these women had turned to their creative process, using paint, photography, collage, fibre arts and sculpture to express their profound experiences of loss (Seftel 2006). Their accompanying artist statements reveal a hidden world of sorrow and resilience.

This chapter will draw from the evocative words and images of the Secret Club artists to help illustrate key aspects of the pregnancy loss experience. We will also review the innovative ways in which the arts and creative rituals – in both therapeutic and self-directed settings – are being used to support families coping with infertility, miscarriage and stillbirth.

As I speak with families who have experienced more recent pregnancy losses, I see that 27 years later we are not nearly as far along as I had hoped. Yes, there is currently a bit more awareness, more permission to speak of pregnancy losses – there is now even a Hallmark condolence card for miscarriage. Yet despite hundreds of articles, editorials and memoirs proliferating on social media and news outlets, bereaved parents still enter a 'secret club' when they experience pregnancy loss. There continues to be a surprising lack of clear and compassionate societal responses: 'Miscarriage is a traditionally taboo subject that is rarely discussed publicly – even though nearly one million occur in the U.S. each year' (Montefiore Medical Center 2013). We know that at least one in six pregnancies end in miscarriage (and likely more); yet despite this prevalence, pregnancy loss remains misunderstood.

Art Therapy and other creative approaches can play an important role in illuminating and supporting this specific form of grief, allowing a woman and her partner to express and make sense of the complex feelings that can arise following pregnancy loss. 'Creative therapies offer grievers a new opportunity for constructing meaning out of their experiences' (Buser, Buser & Gladding 2005). The expressive arts can be a powerful tool to help women and their families re-establish a sense of connection and empowerment, and has even been used as a form of advocacy. One especially important contribution of the arts is that they can make visible the inner world of those who suffer this invisible loss. 'There is something about seeing which makes the loss more tangible and allows grieving to begin' (Kluger-Bell 1998, p. 137).

What is a pregnancy loss?

These losses include a range of experiences including infertility, miscarriage and stillbirth. A miscarriage is defined in the US as a pregnancy that ends spontaneously before 20 weeks. Miscarriage is most likely to occur during the first trimester and, as we have noted, is quite common. Most miscarriages do not have a specific known cause and do not create any future risks.

One less common type of miscarriage is ectopic pregnancy, which occurs when a fertilised egg implants outside the uterus, usually in the fallopian tube – hence the common term 'tubal pregnancy'. An ectopic pregnancy may place the life of the mother at risk, can impact future fertility and requires immediate intervention and more follow-up care.

Stillbirth is defined as the death of a baby in-utero any time after 20 weeks of pregnancy. Sometimes a woman has to go through the birth process even though it will not result in a live delivery. Currently, stillbirth occurs in about one in 100 pregnancies in the United States (CDC 2019). New-born infant deaths are also sometimes included in the discussion of pregnancy-related losses, but will not be the focus of this chapter.

Infertility may also be part of the picture for families who have experienced pregnancy loss. Infertility is usually defined as the inability to become pregnant after a year of actively trying. A newer form of reproductive loss has come into play with *in vitro fertilisation* (IVF). Undergoing IVF procedures can take a tremendous physical, emotional and financial toll; when IVF is not successful it can feel like a significant loss. Some women who struggle with infertility describe waves of grief with each menstrual cycle.

And where does abortion fit into this discussion of pregnancy loss? In the United States it is such a divisive topic that it can hardly be mentioned without feeling like you're putting your foot in quicksand. Is it possible to support a woman's right to choose to terminate a pregnancy while also supporting her right to have a range of feelings about it? Even if a woman is certain that an abortion was the right decision for her, she may still be left with a confusing soup of emotions but few outlets for emotional support. If miscarriage is a secret, abortion is 'top secret', leaving some women reluctant to share with even their closest friends.

Today the line between birth, miscarriage and abortion is more blurred than ever. With new medical technology, we now see the termination of pregnancies due to foetal abnormalities as well as 'thinning out' multi-foetal pregnancies. How excruciating for the woman who has endured endless fertility treatments to be faced with the decision to remove one or more of her embryos to ensure the survival of the remaining others. These medical advances can leave families with agonising decisions – a quandary that has been called the 'dilemma of choice' by author Kluger-Bell (1998, p. 69). Through this lens, miscarriage and abortion can be understood as part of the nuanced and sometimes interconnected spectrum of women's reproductive lives.

A budding attachment

Up until the 1970s it was falsely assumed that women and their families did not mourn the loss of a pregnancy; that assumption is now widely understood to be a myth. Our deepening understanding of attachment theory helps us to envision the quiet connection that is likely forming during pregnancy. The article 'Miscarriage: A Dream Interrupted' (Trepal, Semivan & Caley-Bruce 2005), delves into how an expecting mother begins the developmental process of bonding with her baby well before it is born, and sheds light on the depth of sorrow she may feel when that attachment process is suddenly interrupted.

The article also explores how 'pregnancy is a task that requires women to become accustomed to profound biological, somatic, and psychological changes and involves achieving a maternal identity' (p. 157). Miscarriage interrupts that identity formation, creating a crisis for the woman as well as her family. Messages that a woman has gleaned from her life experiences – including cultural expectations from her family and her partner – may leave her with a complicated blend of beliefs about her worth as a mother and a woman. Women may also carry lingering guilt and doubts about their capacity to carry a pregnancy to term, and may even question their capacity to mother.

Another myth about pregnancy loss is that a woman who feels ambivalent or had not planned to get pregnant will not grieve the end of that pregnancy. On the contrary, a pregnancy that was unplanned or had a complicated beginning can leave a woman feeling 'burdened with guilt as well as sorrow' (Kohn & Moffitt 2000, p. 4). If you scratch the surface, you will find that many expecting parents grapple with a range of hopes, fears and doubts – all normative feelings during the transition toward parenthood. One Secret Club artist, Gabrielle Strong, reflected, 'As women our reproductive lives are filled with mixed emotions. There is no simple response to a confirmation of pregnancy, no matter the desired outcome.'

Because of the developing attachment to the baby, the duration of a pregnancy is not always an accurate measure of the depth of grief experienced by the family (Swanson et al. 2007). Many other factors come into play, including all of the hopes and dreams the expecting parents held for the future. According to some approaches in grief counselling, these bonds of attachment are understood to continue even after the death of a loved one. For some families, grieving is a process of cherishing rather than relinquishing their bonds with those they have lost.

A painting by Secret Club artist Brenda Philips (Figure 3.1) captures the longing and the loss that often appears in artwork after a pregnancy loss. Phillips' painting depicts a grieving woman tenderly holding a pale blue bird, while another image of a bird is seen departing. The artist shared that her artwork was inspired by the infertility and miscarriages she had endured. Her painting is a beautiful representation of the tender bond that had already been established, despite never having had the chance to hold the baby she hoped for.

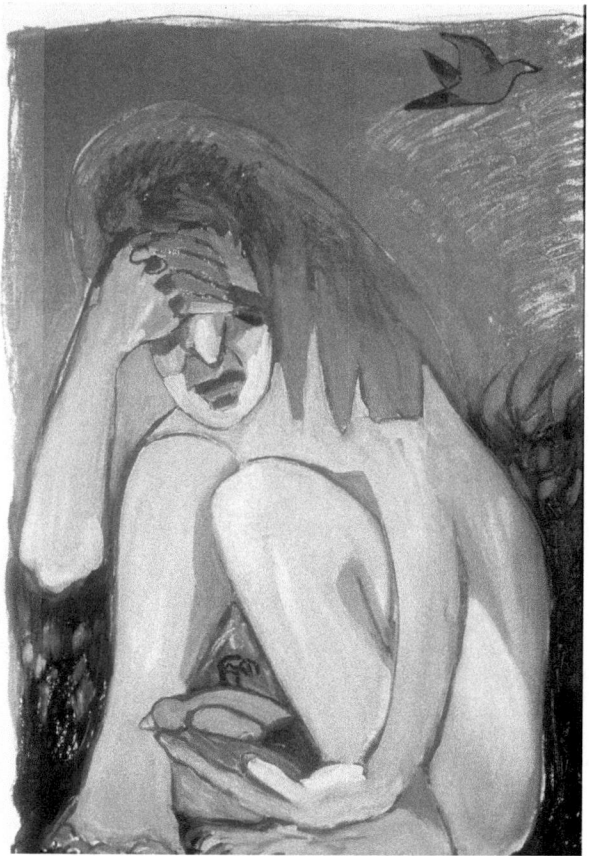

Figure 3.1 Sorrow. Oil on paper, Brenda Phillips.

Viewing pregnancy loss through the trauma lens

Pregnancy loss is not a pretty picture. The reality is that a miscarriage can be a bloody, traumatising event. The physical experience can be painful, with intense cramping and even labour contractions: 'The process can go on for weeks, even months, leaving women in a strange purgatory between pregnant and not' (Kelley & March 2019). Several courageous artists in the Secret Club Project incorporated splatters of red paint in their art to reflect the authentic physical experience of pregnancy loss.

One of those artists, Nona Hatay, shared,

> I can still feel the physical fear and pain. Feeling as if I was going to bleed to death, knowing my hopes and dreams were dead, feeling so helpless and alone in the bathroom all night long. Afterwards, no one really understood how bad it was.

Frida Kahlo, the well-known Mexican artist who suffered a series of pregnancy losses and complications, depicts herself lying on bloody sheets in her surreal painting from 1932, 'Henry Ford Hospital'. To symbolise the impact of their experience, some Secret Club artists have turned to images of skeletons, skulls, or coffins – images so rarely associated with pregnancy and birth.

Reflecting on her piece titled 'The Unexpected', Secret Club artist Mary Flanary says, 'My painting attempts to convey the intense, out of control state of losing a pregnancy and all the unfulfilled hopes' (Figure 3.2). In her discordant painting, random numbers drip with blood, as musical notes careen against a bright red background. The figure's abdomen is a black hole. These kinds of overwhelming experiences and sensations can be seared into a woman's sensory

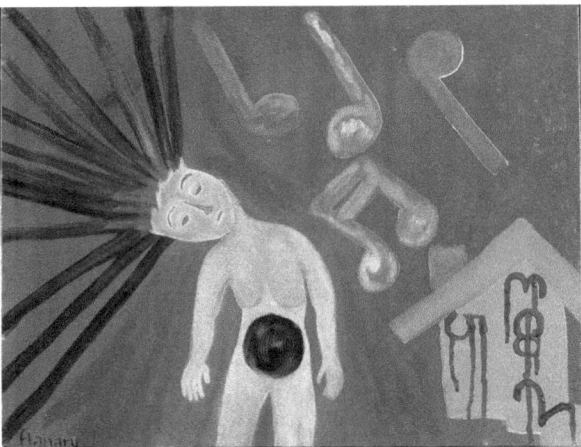

Figure 3.2 The Unexpected. Painting, Mary K. Flanary.

memory. As we learn more about trauma and its impact we can see miscarriage and stillbirth not only as losses, but as potential traumas.

In addition, previous reproductive traumas can have a cumulative impact; a woman may have experienced several pregnancy-related losses in succession, further impacting her emotional state and sense of self. In fact, pregnancy loss can reawaken previous adverse experiences from any point in her life, adding layers of complexity to the grief recovery process.

If a woman experiences her pregnancy loss within an overtaxed and insensitive medical system, she and her partner may experience what has been termed 'medical trauma'. Families frequently express deep dissatisfaction with the management and care of their pregnancy loss. It is often in a sterile room with the ultrasound technician that a couple may become aware that something has gone awry with their pregnancy. This critical moment can be an emotional shock: 'In the few seconds it takes to receive a diagnosis, it can feel like your body shifts from a garden to a graveyard' (Kelley & March 2019).

Subsequent discussions with the treating physician are often dry and clinical, with little attention to the well-documented risk of depression and trauma in women who lose a pregnancy. Even deciding how to handle the 'foetal remains' can be an 'emotional minefield for women and their partners' (Douglas & Fox 2009, p. 90). The language used to discuss follow-up procedures, explanations about what went wrong with the pregnancy and prognosis for future fertility are often unclear, and the medical terminology can be jarring; for instance, medical staff may call a woman over age 35 a 'geriatric mother' or refer to a miscarriage as a 'spontaneous abortion'. Families likely use very different words to describe what they have lost; based on their personal, cultural and religious backgrounds, it may be a pregnancy, a foetus, a baby, an angel.

The responsiveness and sensitivity of medical staff can have a powerful impact on the family's subsequent narrative of loss and recovery. Dr Michael Berman, OB-GYN and former clinical professor at the Yale School of Medicine, notes that when a patient's pregnancy ends in miscarriage, stillbirth or infant death, physicians struggle to find the right approach to break the news to them and console their grief. 'Most of us have not been taught to provide this bereavement care' (Berman 2019). In the face of the losses he witnessed, Berman undertook a rare and moving act: he composed poetry for his bereaved patients (2001).

Like Berman, innovators in the medical field are integrating the arts into training programmes for physicians, nurses and other medical staff to reaffirm the human dimension of healthcare. Engaging with the arts – both making it and viewing it – encourages future healthcare professionals to wrestle with their own conscious and unconscious responses to pain, trauma and loss. These creative explorations in turn prepare providers to authentically witness and support women and their families, while simultaneously reducing their own risk for professional burnout and vicarious traumatisation (Berman 2001; Bertman 1999; Stuart 2004). In the art-infused lectures that I have offered to healthcare professionals, I have seen first-hand that pregnancy loss education and advocacy can be enhanced by the power of the arts.

Mapping the emotional landscape

We now understand that women who have lost a pregnancy will likely experience a range of intense emotions, including sadness, rage, anxiety, shame, emptiness, jealousy and intense self-blame. A groundbreaking study in the early 1990s found that women who have a miscarriage are more than twice as likely to experience clinical depression as other women, especially during the six months immediately following the loss (Neugebauer et al. 1992). This study paved the way for much of the research that followed.

We should also keep in mind that a woman who has been undergoing fertility treatments, experienced a miscarriage or delivered a stillborn infant may be reeling from hormonal shifts that can amplify painful emotions (not unlike a postpartum depression). The lack of clear responses to pregnancy loss can compound the problem.

Feelings of guilt and shame seem almost universal following pregnancy loss: I have yet to meet a woman who did not, on some level, blame herself. In an effort to make sense of this inexplicable loss, a bereaved mother may become preoccupied with guilt-tinged narratives about what she has done wrong. Infertility and pregnancy loss can even be misinterpreted as a punishment for a previous mistake.

A 2013 survey of more than 1,000 adults in the US found that misperceptions about miscarriage and its causes are widespread. While most miscarriages are the result of chromosomal abnormalities and other medical complications, the study revealed that most people falsely believe that miscarriage can be caused by an argument, lifting a heavy object, a previous abortion or even a woman's negative thoughts about the pregnancy. The study's authors concluded, 'the false perceptions and lack of understanding about miscarriage are significant in the US and contribute to many women and couples feeling isolated and alone after suffering from a miscarriage' (Montefiore Medical Center 2013).

Another prominent feeling that can be associated with pregnancy loss is anger. In Tammy LeMasters Gross' digital artwork, the eyes glow red with rage (Figure 3.3). 'The outpouring of anger may be a response to the unfairness of life, a woman's feelings of incompetence, her inability to control what has happened within her own body, the lack of sensitive medical response, or other frustrations' (Speert 1992, p. 124). A bereaved parent may be angry at God for allowing the pregnancy loss to happen or feel resentful of friends who appear to have so effortlessly produced perfectly healthy children. Yet women are often socialised not to express anger directly because it is not considered feminine or attractive.

All of these emotions may be a normal part of grief, but they often remain underground. In a recent editorial in the *New York Times*, the authors posit that, 'Miscarriage might just be the loneliest experience that millions of women have faced' (Kelley & March 2019). The isolation and silence associated with pregnancy loss brings to mind the concept of 'disenfranchised grief', which is defined as grief that is not socially accepted and therefore hidden (Doka 1989). Examples of early losses that may be 'disenfranchised' include a miscarriage or stillbirth, a

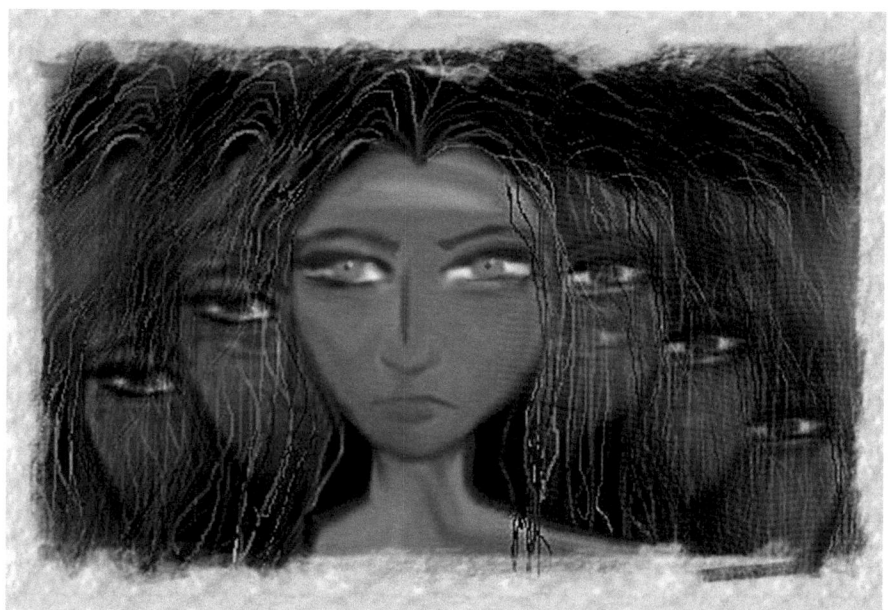

Figure 3.3 Self-portrait (Anger). Digital art, Tammy LeMasters Gross.

secret adoption or an abortion. Doka has found that when grief is not acknowledged, grief resolution cannot occur. It is no wonder that many women turn to their own creative process in the face of secrecy and isolation.

Expanding the circle: the impact on the couple and the family

While some women may be embarking on the path to parenthood on their own, most women have a partner – male, female, or identifying as non-binary – who is also touched by the loss. Several studies over the past few decades point to the increasing involvement of expectant partners in the excitement around a pregnancy. 'The entire family unit is drawn into a closer experience of the pregnancy due to early home pregnancy test, heartbeat monitors, and other advanced technology such as ultrasound' (Douglas & Fox 2009, p. 91).

With a stronger early attachment being formed, it makes sense that partners may feel the impact of a miscarriage more profoundly. One study of Irish fathers coping with pregnancy loss found that 'men who have strongly visualised their baby will have a deeper experience of grief' (McCreight 2004, p. 346). These findings, highlighting the father's visualisation process, raise interesting ideas for the potential use of Art Therapy in support of the non-pregnant partner.

This same study found that after a pregnancy loss, male participants reported feelings of self-blame, confusion around their identity as a father, and pressure to appear stoic and strong. Bereaved fathers may be at risk for a delayed onset of grief. Yet because men may not appear to be 'actively' grieving, their friends, family and professionals can inadvertently overlook their emotional needs and direct most of their attention to the mother.

I was heartened to come across a piece in *The Guardian* newspaper highlighting an art exhibit by London-based artist Andrew Foster. His monumental 75ft scroll painting titled 'Pain Will Not Have the Last Word' imagines the lives of the children he dreams of after he and his wife lost three pregnancies to miscarriage. Figure 3.4 offers a detail from his scroll; above three figures he writes, 'Why did you leave me without saying goodbye?' In the article he shares how devastated he was by the losses, adding: 'There's a need for it to be recognised that men grieve too.' He continues, 'I was surprised how little people asked me how I felt at the time' (Goodchild 2015). During his exhibit, Foster partnered with a pregnancy loss advocacy group to help raise awareness about the impact of miscarriage on men.

Disappointments and differences in grieving experiences can also emerge in lesbian couples. Following a pregnancy loss, one partner may be more expressive, presenting as tearful and seeking emotional connection, while the other partner may appear more stoic, preferring to spend time alone doing practical tasks. This potential gap in grieving styles has been called 'incongruent grieving' and can lead to miscommunication and resentment (Kohn & Moffitt 2000, p. 34). I have

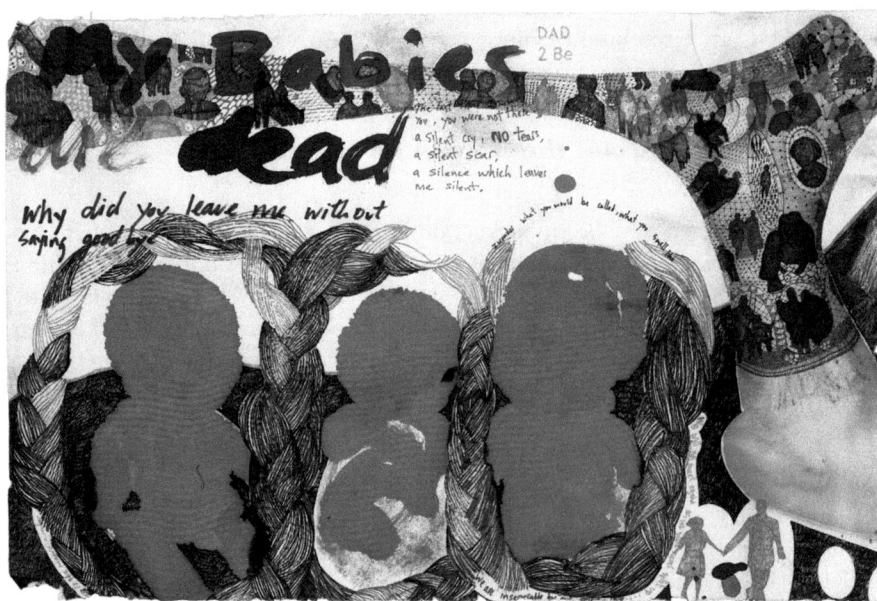

Figure 3.4 Pain Will Not Have the Last Word. Detail of scroll painting, Andrew Foster.

also had female clients in same-sex relationships share that they were envious of their partner's ability to bear a healthy child when – due to infertility or other complications – they could not.

The work of one Art Therapy student acknowledges the toll that pregnancy loss can take on a relationship (Faulkner 2003). For her thesis project, Alexis Faulkner designed a series of art exercises for couples to engage in together. In one of the art exercises, parents are offered three-dimensional materials, including clay, fabric and chenille stems to create an object together that represents their lost child. The art directive allows for 'a tangible object to be made that can be seen and held by the couple' (pp. 11–12). Another exercise offers a chance for the partners to decorate a box in which they can place mementos. This conjoint creative process provides more opportunities for the couple to validate their loss, communicate their feelings and to honour each other's manner of grieving.

Art experiences and rituals can also be designed to include children of families coping with pregnancy loss. Siblings need to have their questions met with age-appropriate and honest information. Stephanie Paige Cole, bereaved parent and pregnancy loss advocate reminds us, 'The death of a baby can be very difficult on our surviving children, and even our subsequent children. These kids witness their parents wrestling with overwhelming grief, and struggle with their own feelings of sadness and confusion.'

Stephanie founded the Sweet Pea Project in Lancaster, Pennsylvania, for families who have experienced pregnancy loss. Among other services, they host an annual event for siblings, which includes an opportunity to engage in a creative project. One year the children jotted messages on wildflower seed papers which were then planted in flower pots they had decorated. Another year they painted paper butterflies to add to an enormous 'butterfly tree' that now resides in a nearby hospital. Other projects include sculpting garden stones out of clay and hanging colourful paper birds from the ceiling of their local children's library.

Pregnancy after loss

How do families who have survived pregnancy loss manage the hopes and fears that arise around the idea of trying again? A woman may no longer be able to envision or believe in the arrival of a healthy baby. In her painting, 'Response to a Subsequent Pregnancy', Stephanie Paige Cole mapped out her overlapping hopes and worries (Figure 3.5). If the family does successfully bring a baby to term, they may experience amplified anxiety about the child's wellbeing. After losing a baby, finding a way to feel safe in the world – or safe enough – can be an ongoing challenge.

Susan Jacobsen, an Art Therapist who practices in Colorado, has grappled with these kinds of worries after her traumatic experiences. Toward the end of a normal pregnancy, Susan found herself suddenly fighting for her life due to a misdiagnosis of a high-risk medical condition. Her full-term son Henry did not survive. Traumatised by her loss, Susan endured two more miscarriages and years of struggling with infertility. Finally, she and her husband had their son

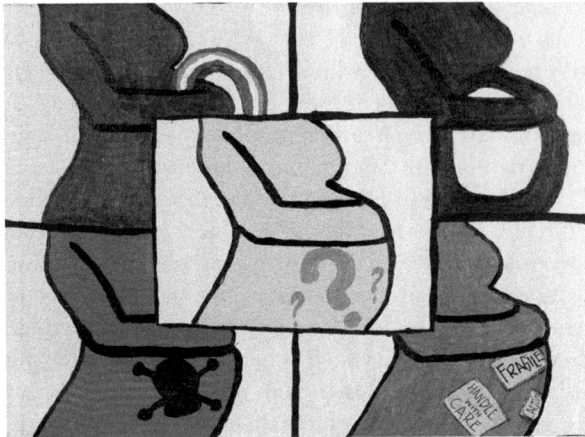

Figure 3.5 Response to a Subsequent Pregnancy. Acrylic on canvas, Stephanie Paige Cole (first published in the book *Still*, 2010).

Jens when she was 42 years old. Susan savours time with her son, but she also has moments of significant anxiety about his wellbeing, wondering, 'What if something terrible happens again?'

Sending her son to kindergarten was particularly anxiety provoking and she used art making to help manage her fears. Throughout her motherhood journey – encompassing grief and trauma, infertility, and finally parenting a healthy child – Susan has used art to support her recovery and growth. As part of that process, she occasionally creates self-portraits centred on specific themes. These drawings allow her to both explore and contain her worry, which in turn frees her to be more present as a parent (Figure 3.6).

Today Susan offers Art Therapy groups to support expressive avenues for other women. In her 'Pregnancy after Loss' group, participants engage in their own creative process as they 'navigate the road to and through motherhood'.

Creative expression in response to pregnancy loss

There is a significant body of literature exploring the use of creative Arts Therapy to support clients coping with more common forms of grief. Over the past 30 years, research studies utilising music, visual arts, videography, writing, movement and theatre arts have blossomed, demonstrating the benefits of expressive Arts Therapy (Berman 2001; Duffey 2005; Rogers 2007). 'The creative arts can enable an expression of emotion that transcends the usual verbal exchanges of therapy' (Buser et al. 2005, p. 177). By engaging in creative Arts Therapy, grieving clients can move beyond despair to discover inner strength, hope and new meaning.

However, there are only a few studies on using creative Arts Therapy to specifically address the unique grief associated with pregnancy loss. Ellen Speert's

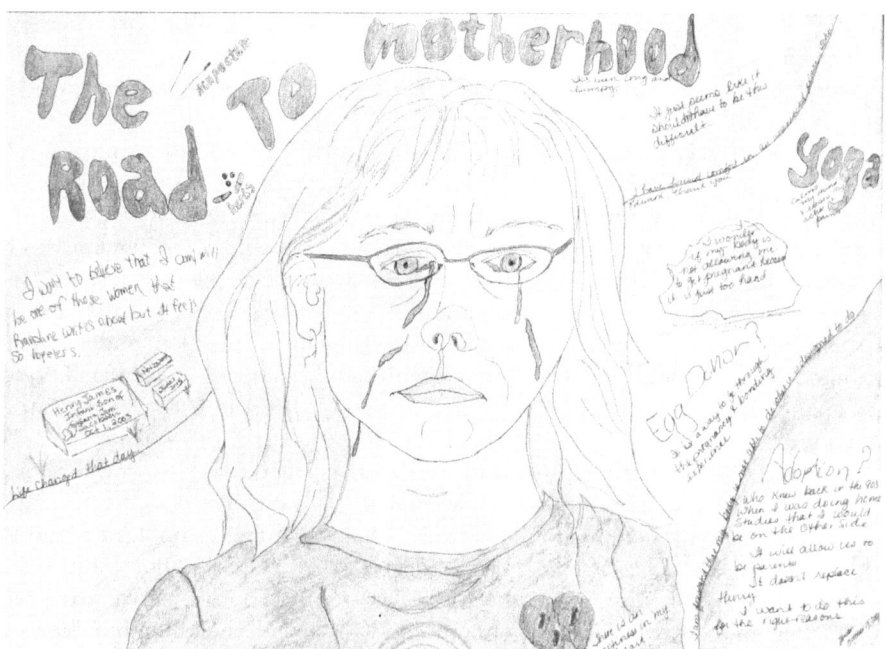

Figure 3.6 The Road to Motherhood. Blind contour drawing, Susan Jacobsen.

groundbreaking article, published in 1992, explores the use of Art Therapy with a group of women who had experienced miscarriage, abortion or stillbirth. After my own miscarriage, Speert's work was the only relevant Art Therapy article I could find (I was happy to learn recently that she continues to offer healing workshops for pregnancy loss in Encinitas, California).

A more recent article by Douglas and Fox (2009) recommends the use of creative interventions – in this case writing and drawing in a personal journal – to cope with grief following a miscarriage. One of the authors found that engaging in art journaling offered 'profound and meaningful creative expression of grief leading to self-awareness, emotional release of great turmoil, a degree of peace with the loss, and hope for the future' (p. 96).

Streeter and Deaver (2018) conducted research using Art Therapy to address the depression frequently associated with infertility. The loss of control over the capacity to have a baby is one of the most hidden losses in the range of reproductive crises. The study offered participants six Art Therapy experiences, including inside/outside boxes, process painting, clay modelling and large-scale body maps. Following the Art Therapy interventions and discussions, the women in the study experienced a significant decrease in their depressive symptoms and reported less panic and anxiety. The participants also reported that the Art Therapy exercises increased their sense of validation, self-awareness, the development of new coping skills, and improved communication with spouses and family members. Speert noted some similar experiences in her Art Therapy group for perinatal loss; her participants spoke of 'experiencing greater energy and less depression during art making, despite the sad content of their work' (1992, p. 124).

Art Therapy can also play a role in assessing the traumatic impact of pregnancy loss, although there is thus far scant research to guide us. Art Therapists who are trained in trauma-informed treatment are likely to pick up on the signs of distress in the art productions of clients who are struggling after a miscarriage or stillbirth. Indicators in the artwork of hopelessness, lingering pervasive fears, dissociation or dissolution of a cohesive sense of self may point to a need for more intensive support. Assessing for depression and trauma should be a part of any provider's work with families coping with infertility or pregnancy loss, while being careful not to pathologise the bereaved parent's response.

Alongside the professional literature on creative arts therapy we can find examples of bereaved parents who followed their own creative paths to healing, outside of a formal therapeutic relationship. One of the first examples I found is the book, *Creative Acts of Healing: After a Baby Dies* by Dutch author Judith van Praag (1999). In her memoir, the author turns to writing, textile arts, papermaking and other expressive modalities to wrestle with the unfathomable loss of her stillborn daughter. Other parents have employed 'crafts' to help express and heal the grief of pregnancy loss, finding solace in creating scrapbooks, needlepoint, quilts, jewellery and memory boxes to honour the pregnancies they carried. Some parents find relief in designing memorial tattoos to 'give shape and form to the grief of pregnancy loss' (Hill 2014, p. 203).

I have noticed an open-ended process in which many artists impacted by pregnancy loss trusted and followed their creative intuition. Stephanie Paige Cole, in her brief but powerful book of art and poetry titled *Still*, relates a similar process after the loss of her daughter:

> I began painting and sculpting and writing out everything I felt. Sometimes I would begin a piece with a specific idea in mind, but most of the time I just sat down at the canvas with a brush in my hand and tears in my eyes, and I just let it happen. I can't even begin to explain how good it feels to release those toxic feelings from my body and spread them all over the canvas.
>
> (Cole 2010, p. 34)

Whether in an Art Therapy setting or on one's own, the creative process offers unique benefits: the development of symbolic imagery that allows for the expression of complicated feelings; the physical release achieved through the manipulation of the art materials; and the creation of a tangible marker of the existence of this loved one, allowing bereaved parents to share their loss with others.

Body-based grief: loss from the inside out

> My paintings deal with feminine grief. It is a function of the body. It lives
> and breathes in every fibre.
>
> Kathy Ann Fleming, Secret Club artist

It has always made sense to me that pregnancy loss, which occurs in the body,
would need to be expressed through the body by visceral, tactile means. The
power of the creative process is that it allows us to bring forth what is so hard to
articulate with words: the flowing out, the emptiness, the sense that your own
body has betrayed you. Expressive modalities can capture the dark messiness of
pregnancy loss, that passage between birth and death. Secret Club artist Malinda
Ann Hill shared, 'After my own pregnancy loss, when words could not express
the depth of my emotions, I began to create art to capture the intensity of my
pain' (2014, p. 203).

Speert describes this embodied process in the Art Therapy groups she designed for women who had suffered perinatal loss. Her clients spoke of their
yearning and 'deep physical pain, aching arms and/or chest during the months
following perinatal loss' (1992, p. 124). Speert reports that participants found
both symbolic and physical release in the use of clay, tissue paper and other
tactile media. The three-dimensional, resistive materials seemed particularly
helpful in working out their unspoken rage, grief and emptiness, and ultimately
creating a new sense of connection with self and other. Streeter and Deaver
found similar benefits of three-dimensional art materials in their work with
women coping with infertility (2018, p. 65). The authors also point to the 'create,
destroy, renew' process that three-dimensional materials allow.

But creation doesn't always come easy. Stephanie Paige Cole shared (in a
personal correspondence) that after her stillbirth she found herself only able to
destroy:

> At first, after Madeline died, I felt so thoroughly broken that all I could do is
> break things – mostly clay pots in the driveway. I would smash them and
> shout and cry. My husband would clean them up after I went back inside.
> But one day, I picked up a few of the pieces. I saw so much of myself in their
> jagged edges, in their irreparableness, and I wanted something more for
> them. Using cement and paint, I sculpted the broken shards into a heart. It
> felt good. It felt like me. Badly broken, but somehow, still here.

That moment was a turning point, as she saw the 'potential of creation coming
from destruction'.

Artist and university lecturer Lucy O'Donnell, who is based in Yorkshire,
describes working on a series of large drawings which emerged from her experience of infertility and multiple miscarriages. In her art-making process she
drew and smudged graphite on paper, rubbing it raw in places. She explains how
the process involved her hands – the hands that expected to touch and hold a

baby and instead remained empty and longing. In an excerpt from an accompanying poem, she writes, 'The wanting the waiting/The void and the aching'.

That sense of emptiness that follows pregnancy loss, that persistent feeling that something is missing or has been stolen, appears again and again in the art of pregnancy loss. Some bereaved artists reflect their palpable loss through depictions of barren landscapes or quiet interior scenes featuring an empty crib or toys that will never be played with. It is not unusual for a woman to also portray that emptiness by creating an image of a female figure with a void where there was once a pregnancy (Seftel 2006; Speert 1992). Symbolic representations of empty wombs can be seen in paintings in Figures 3.2 and 3.5.

Containers/containment

Many women who make art after pregnancy loss seem to intuitively create images reminiscent of uterine and embryonic forms, resulting in expressive works not often seen in the mainstream, male-dominated art world. Some of my own art can only be described as images of angry or wounded vulvas and wombs

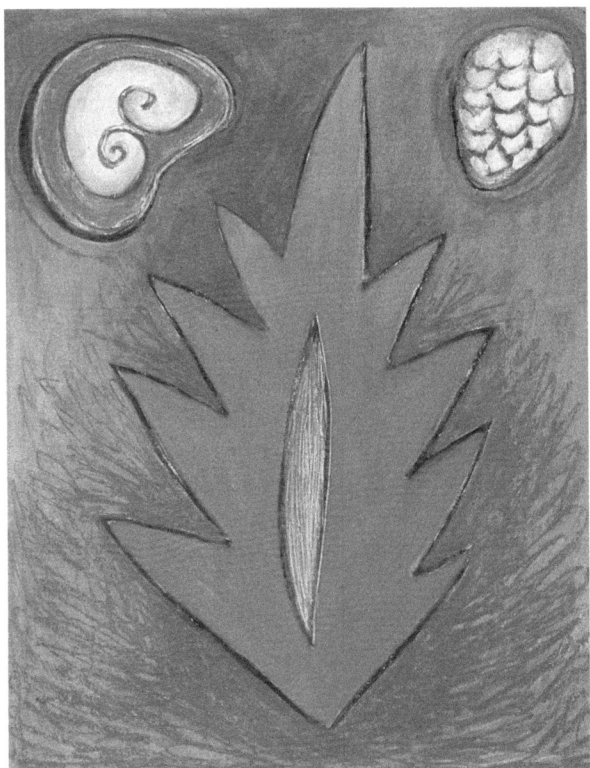

Figure 3.7 Untitled. Oil on paper, Laura Seftel.

(Figure 3.7). Like many of my pieces about miscarriage, this painting reflects an internal bodily experience of loss; it remains beyond spoken language for me – I was never able to title it.

The symbol of a vessel or container – which mirrors the form and function of the uterus – emerges as a seemingly universal image of pregnancy loss. Vases, jars, bowls, teapots – all show up in two-dimensional and three-dimensional art, not only in our contemporary depictions of pregnancy loss but in traditional rituals around the world. Perhaps the image of a container can also serve to 'contain' the bereaved mother's overwhelming grief and yearning. Vessels that are broken, scarred or shattered also sometimes represent a lost pregnancy – and the accompanying broken dreams.

For Alina, an Art Therapy client who worked with me following a miscarriage, the image of a vessel became a key symbol of healing. First, in the initial phase of therapy, she used paint and collage to explore layers of her traumatic experience. As treatment progressed, she spent several sessions creating the image of an iconic vase with a burning candle in its centre. The shape of the vessel echoes the female form. Behind it, she pieced together a fragmented background cut from Impressionist landscapes taken from an old calendar; this new landscape re-sembles a pastel-coloured mosaic. The vessel appears to hold a hint of hope and healing, and she is feeling ready to embrace another pregnancy.

Alina's pieced-together collage reflects a pattern of destruction and recon-stitution seen in artwork by other women who have experienced pregnancy loss. A renewed sense of wholeness or integration is possible – but only if it takes into account that which has been lost or broken. In the case of Alina's collage, she pieces together a welcoming landscape, yet it retains a sense of disjointedness.

In addition to images of vessels, other notable themes may emerge in preg-nancy loss art and poetry. Often a winged being – a bird, a butterfly, an angel – appears in the work, perhaps taking flight (as seen in Figure 3.1). Empty nests may also be depicted. Occasionally artists create a scene in which they are holding a representation of their baby or depict an infant cradled in the hands of God. Bereaved mothers may also create dolls or sculpt figures representing their lost babies – a creative act found in many traditional cultures following the loss of a pregnancy (Kluger-Bell 1998, p. 138; Sha 1990, p. 34). While many of these symbols have a universal quality, each work of art represents the unique, per-sonal story of one bereaved parent.

A more systematic review of symbolic imagery that emerges following preg-nancy loss could be an area for future study. For now, the expressive themes that arise in Art Therapy settings, research studies and arts projects can help us attune to the emotional landscape of grieving mothers and their families as we witness and validate their experience.

Breaking isolation: group work

In her article on Art Therapy and pregnancy loss, Ellen Speert found the group setting to be well-suited to meet women's psychological need for connection as viewed through a relational model of identity development. She found that 'the group therapy format provides more reflective surfaces to both contain and mirror each woman's experience of loss and validate her sense of self' (Speert 1992, pp. 127–128).

Parents fortunate enough to live in communities that offer pregnancy loss support groups have opportunities to ease their sense of isolation. For example, Empty Arms in western Massachusetts, (founded by a bereaved mother) offers groups for miscarriage support, subsequent pregnancy support and parenting after a loss, and support around infertility. This non-profit agency's network of services also includes immediate peer support available in local hospitals, help with memorial planning and lactation support after loss.

Empty Arms has occasionally sponsored events for bereaved parents to make art together. At one art gathering, participants assembled tactile materials such as coloured tissue paper, wood shapes, even sand paper and wire, to create personal objects representing their loss and their recovery. In similar fashion, Speert offered her group participants materials for collage and assemblage such as feathers, cloth, glitter, paint and clay. She also ended her Art Therapy group with a group mural experience, highlighting the connection and intimacy that had been established (Speert 1992, p. 127).

One of my favourite group art experiences to support pregnancy loss is creating 'comfort pillows' – simple canvas or muslin squares that can be embellished with healing images and then filled. A special message or prayer can also be placed inside.

While pregnancy loss groups can be profoundly supportive, juggling the specific needs of participants requires facilitators to be sensitive to the unique story of each member. Group leaders may choose to design pregnancy loss support groups geared specifically for participants in different phases of recovery. However, if a group is heterogeneous it is best practice to name the differences in participant's experiences while working to ensure that all losses are honoured.

Parents who have lost a pregnancy or new-born may also appreciate opportunities to gather on special occasions such as holidays or Pregnancy Loss Remembrance Day (October 15), which is observed in many countries around the world. These community rituals often incorporate a creative, hands-on commemorative experience, offering another opportunity to break through the isolation that can surround these early losses.

Creating rituals and memorials: interface with Art Therapy

Pregnancy losses reside on the border of life and death, a realm that for many families has deep cultural, spiritual or religious meaning. Yet there are few established rituals in Western culture to acknowledge these losses. Part of the healing process, therefore, may include supporting families to develop grief rituals. In my research of traditional responses to pregnancy loss around the world, I found many cultures have developed rituals and sacred objects to actively mark the milestone of a pregnancy that is interrupted (Sha 1990). Because there is considerable overlap between creating a ritual and creating expressive art, many traditional cultures do not even make a distinction between the two.

Common elements in rituals, both past and present, involve symbolic objects, song or prayer, movement and elements from nature (earth, fire, water, air). For example, a memorial candle-lighting ceremony might involve decorating candles and then floating them in a stream or bowl of water.

One recent study on the use of rituals for recovery from grief (not specific to pregnancy loss) highlights the benefits of the ritual being designed by the mourner as a unique personal expression (Sas & Coman 2016). Mourners were supported to create meaningful ritual objects in a process that drew on an Art Therapy approach, allowing for making, handling and showcasing symbols. Rituals may also have a place in the family life cycle, as they move through holidays, anniversaries or missed milestones.

Another bridge between art and spirituality is the making of altars, shrines or votives, which may serve as a tangible marker of a lost pregnancy. Having something to see, to touch and to return to helps externalise the healing process. Several years after my own early miscarriage, I created a small wooden shrine to mark the loss; the shrine is painted shades of blue, with a pinkish-red vessel at the centre (Seftel 2006, p. 171). For me, it was not intended to memorialise a baby – I never really thought of my pregnancy as a fully formed person – but was an acknowledgement of a sacred milestone in my life.

A recent *New York Times* article describes parents creating 'memorial videos' after they lost babies at birth. These videos, which often follow a specific format, are examples of new rites of passage being created by grieving parents. They allow families to engage their creativity, and often include music, photography, footprints of the baby and other mementos. One mother says of her stillborn daughter, 'I think without the video it may have been more difficult for people to comprehend that she was here' (Ro 2019).

Conclusion: healing benefits of the arts

When expectant parents experience a miscarriage or other reproductive loss, hopeful new beginnings collide with shock and grief. Art making and creative rituals can help navigate these turbulent emotions and open up new possibilities for healing. Integrating the expressive arts into the grieving process allows bereaved parents to reveal hidden layers of experience and honour all of their stories.

As we have seen, several research articles and case studies point to the use of Art Therapy techniques to deepen the healing process for families coping with infertility, reproductive losses, and stillbirth. The arts can be integrated into individual counselling, couples work, family rituals, group therapy and support groups, all with a focus on pregnancy loss.

The creative process can reflect the painstaking work of putting oneself back together after a potentially shattering experience. Author Judith van Praag reminds us, 'healing lies in patching the pieces together' (1999, p. 169). As a creative act, art making moves us from a passive stance to one of life-affirming self-expression. The creative arts can help bereaved parents break their isolation, enhance emotional communication, mark their 'invisible' losses, reconfigure their identity as parents and even transcend despair.

We are left with the question: how do we help society respond more sensitively to pregnancy loss and other reproductive complications? The emotional impact of pregnancy loss can hit hard and last for years – maybe even a lifetime – yet too much secrecy and misinformation still surround it. Through advocacy and education, a groundswell of re-visioning and re-imagining is already underway and the expressive arts can be a powerful part of that movement. When artists reveal their personal narratives of grief, they are educating us in a way that instruction manuals cannot – they wake us up and open our hearts. When art shines a light on this invisible loss, the Secret Club becomes a little less of a secret.

References

Berman, M. R. 2001. *Parenthood Lost: Healing the Pain After Miscarriage, Stillbirth, and Infant Death*. Westport, CT: Greenwood Publishing Group.

Berman, M. R. 2019. *Hygeia for Perinatal Loss*. Available at: https://p10.secure.hostingprod.com/@ombudu.com/ssl/Poetry_Metaphor_Medicine_2019.pdf (accessed October 2019).

Bertman, S. L., ed. 1999. *Grief and the Healing Arts*. London: Routledge.

Buser, T., Buser, J., & Gladding, S. 2005. Good Grief: The Part of Arts in Healing Loss and Grief. In T. Duffey (ed.), *Creative Interventions in Grief and Loss Therapy* Binghamton, NY: Haworth Press, Inc., pp. 173–183.

CDC (Centers for Disease Control & Prevention). 2019. What is Stillbirth? Available at www.cdc.gov/ncbddd/stillbirth/facts.html (accessed September 2019).

Cole, S. P. 2010. *Still*. Durham, CT: Eloquent Books.

Doka, K. J. 1989. *Disenfranchised Grief: Recognizing Hidden Sorrow*. Lexington, MA: Lexington Books.

Douglas, K. I., & Fox, J. R. 2009. Tears of Blood: Understanding and Creatively Intervening in the Grief of Miscarriage. In G. R. Walz, J. C. Bleuer, and R. K. Yep (eds.), *Compelling Counseling Interventions: VISTAS 2009*. Alexandria, VA: American Counseling Association, pp. 89–100.

Duffey, T., ed. 2005. *Creative Interventions in Grief and Loss Therapy: When the Music Stops, a Dream Dies*. London: Haworth Press.

Faulkner, A. F. 2003. *Art Therapy with Couples Who have Lost a Child Through Miscarriage*. Master's thesis, Eastern Virginia Medical School.

Goodchild, S. 2015. Bereaved Father Uses His Art to Show How Men Share the Pain of Miscarriage. *The Guardian*, 23 May. Available at: www.theguardian.com/lifeandstyle/2015/may/23/artist-men-also-suffer-agony-miscarriage-lose-baby (accessed November 2019).

Hill, M. A. 2014. Memorial Tattooing: Making Grief Visible. In B. E. Thompson & R. A. Neimeyer (eds.), *Grief and the Expressive Arts: Practices for Creating Meaning*. London: Routledge, pp. 202–204.

Kelley, L., & March, L. 2019. You Know Someone Who's Had a Miscarriage. *New York Times*, 10 Oct. Available at: www.nytimes.com/interactive/2019/10/10/opinion/miscarriage-pregnancy.html (accessed October 2019)

Kluger-Bell, K. 1998. *Unspeakable Losses: Understanding the Experience of Pregnancy Loss, Miscarriage and Abortion*. New York: W. W. Norton and Co.

Kohn, I., & Moffitt, P. 2000. *A Silent Sorrow: Pregnancy Loss Guidance and Support for You and Your Family*, 2nd ed. London: Routledge.

McCreight, B. S. 2004. A Grief Ignored: Narratives of Pregnancy Loss From a Male Perspective. *Sociology of Health & Illness*, 26(3): 326–350.

Montefiore Medical Center. 2013. Miscarriage Perceptions vs. Reality: Public Understanding Not in Sync with Facts. News release. Available at: www.montefiore.org/body.cfm?id=1738&action=detail&ref=1087 (accessed September 2019).

Neugebauer, R. et al. 1992. Depressive Symptoms in Women in the Six Months After Miscarriage. *American Journal of Obstetric Gynecology*. 166. pp. 104–109.

Ro, C. 2019. Parents Mourning Stillbirth Follow Familiar Patterns on YouTube. *New York Times*, 16 April. Available at: www.nytimes.com/2019/04/16/well/family/parents-mourning-stillbirth-follow-familiar-patterns-on-youtube.html (accessed September 2019).

Rogers, J. E., ed. 2007. *The Art of Grief (Series in Death, Dying and Bereavement)*. London: Routledge.

Sas, C., & Coman, A. 2016. Designing Personal Grief Rituals: An Analysis of Symbolic Objects and Actions. *Death Studies*, 40(9): 558–569.

Seftel, L. 2001. The Secret Club Project: Exploring Miscarriage Through the Visual Arts. *Art Therapy: Journal of the American Art Therapy Association*, 18(2): 96–99.

Seftel, L. 2006. *Grief Unseen: Healing Pregnancy Loss through the Arts*. London: Jessica Kingsley Publishers.

Sha, J. 1990. *Mothers of Thyme: Customs and Rituals of Infertility and Miscarriage*. Ann Arbor, MI: Lida Rose Press.

Speert, E. 1992. The Use of Art Therapy Following Perinatal Death. *Art Therapy: Journal of the American Art Therapy Association*, 9(3): 121–128.

Streeter, K., & Deaver, S. 2018. Art Therapy with Women with Infertility: A Mixed-Methods Multiple Case Study, *Art Therapy: Journal of the American Art Therapy Association*, 35(2): 60–67.

Stuart, E. 2004. Art and Grieving: A Reflection on Just-in-Time Education. *Journal of Palliative Medicine*, 6(2): 270–275.

Swanson, K. M. et al. 2007. Contexts and Evolution of Women's Responses to Miscarriage during the First Year After Loss. *Research in Nursing & Health*, 30(1): 2–16.

Trepal, H. C., Semivan, S. G., & Caley-Bruce, M. 2005. Miscarriage: A Dream Interrupted. *Journal of Creativity in Mental Health*, 1(3/4): 155–171.

Van Praag, J. 1999. *Creative Acts of Healing: After a Baby Dies*. Seattle, WA: Paseo Press.

4 Overcoming severe fear in late pregnancy

The use of Art Therapy in maternal healthcare, in the south of Sweden

Helén Wahlbeck

Introduction

This chapter describes how to use Art Therapy in maternal healthcare, to facilitate attachment to the baby and for treatment of severe fear of childbirth. It describes a single case in a care situation and how the picture becomes the solution. It also contains a description of a scientific project in a maternal healthcare clinic in Sweden. The project had the intention of finding out if Art Therapy could work as a good tool in severe childbirth fear and trauma, and this is a discussion of the results.

The birth rate in Europe is 5.2 million a year, and in Sweden it is 115,000 (Eurostat 2019; SCB 2019). Most of the pregnancies can be seen as normal, but around 12–20 per cent of these pregnant women are suffering from mental illness of some kind, which is similar to other parts of the world (Rubertsson et al. 2014; Jha et al. 2018; Kassada et al. 2015). The most common illness is anxiety and depression. The reported prevalence of fear of childbirth, *tokophobia*, varies from 6 per cent to 30 per cent in international studies depending on definitions, methodology and cultural contexts of the studies (Adams, Eberhard-Gran & Eskild 2012; Laursen, Johansen & Hedegaard 2009; Nieminen, Stephansson & Ryding 2009). Secondary tokophobia occurs in parous women who in many cases have previously experienced a traumatic birth. About 2.5–6 per cent of new mothers met diagnostic criteria for post-traumatic stress disorder (PTSD) after childbirth (Susan et al. 2009; Alcorn et al. 2010). These women are not able to function properly and, as a result, the mother and child attachment, development and growth will be adversely affected (Christie et al. 2019).

Here we need an intervention of a different kind. Maternal mental health is very important and mental illness/disorders must be treated. Pregnant women with anxiety, depression or PTSD who suffer severe fear of childbirth are a vulnerable group and not homogeneous. Primary tokophobia can occurs in nulliparous women who may be so afraid that they don't dare to become pregnant. It can be about losing control in pain, but also about the body. They can be afraid of being damaged, experiencing body changes or have a history of being sexual abused. The women fear uncontrollable aspects, the pain of childbirth, parenthood, loss of self-confidence and even death (Areskog, Kjessler

& Uddenberg 1982; Saisto & Halmesmaki 2003; Hofberg & Ward 2004). Therefore, there is a need for different types of treatment options to manage this heterogeneous group.

In Swedish maternal healthcare, women see the midwife at specified intervals. Many problems experienced by women in early pregnancy can be solved by the natural maturing process and with knowledge and support from her midwife. But in more severe cases, there is a need for other interventions. The most common way to take care of these women is to refer them to a psychologist for counselling and cognitive behavioural therapy (CBT) or a specialist midwife/physician at the hospital, or a combination. The team and the individual woman plan together how birth care should be given. This includes a discussion of the woman's fears, a review of past obstetrical case notes, if such exist, information about childbirth and a visit to the birthing environment. The psychologist can be helpful with preparing her for motherhood, reducing her anxiety and level of depression. Despite this, some women are still unable to mentally prepare for childbirth and parenting. It results in a rising rate of planned caesarean sections and post-partum depressions (Rauh et al. 2012). In Sweden, there is not yet a tradition for using Art Therapy as an intervention during pregnancy. A brief literature review in 2017 includes several studies about different way to use Art Therapy in ante-natal and post-natal care (Hogan et al. 2017).

History of patient 'EM'

Some years ago, a situation arose in my work in maternal healthcare that would lead me to see art as an excellent therapeutic tool during pregnancy. A young woman was expecting her first child. She previously had a severe eating disorder (bulimia nervosa), and, as a result, she had a very dysfunctional attitude to her growing stomach. Despite intensive efforts to establish a connection between the mother and her unborn child, we failed. She felt a deep disgust over her body and was unable to visualise a child in it. As the pregnancy weeks went on, a psychologist was contacted but this also failed to have a positive impact.

As part of her check-up, I asked her to go home and draw a picture of the child and bring it to her next appointment. At our next meeting, she presented a good representation of her child on the paper I gave her. A colourful picture of a baby. She smiled for the first time when we talked about the picture and it even led to her giving the child a name. The image she made became a transitional object, to which she was able to relate, and start her process of becoming a mother. She finally let her anxiety-laden body be. This made me realise what a powerful tool the image is.

The body as a barrier between mother and child

Pregnancy is a tangible, physical process that shakes the mental compass con-siderably. Body control is challenged by changes and rapid growth, and the child 'tapping' to advertise its presence. The unborn child should ideally be integrated with the woman's body and psyche, so that a first attachment will be established.

Body image experiences of women progressing through pregnancy showed that, normally, women are able to accept the body changes as long as they recognised the functionality of the pregnant body (Watson et al. 2016).

In the case of disturbed body perception with lack of coherent sense of body, or a history of sexual abuse, where the body is initially an 'enemy or battlefield' invaded by someone, this important process does not work (Levens 1995). Nor does it work when there is previous physical trauma or severe illness where the body is perceived to have failed. Instead of the body, child and psyche, being integrated with each other, the body becomes a 'mental barrier' between mother and child, that makes pregnancy, childbirth and motherhood difficult. In the case of pregnancy and eating disorders or other body obstacles, time is limited by pregnancy, and it can be more about separating the negative feeling of the anxiety-laden body from the expectant child and helping the woman to distinguish her feelings. It is important to make her understand that she can allow herself to have positive feelings for her child, even if she is struggling with her body, and help her to clarify and visually picture her child.

Giving birth forces women to concentrate on specific parts of her body. In cases of historical sexual abuse, this can provoke feelings of nausea, disgust and severe anxiety. It can be a significant part of the problem in severe childbirth fear. In 2011, I started my research work to offer women Art Therapy for the treatment for severe fear of labour.

Art Therapy as an intervention in severe fear of childbirth: a research project

The intention of the study was partly to explore the possibility of using Art Therapy as an intervention during such a limited period as the pregnancy offers, but also an opportunity as a midwife to get a deeper look into the importance of motherhood in relation to childbirth.

In this study, the women were identified as having fear of childbirth by their midwife in ante-natal care. It was aimed at both nulliparous and multiparous and their fear rested on very different grounds.

> Women expressed fear linked to the birthing environment and of suffering traumatic hospital experiences through abusive and negligent encounters with professionals, which had left deep emotional impressions. In some cases it was expressed as a general fear of hospital and about what can happen there. Fear of being torn apart or physically damaged during the birth was often vividly expressed. The women had lost confidence in their body's ability. They were afraid of losing control in extreme pain and afraid that the baby would be injured or even die.
>
> (Wahlbeck, Kvist & Landgren 2018, p. 4)

The women who were randomised for Art Therapy as part of the treatment for childbirth fear received five sessions of Art Therapy, either one-to-one or in a group setting as an adjunct to usual care (counselling). The decision to treat them in parallel was based on the fact that the usual counselling has a different function. The goal of this counselling is to work with the woman to create a care plan for the birth in a way that she can accept and to make her and/or her partner feel more secure. Art Therapy is more about exploring the origin of their fear, identifying it and clarifying it. The pregnancy limited the possibility to have flexible number of treatments, as is usually offered in Art Therapy. But there are studies in populations with PTSD that show short-term Art Therapy can work well (Gantt & Tinnin 2007). The women in this study started the treatment with Art Therapy between 20 and 35 weeks of pregnancy. Sometimes the pregnant woman suppresses her fear until late in pregnancy, which makes it more complicated to offer her support in time. In this case, the support has continued after birth.

All participants got five sessions of 1.5–2 hours depending on the size of group. Their experience of limited therapy was followed up via a questionnaire and none of the participants felt that there were too few treatment occasions or that the treatment time/duration was too long or short. All women were free to decide if they wanted one-to-one therapy or to be in a group. Most of them chose to be in a group. To have the possibility to share experiences with others was very important. Taking part in and experiencing other people's images gave rise to insights about themselves and ideas of how to relate to fear. Because of the time limit in pregnancy, and to make it possible to compare and measure quantitatively, the choice of using fixed pregnancy-linked themes was made. Core themes included child, body and control, delivery-room, and frameworks such as 'Where am I going?', 'What is hindering me?', and 'How can I get through this?'

Nineteen participants who had undergone Art Therapy were interviewed during 2011–2013 about their experiences of the treatment. Interviews were conducted three months after childbirth. In the analysis, a main theme of gaining hope and self-confidence emerged from the women's experiences of being treated with Art Therapy for their fear of childbirth (Wahlbeck et al. 2018).

The origin of fear

The fear of giving birth was often disguised and difficult to grasp at the beginning of treatment and therefore difficult to understand and process. The women in this study described barriers hindering emotional communications, such as bad experiences of earlier meetings with health professionals and of medical procedures. They spoke about mental defence mechanisms, the difficulty of identifying the origin of their fear and understanding it. They also expressed feelings of loneliness in their fear and the inability to communicate it to partners, midwives and other professionals.

Therefore, an important part of the treatment was to uncover the origin of the fear and to help the woman understand it. She needed to emotionally discover her problem to go further. By giving the woman the opportunity to express herself in the picture of the child/motherhood, the body and the delivery room, she is offered a visual space in which it is possible to live out her fear, gain perspective and describe her fear in words. Then the anxiety and fear become something that can be dealt with and resolved.

Attachment to the baby

The women described how fear and anxiety prevented them from creating a mental picture of themselves giving birth and becoming a mother. Women expressed that they had a negative self-image and could not identify themselves with becoming a parent and being able to bond with the baby. Fear and anxiety about giving birth can negatively affect motherhood and therefore it is very important to gain a view, reflect and help the mother to start her child bonding process. The pictures that were created by the women were very different in character. The women were not always able to make a picture of a baby, but they tried to create a sense of it with the help of colour, form and expression. The reactions of the women with difficulties to connect with their babies were usually very direct in their expression, featuring feelings of sadness and horror due to the 'threatening' motherhood. For women who had a normal attachment, it could be reassuring and important to have it confirmed, and the expected baby could be used as a positive driver in the work with the fear of childbirth.

Understanding an inability to visualise the child may trigger feelings of shame and guilt, or perhaps this is the first time a woman has had the opportunity or been forced to express any form of emotion regarding or picturing the expected child. This reflection is the starting point to continued work with the bonding process and future motherhood (see Figure 4.1). The child will become *someone* on the paper, someone to relate to. The non-child 'is'. Whether associated with good or bad feelings, the baby exists.

The body's emotional map: mind and body mapping and control

Pregnancy and fear of giving birth, is strongly linked to the physical. To understand and make visible the women's emotional body maps, the use of the mind and body mapping technique was a conscious choice to understand which emotions are strongest, most important and take up the most space. The women were given some suggestions of feelings that could be positively or negatively linked to childbirth fear – worry, fear, control, joy, trust, strength – and they were also free to choose others. These sentiment terms were picked from a Wijma Delivery Expectancy/Experience Questionnaire (W-DEQ), which measures feelings and thoughts women may have before or after childbirth using a Likert Scale approach (Wijma, Wijma & Zar 1998). For example, if the woman cannot map the feeling of 'trust' then it helps her to understand that she finds it difficult to trust – either her own body to successfully deliver the child, or it may indicate a lack of trust in the birthing environment. Alternatively, the woman

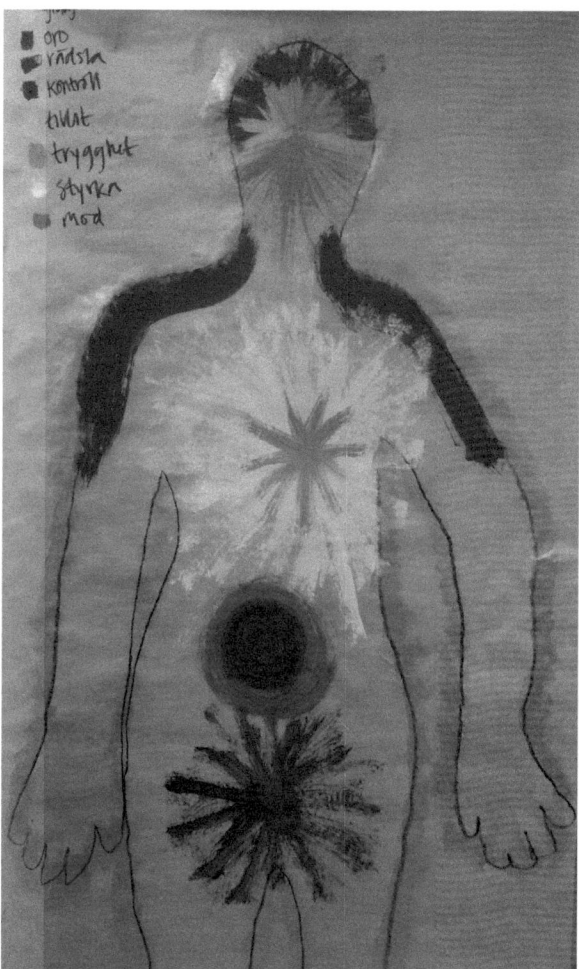

Figure 4.1 The Origin of Control, 2016.

may choose to map 'control' in the area of the head and body, identifying control as an important factor in the root cause of her fear. Mapping control in the head could mean that she is afraid to lose control of the situation, whereas mapping control in the body could mean a fear of examination or not wanting to lose control of herself physically during childbirth. In this way it will allow the woman to see and experience the fear.

Fear of losing control during childbirth may be an effect of the liminal status that pregnancy in itself is, but working with the image of one's own body also arouses many feelings about the birth itself and the fear of breaking apart when the child is to emerge. It can also be clear, for example, that the joy of the child is contained in the body despite the worry of being injured. This is a good starting point to navigate through these difficulties, and mind and body mapping is a perfect tool in the early stages of fear of childbirth counselling.

So now the woman understands her feelings about being a mother more, and what feelings are important relative to her body. These are two important guidelines when considering how to continue to support her. Since exaggerated sense of control or fear of losing control is very common, we worked with the themes of having control, losing control and letting go of control, to turn and twist the concept of seeing them from different perspectives and to get a feel for it figuratively. How does it feel when I have control? How is my experience of loss of control? What happens then? What would I need to dare release the control? How did I feel to make that picture? These themes generated good conversations about the fear of loss of control (see Figure 4.1).

Identifying the trauma

For women who have previously suffered severe birth trauma or other types of trauma that may be closely associated with the fear of giving birth, one important element is to identify the trauma: *Where* did it happen? *Why* did it happen? *What* exactly happened, and *how*? (Murray, Merritt & Grey 2016).

In order to help the woman dare to enter the trauma, understand what happened and confirm her experience, the theme of the delivery room was used. The woman entered through her picture either into the mental room she had been in during her last birth, or the worst delivery room she could imagine being in. Here her vulnerability became clear, the role of the partner, the roles of the staff and all the difficult feelings that came back, and we could talk about them and 'lock' them into this particular event.

Here pictures of old non-birth-related hospital experiences also appeared. To have been forced into infirmity as a little child and forced to leave the family, or suddenly realise that the visual room on the picture shows a situation with a dying relative (Figure 4.2). This makes the pregnant woman understand that that was a girl's memories there and then, easing the burden, and allowing a new adult perspective to be constructed. It is so important to understand what mental room the woman is carrying in her head and emotionally referring to. This helps her separate that event from what lies ahead. Pictures help to visualise the actual trauma, the before setting, the general scene, while an 'after picture' helps to move beyond the trauma (Gantt and Tinnin 2007).

Image as a navigation instrument

Several women in the study expressed how the image became like a 'container' where emotions from a previous memory could be expressed, discovered, processed and finally dumped, given the opportunity to find a new direction to cope with their fear. It was expressed as a relief and decreased anxiety during the pregnancy.

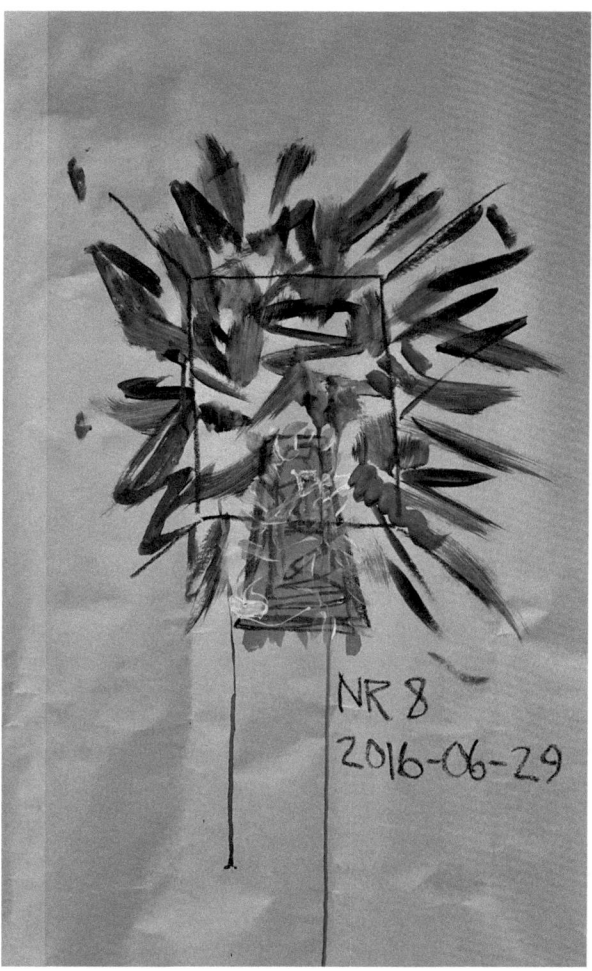

Figure 4.2 The Room, 2016.

The women could, by recalling their entire process at the end of the treatment, put words on which images were most important, which ones were emotionally difficult to deal with, and how the feeling for the images could change as they were processed. During the entire period of Art Therapy, there was also a dynamic relationship with the specialist midwife and the ordinary midwife in maternal healthcare, where the actual delivery planning would take place. The image also proved to have a great intrinsic value in that it was actually created by the woman herself. It could be shown to the partner who at home could facilitate conversations about her fears and possibly previously shared birth trauma. The value of the picture could be so great for the woman that she framed important ones and put it above the baby's bed.

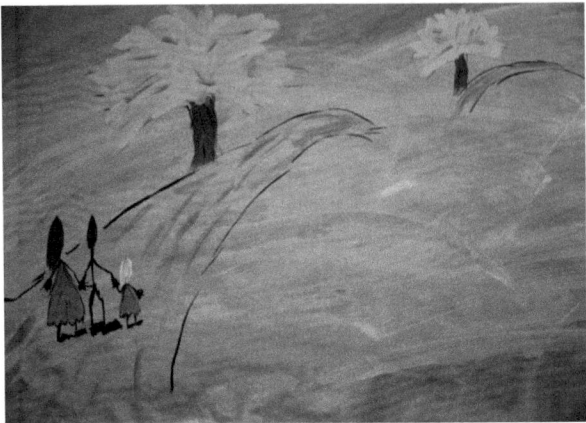

Figure 4.3 The Family/Target Image, 2013.

Part of the treatment was to create target images to mentally stick to. It was both the image of how it should be and the image of how she wants it to be. Target images were important and sometimes contained self-awareness elements representing climbed mountains, conquered obstacles, but the image of the future family was the most common here. To rest in parenthood when everything is over, 'I came out the other side!', 'I/we survived!', 'Now life can begin!' Something to really long for. Something to dare to believe in. These image represented visual encouragement of parenting and the new life coming into the world.

The future use of Art Therapy in tokophobia and motherhood

Based on my experience of using Art Therapy as an alternative treatment for childbirth fear, I would like to summarise it as follows. Becoming a mother/ parenthood is closely linked to fear of giving birth, and this needs to be resolved. The image is a fantastic medium for processing trauma, using the work to un- cover and identify the parts of the birth fear, and to clarify and facilitate the connection process between mother and child. Further studies should consider the use of the arts within health in pregnancy, birth and new parenthood.

To avoid women entering a new pregnancy with severe childbirth fear due to previous birth trauma, it would be optimal to offer both the woman and her partner Art Therapy within six months of giving birth.

For the first-time mother or a multipara already pregnant again, it may be best for the woman if she completed the Art Therapy one month before giving birth. There will always be a risk that the woman gives birth earlier than expected, or that there will be complications. She also needs to prepare herself mentally and practically for the child to come. Every woman is to have a follow-up post-partum.

Based on my experience, Art Therapy should be seen as a complement to the usual maternity care support team that handles practical planning for childbirth. It is optimal if the therapy is completed before the planning with the support team begins. This is because Art Therapy in this study was about exploring the origin of their fear, sorting it out and making it clear, and the goal of special care support is more to make a care plan acceptable to the mother for the birth. Together it can be a more comprehensive support.

It would be exciting to include work with image and/or clay in group therapy around the theme of the child/parenthood during pregnancy as an extra option available to all mothers. I believe that it is a perfect tool for mothers with problems visualising bonding, and there are already several good examples of how to use Art Therapy with the purpose of strengthening the self-image of the mother and attachment to the child (Hogan, Sheffield & Woodward 2017; Arroyo & Fowler 2013; Swan-Foster 1989). Finally, there is great need for more extensive cross-cultural studies within this research area, to secure the evidence of usability in the field of Art Therapy.

References

Adams, S. S., Eberhard-Gran, M., & Eskild, A. 2012. Fear of Childbirth and Duration of Labour: A Study of 2206 Women with Intended Vaginal Delivery. *Bjog*, 119: 1238–1246.

Alcorn, K. L., O'Donovan, A., Patrick, J. C., Creedy, D. & Devilly, G. J. 2010. A Prospective Longitudinal Study of the Prevalence of Post-Traumatic Stress Disorder Resulting from Childbirth Events. *Psychological Medicine*, 40: 1849–1859.

Areskog, B., Kjessler, B., & Uddenberg, N. 1982. Identification of Women with Significant Fear of Childbirth during Late Pregnancy. *Gynecologic and Obstetric Investigation*. 13: 98–107.

Arroyo, C., & Fowler, N. 2013. Before and After: A Mother and Infant Painting Group. *International Journal of Art Therapy*, 18: 98–112.

Christie, H., Hamilton-Giachritsis, C., Alves-Costa, F., Tomlinson, M., & Halligan, S. L. 2019. The Impact of Parental Posttraumatic Stress Disorder on Parenting: A Systematic Review. *European Journal of Psychotraumatology*, 10: 1550345.

Eurostat. 2019. *Births and Fertility*. Eurostat. Available at: https://ec.europa.eu/eurostat/documents/2995521/9648811/3-12032019-AP-EN.pdf/412879ef-3993-44f5-8276-38b482c766d8 (accessed April 2020).

Gantt, L., & Tinnin, L. 2007. Intensive Trauma Therapy of PTSD and Dissociation: An Outcome Study. *The Arts in Psychotherapy*, 34: 69–80.

Hofberg, K., & Ward, M. R. 2004. Fear of Childbirth, Tocophobia, and Mental Health in Mothers: The Obstetric-Psychiatric Interface. *Clinical Obstetrics and Gynecology*, 47: 527–534.

Hogan, S., Sheffield, D., & Woodward, A. 2017. The Value of Art Therapy in Antenatal and Postnatal Care: A Brief Literature Review with Recommendations for Future Research. *International Journal of Art Therapy*, 1–11.

Jha, S., Salve, H. R., Goswami, K., Sagar, R., & Kant, S. 2018. Burden of Common Mental Disorders among Pregnant Women: A Systematic Review. *Asian Journal of Psychiatry*, 36: 46–53.

Kassada, D. S., Waidman, M. a. P., Miasso, A. I., & Marcon, S. S. 2015. Prevalência de transtornos mentais e fatores associados em gestantes. *Acta Paulista de Enfermagem*, 28: 495–502.

Laursen, M., Johansen, C., & Hedegaard, M. 2009. Fear of Childbirth and Risk for Birth Complications in Nulliparous Women in the Danish National Birth Cohort. *Bjog*, 116: 1350–1355.

Levens, M. 1995. *Eating Disorders and Magical Control of the Body*. London: Routledge.

Murray, H., Merritt, C., & Grey, N. 2016. Clients' Experiences of Returning to the Trauma Site during PTSD Treatment: An Exploratory Study. *Behavioural and Cognitive Psychotherapy*, 44: 420–430.

Nieminen, K., Stephansson, O., & Ryding, E. L. 2009. Women's Fear of Childbirth and Preference for Cesarean Section: A Cross-Sectional Study at Various Stages of Pregnancy in Sweden. *Acta Obstetricia et Gynecologica Scandinavica*, 88: 807–813.

Rauh, C., Beetz, A., Burger, P., Engel, A., Haberle, L., Fasching, P. A., Kornhuber, J., Beckmann, M. W., Goecke, T. W., & Faschingbauer, F. 2012. Delivery Mode and the Course of Pre- and Postpartum Depression. *Archives of Gynecology and Obstetrics*, 286: 1407–1412.

Rubertsson, C., Hellstrom, J., Cross, M., & Sydsjo, G. 2014. Anxiety in Early Pregnancy: Prevalence and Contributing Factors. *Archives of Women's Mental Health*, 17: 221–228.

Saisto, T., & Halmesmaki, E. 2003. Fear of Childbirth: A Neglected Dilemma. *Acta Obstetricia et Gynecologica Scandinavica*, 82: 201–208.

SCB. 2019. *Födda i Sverige*. Available at: www.scb.se/hitta-statistik/sverige-i-siffror/manniskorna-i-sverige/fodda-i-sverige/ (accessed April 2020).

Susan, A., Harris, R., Sawyer, A., Parfitt, Y., & Ford, E. 2009. Posttraumatic Stress Disorder after Childbirth: Analysis of Symptom Presentation and Sampling. *Journal of Affective Disorders*, 119: 200–204.

Swan-Foster, N. 1989. Images of Pregnant Women: Art Therapy as a Tool for Transformation. *The Arts in Psychotherapy*, 16: 283–292.

Wahlbeck, H., Kvist, L. J., & Landgren, K. 2018. Gaining Hope and Self-Confidence: An Interview Study of Women's Experience of Treatment by Art Therapy for Severe Fear of Childbirth. *Women and Birth: Journal of the Australian College of Midwives*, 31: 299–306.

Watson, B., Broadbent, J., Skouteris, H., & Fuller-Tyszkiewicz, M. 2016. A Qualitative Exploration of Body Image Experiences of Women Progressing through Pregnancy. *Women and Birth: Journal of the Australian College of Midwives*, 29(1): 72–79.

Wijma, K., Wijma, B., & Zar, M. 1998. Psychometric Aspects of the W-DEQ: A New Questionnaire for the Measurement of Fear of Childbirth. *Journal of Psychosomatic Obstetrics & Gynaecology*, 19: 84–97.

5 Lost and found

Locating meaning within the landscape of perinatal loss

Claire Flahavan

> She was a clay vessel
> imagining its spaces
> dreaming of its contents…

This chapter concerns the spectrum of losses that can occur in relation to pregnancy, and elaborates particular ways of supporting these experiences in therapy. These losses include miscarriages, stillbirths, terminations, ectopic or molar pregnancies, and infertility, among others. There are particular dimensions to these losses that can make the grieving process especially difficult to resolve. In each of these circumstances the expected horizons of a life shift or sometimes rupture catastrophically, leaving the woman or couple in an altered landscape. In certain respects, perinatal losses occupy realms of time, place and space that defy our everyday language. These are situations for which there may seem to be no words, or in which 'ordinary words' lack sufficient scope or traction.

Cartwright (2015) notes that

> we can experience only that for which we have a language, so we [must] expand our language. We look for the enabling metaphor and the resonant simile to recognise ourselves, to tell [ourselves...] how we feel and how we perceive the world.

Metaphors extend our language, enabling us to encompass the intangible and the ineffable, stretching our imaginative capacities and allowing complex subjective experiences to be shared. Writer Robert Macfarlane describes in a radio interview the necessity of being able to imbue language at times of crisis with a particular kind of palp and heft: 'to be able to give to language aspects of matter... and to matter aspects of language' (Macfarlane 2019). This is the challenge with which we are confronted within the therapy space when meeting experiences of perinatal loss: that of finding an 'extra-ordinary language' in order to support our clients to articulate and bear the 'matter' of their experience. The image-making process and other creative acts or 'leaps of imagination' afford access to alternative ways of apprehending, expressing and shaping difficult experiences, even when these very experiences may feel ephemeral or fugitive.

This chapter explores the ways in which the discovery or shaping of 'an enabling metaphor' through imagery and words, to represent experiences of perinatal loss, can be therapeutically useful.

The chapter starts with an overview of the complexities that underpin the impact of perinatal loss, looking at early and late pregnancy losses, as well as the experience of infertility. The key tasks in mourning are then discussed, bearing in mind the unique features of perinatal loss, which differentiate it from other kinds of bereavement. The concept of the 'enabling metaphor' is elaborated as a potentially useful avenue for anchoring experiences of perinatal loss, especially where themes around ambiguity are to the fore. These issues are illustrated using a series of anonymised short vignettes, with consent from the individuals involved, alongside images made by the author in response to this work, as part of her own supervision process.

The impact of perinatal loss

> [This landscape seems] to return the eye's enquiries unanswered, or swallow all attempts at interpretation. [It confronts] us with the problem of purchase: how to anchor perception in a context of vastness, how to make such a place *mean*. We have words we use for such places, half in awe and half in dismissal – stark, empty, limitless. But we find it hard to make language grip [these] landscapes [... that] excel in expanse, reach and transparency.
>
> (Macfarlane 2008, p. 78)

Macfarlane is describing here the difficulty of coming to grips visually with flat open terrain: landscapes that offer up no texture, contour or detail to catch and engage the eye. His description also captures, however, something of the terrain of perinatal loss: a baby, or the idea of a baby, or the hope for a baby is lost, but how does one make language or imagination 'grip' this difficult reality? The loss may be entirely invisible to others, difficult for the woman to conceptualise or may abruptly interrupt a healthy pregnancy in such an unexpected way that it seems difficult to 'make real'.

The specific meaning of any experience of perinatal loss will be unique to the individual or couple, resting on their subjective sense of what it is or who it is that has been lost, or whether indeed the state of pregnancy was expected, achievable or wanted at all. Where a sense of loss is to the fore, however, there are particular issues that may be especially impactful. The trajectory of the parent or couple's own developmental process may feel derailed, sometimes abruptly. An embodiment of one's hope for the future has been lost (Leon 1990, p. 26). There may be a sense that one's body has failed, perhaps catastrophically (see Figure 5.2). Leon notes that this sense of disruption may be partial or temporary, as prior or subsequent pregnancies may facilitate a sense of repair (1990, p. 27). In other cases, the client may be grappling with the likelihood (or certainty) of never being able to have children.

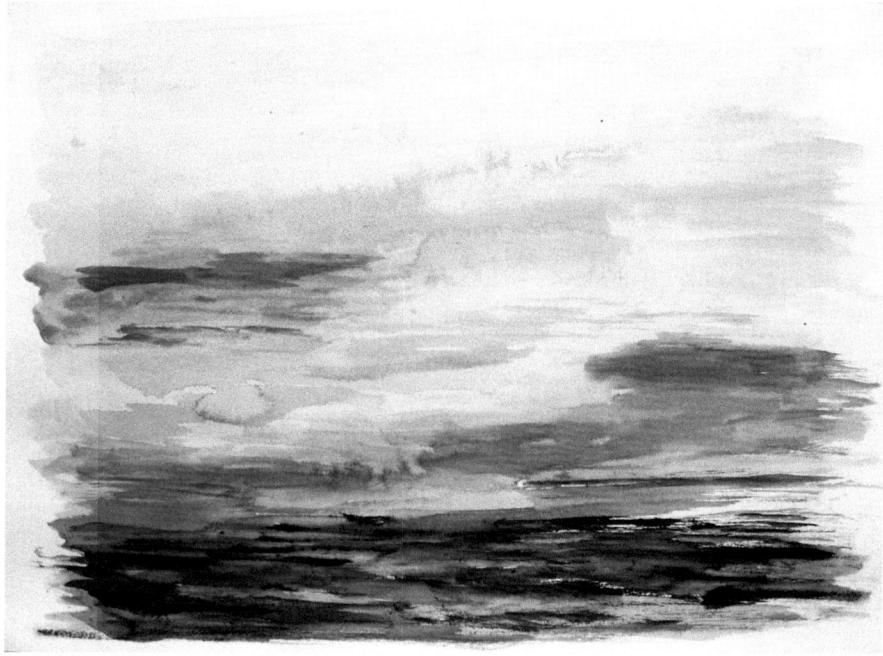

Figure 5.1 Adrift. Claire Flahavan.

Early losses

> The doctor says it's an empty room in there
> And it is
> A pale sack with no visitors.
> I have made it and surrounded it with my skin
> To invite the baby in
> But he did not enter...
>
> (Lasky 2018)

Early pregnancy losses may feel especially intangible and unreal. Lisa, describing the impact of a succession of early miscarriages across her thirties, articulated this eloquently, saying that she was grieving multiple losses, and yet had 'nobody' and nothing to grieve. She spoke in therapy about her sense that people didn't realise that for her, having a miscarriage meant losing *a baby* not 'just a pregnancy' each time. She felt that even family and friends expected her to 'move on', but described an absolute feeling of stasis, a sense of being drained of any appetite for work or for socialising, and a kind of unravelling within herself. This 'unravelling' encompassed both her sense of her body

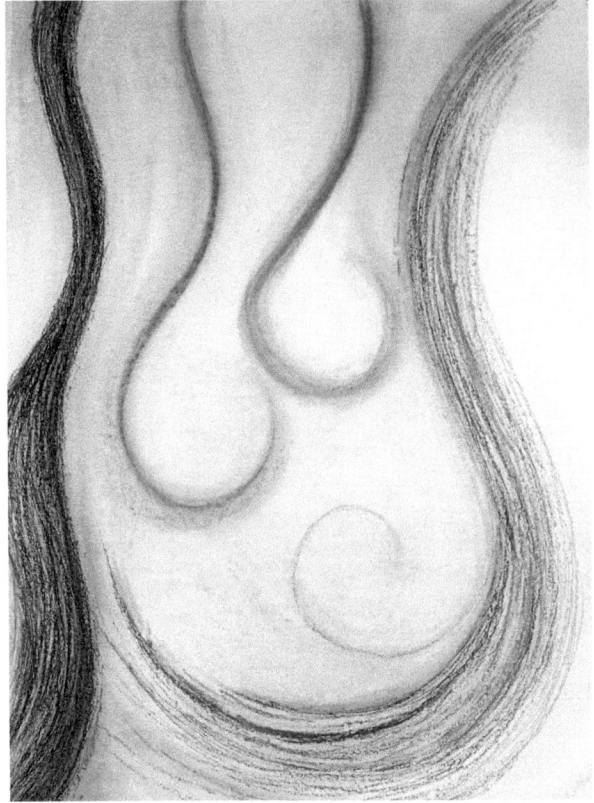

Figure 5.2 Unravelling. Claire Flahavan.

having failed to 'hold her pregnancies', as well as wider themes around the disruption to the predicted 'shape' or weave of her life.

There is a considerable literature investigating the psychological effects of miscarriage, with a frequent emphasis on whether the gestational stage of the pregnancy is important in predicting the severity of the psychological response. McCarthy (2016) notes that what is so often missing here is the key subjective question for the woman: what is it that I have lost? Was it a pregnancy, a cluster of cells, an inconvenience or a baby? For some women, a loss at six weeks may feel catastrophic, depending on the personal history underpinning their experience of pregnancy and the hopes invested within it. An early miscarriage occurring against a backdrop of multiple cycles of fertility treatment may well be devastating for example (see Figure 5.3). The advent of better-quality, high-resolution scanning also permits attachment and investment in a pregnancy, even at very early stages.

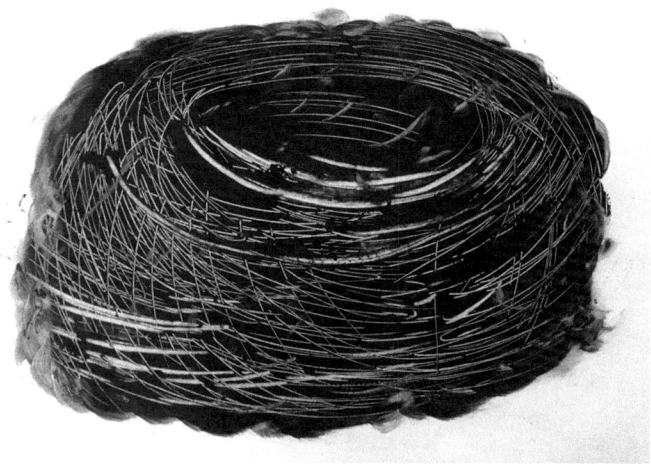

Figure 5.3 Empty Nest. Claire Flahavan.

Later losses

Losses later in pregnancy lack the ambiguity or 'invisibility' of early losses, but pose a different set of challenges. Here, the 'full feelings' of advancing pregnancy become inextricably interwoven with death. Maggie (36) described her experience following a medical termination at 22 weeks for a fatal foetal anomaly: 'I can still feel the kicks, as if I'm still pregnant ... I know it can't be possible, but it's as if my body is remembering ... as if it wants to remember – to hold on to whatever it can of her.' Maggie also articulated a distressed awareness of an emptiness inside her, in the months following the delivery of her baby superimposed painfully on her somatic memories of the baby's movements.

One of the most significant regrets for Maggie and her husband was that their extended family did not have a chance to meet their daughter, whom they had named Marie. The absence of shared memories of Marie made it difficult for Maggie's family to find a language with which to speak about her, and this added significantly to Maggie's distress. She spoke about her sense that her pregnancy had not translated into an 'actual baby' in the minds of others: almost as if Marie had never existed at all.

Maggie spoke of the importance of being able to recall the actual shape and feel of Marie's body and facial features, including her mouth and chin, in terms of 'making real' Marie's memory. The similarity of her baby's features to her own was something that she cherished in particular, allowing Maggie to hold and place her baby more fully within a sense of the family line.

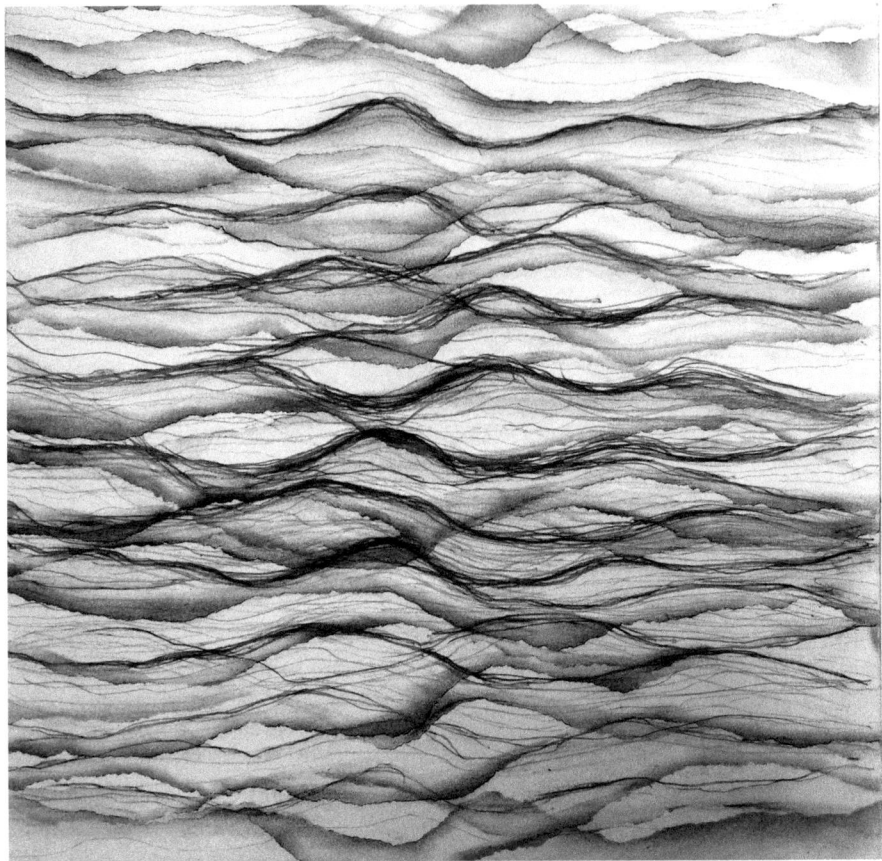

Figure 5.4 I Can Still Feel Her Kicking. Claire Flahavan.

Infertility

In the case of individuals or couples coming to terms with infertility or childlessness for other reasons, the losses experienced may be more covert and invisible, remaining unspoken, even to close friends or family. There is an absence of a wished-for baby as in other cases of perinatal loss, but in some cases without a 'discrete' or specific loss to mourn. For others there may be multiple iterations of intense hope and disappointment as they progress through successive cycles of failed fertility treatment (Figure 5.5). To the woman who is grieving childlessness, the world may feel 'full of babies', an ever-present reminder of what she cannot have, and where she cannot go.

Danielle was referred for therapy following a hysterectomy at the age of 38 due to the presence of large fibroids (benign tumours). She had always wanted children, but this possibility was now biologically closed to her. She described

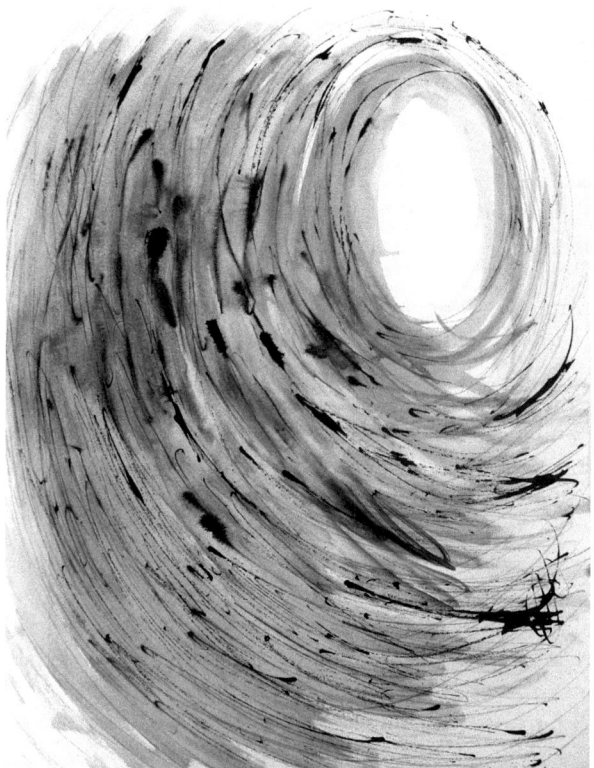

Figure 5.5 Wound. Claire Flahavan.

feeling lost and battered, 'like someone who has washed up on a beach somewhere, where they don't know where they are'. Her words are echoed by O'Neill's delicate rendering of the landscape of grief (2009, p. 160):

> [We] have drowned and been washed up on the shore of a strange country. We do not recognize this land and we feel numb... the world has become unreliable and strange, we do not know where we are going. [We are] adrift in a landscape of death where we feel marked. [W]e stand on the shore, and hear the water rushing over the pebbles, clinking the little stones together before rushing out again and we wait and we watch.
>
> (O'Neill 2009, p. 160)

Danielle recovered well from the hysterectomy procedure itself, but described a sense of estrangement from friends and colleagues as she grappled privately with the reality of her childlessness. She spoke in particular of the difficulty of trying to show up with her partner for family occasions, like christenings or birthday parties for nieces and nephews. She spoke about childlessness as a kind of harsh reality that revealed itself abruptly following her surgery, and yet the invisible nature of the loss made it difficult to talk about or to acknowledge.

The grief process

In her beautiful memoir *The Fish Ladder*, author Katherine Norbury articulates something of the grief that accompanies perinatal loss, describing her experience of a miscarriage:

> When summer came, and brought with it the realisation that our baby should have been with us, I found that I was struggling … the world had closed around me in a tight, hard sphere. […] I searched for something that would keep the air breathable, the sound of the wind audible, the smell of a bonfire or the smart tang of sea salt sharp on my lips and tongue. That might shut out the possibility of stasis. […] I discovered that there were places, empty spaces, places in the heart, that I simply hadn't imagined could exist.
>
> (Norbury 2015, pp. 6–7)

In her book Norbury sets out on a quest to follow a river from the sea to its source, and we become companions on her journey through dual landscapes: internal and external as she navigates grief. She documents an encounter with 'Another Place': an installation by sculptor Antony Gormley at Crosby beach in Liverpool. One hundred life-size casts of the artist stand along the beach, alternately revealed and submerged by the sea, as the tides ebb and flow. In Norbury's words:

> The metal men became apparent, one by one, stretching into the distance. I stood next to one of [them] and tried to follow his gaze. Looking out to sea. My task this summer, the task I had set myself, was to look back. To turn my back on the sea [… and to] walk back into myself.
>
> (Norbury 2015, p. 36)

In some ways, this too is the central task of therapy: to support the individual to 'walk back into themselves', so that they can anchor the loss they have experienced, and weave it into the narrative of their life story. The loss of a pregnancy can be viewed in terms of the bereavement response outlined in other situations: there may initially be a sense of shock or numbness, followed by a period of active grieving where themes around yearning and emptiness predominate. Recovery is gradual, signalled by a resumption of everyday activities and a restored capacity to experience pleasure. However, there are unique features to this kind of loss, which differentiate it from other bereavements. Mourning a perinatal loss requires painful contact with *fantasies* about the imagined child-to-be, rather than actual memories. In some circumstances (e.g., in the case of early losses) there may be little tangible evidence that a baby existed. In situations of infertility or childlessness for other reasons, there may never have been a pregnancy at all, and the onset of grief may be heralded by advancing age, or the gradual realisation that a successful pregnancy is not to be. Perinatal bereavement is thus a kind of prospective mourning – a letting go of wishes and hopes about one 'who could have been, but never was' (Leon 1990, p. 35).

Perinatal loss represents a loss of part of the self (Figure 5.6). As such, Leon (1990, p. 40) notes that there may be multiple wounds to a woman's sense of omnipotence, femininity and selfhood, as well as the deprivation of lifelong developmental aspirations towards motherhood. Themes about the body are frequently to the fore in therapy; for example, themes around the failure of the body to support the pregnancy and allied feelings of inadequacy – a sense of somehow 'not being motherly or womanly enough'. It is not uncommon to encounter feelings of guilt and self-blame within this: a sense of responsibility for the pregnancy loss (worries about exercise or lack of exercise, diet, medications taken during the pregnancy, etc.). The absence of culturally sanctioned mourning rituals in some situations of perinatal loss may also be keenly felt, leaving the individual or couple with a sense of having no tangible 'place' to locate what has been lost – intra-psychically, spiritually or geographically.

Reconstructing a sense of significance in the aftermath of any loss frequently involves an active process of self-organisation, and adaptation to an altered life-story. Bertman (1999, p. 3) reminds us that we are 'kaleidoscopic creatures', made up of past experiences, family kinships, culture, secret lives, perceived futures, as well as transcendent dimensions. The central therapeutic endeavour is

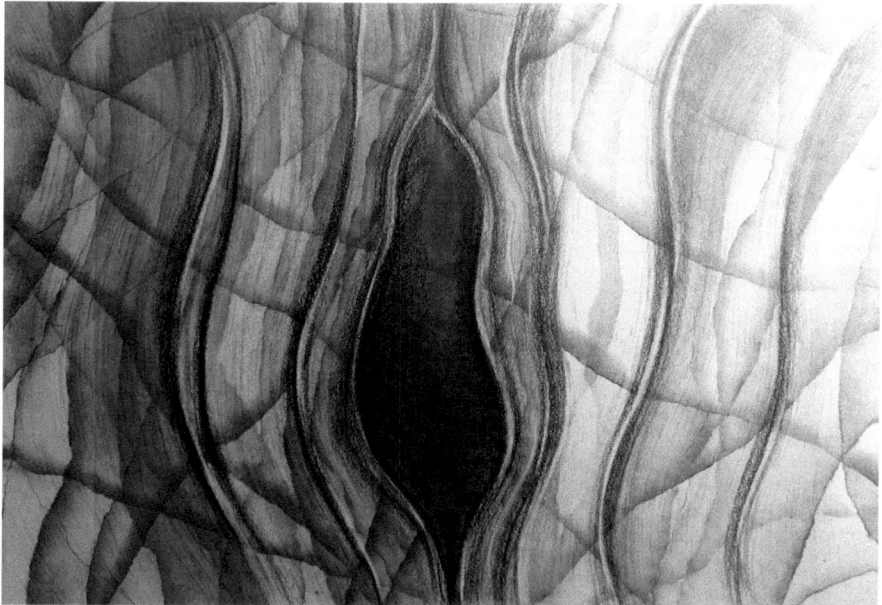

Figure 5.6 The Bud that Does Not Flower. Claire Flahavan.

perhaps to engage with the unique meaning of a particular loss or losses for the client, in the context of their particular life history and trajectory. The wishes and fantasies in relation to the child or children who will never be, must be surfaced, articulated and mourned. Holmes (2008, p. 169) notes that the therapy space offers the client a chance to focus on tiny fragments of experience: 'to slow them down, to replay them, tracing their emotional links backwards in time and sideways with other sets of experiences and emotions'. The development of a positive transference to the therapist is an important ingredient in creating the kind of holding environment that is necessary for this work (Figure 5.7). The ending of therapy, with the dissolution of the therapeutic relationship, offers additional opportunities for working through the initial loss.

Locating meaning in landscapes of loss: the role of the enabling metaphor

Carey (2018, p. 16) writes that in order to bear absence – an element of the mourning process, we must facilitate our clients in the process of developing a

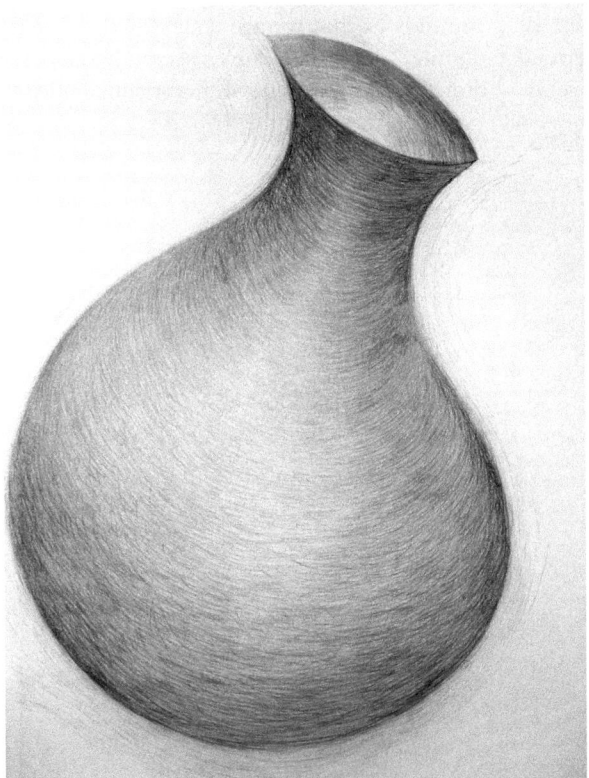

Figure 5.7 Vessel. Claire Flahavan.

sense of internal space. Within this space, absent objects can then be held imaginatively, and symbolised 'as part of a growing personal internal landscape with a developing emotional and imagistic vocabulary'.

Levine (2009, p. 26) notes that there are different ways of telling stories: 'one of them is through "poiesis", making or shaping. We know something by shaping it, by giving it a form'. The creation of 'form' or substance from the formlessness of perinatal loss can assist in 'making real' the loss, particularly where themes about ambiguity have been to the fore. For some clients, this kind of 'poiesis' may come about through the discovery or creation of a metaphor or symbol that captures the particular quality of their experience in a personally meaningful way. Writer Jennifer Cheng (2019) reminds of us Emily Dickinson's words, 'Tell it slant', and the need for 'angled articulations' at times of trauma and personal crisis which allow personal losses to be approached obliquely rather than head-on.

Three short clinical vignettes now follow, to illustrate the uncovering of 'enabling metaphors' in Art Therapy that allowed for 'angled articulation', grieving, meaning-making and movement in various situations of perinatal loss.

Vignette 1: Mary

Mary sought therapy, after a late miscarriage at 16 weeks during her first pregnancy, which had been conceived via IVF. Mary was 41 at this point, and her grief was compounded by a sense of 'time running out'. She had delighted in the early stages of her pregnancy, and recalled in therapy her sense at the time that 'finally she was doing what her body had always wanted to do'. Following the miscarriage, she described her memories of the pregnancy feeling increasingly unreal, and spoke about the importance of her printed ultrasound images, as 'proof' that she had been able to hold and carry a baby inside her.

Mary's family had a holiday home in the southwest of Ireland, and she and her partner had spent time there during her pregnancy. She recalled walking by the sea and feeling a sense of connection with the baby and her own capacity for motherhood. Mary was a keen photographer and had taken beautiful images of the wild landscape during her pregnancy. Across the course of therapy, she returned on a number of occasions, to revisit and photograph this rugged landscape, as a way of 'making real' in some way, her connection to the lost pregnancy, and to that part of herself that needed to own the experience of having been a mother, however transiently. It was almost as if this landscape became a vessel that could hold her memories and feelings. Images of rain-heavy skies, swollen rivers and turbulent seas echoed Mary's grief sympathetically, alongside light-filled images of sea and sky, that offered horizon-lines against which to steady herself.

Macfarlane describes the importance of particular landscapes that hold parts of our 'self' or our story. These are landscapes that we bear with us in absentia, places that live on in memory, long after we have left them:

Most of these places [are] not marked as special on any map. But they become special by personal acquaintance. A bend in a river, the junction of four fields, a climbing tree, a stretch of old hedgerow or a fragment of woodland glimpsed from a road regularly driven along – these might be enough. Or fleeting experiences, transitory, but still site-specific.

(Macfarlane 2008, pp. 236–237)

Macfarlane notes that these landscapes catch and absorb something of the experiences we have passed through, and how these experiences have changed us, perhaps permanently. For Mary, there was a kind of comfort in knowing that she could access precious memories of her pregnancy via her photographs, rather than feeling that this experience had slipped away from her entirely. This sense of being able to hold her pregnancy experience safely and tangibly, in a way that could not easily be erased, allowed Mary to begin to confront difficult decisions about whether or not to embark on a further IVF cycle.

Vignette 2: Richard

Richard attended therapy along with his wife Christine, after a significant pregnancy loss at 13 weeks. He spoke of identifying a lakeside weeping willow tree in a park on his way to and from work, which became linked in his mind with their loss. The shape and form of the tree – flowing softly over water – spoke to him initially of the sense of sadness that permeated their home at that time (Figure 5.8). The poet Sean Hewitt writes beautifully about the experience of entering nature in this way, of observing it, and finding aspects of our selves reflected therein: in 'places where words extinguish/themselves and leave all the things/that cannot be fixed or forgotten' (Hewitt 2019). Extracts from Hewitt's poem 'Petition' were used in therapy to support and mirror Richard's experience:

> Just now,
> it starts to rain: I watch the pond
> pock and sting [...]
> and I, down
> on my knees [...],
> watch it breaking;
> and the world is down on its knees
> beside me – the sky, the rain shattering
> its own image and mine.
>
> (Hewitt 2019)

Over time Richard's relationship with the willow-tree shifted and changed. He described a sense of the tree 'giving him permission to grieve': offering a small resting-place or pause on morning and evening commutes, punctuating his busy weekdays.

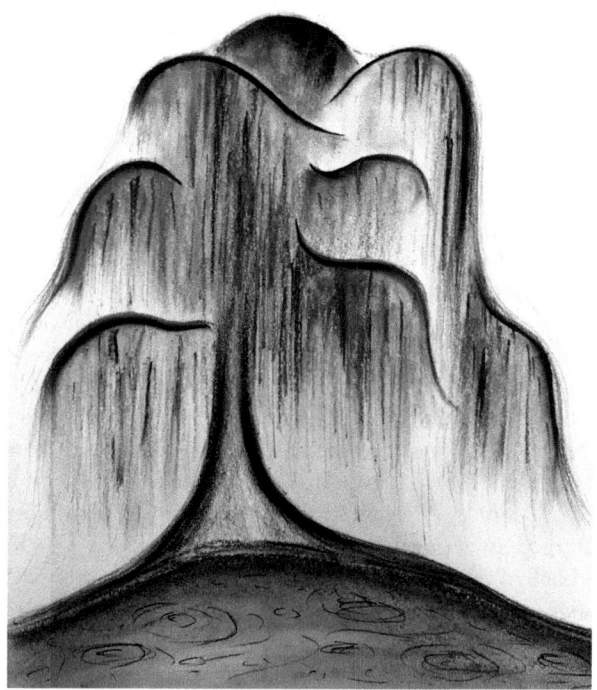

Figure 5.8 Willow. Claire Flahavan.

I came here to see myself shattered
and remade [...]
and the willow with its head laid down
on the water is whispering something.
(Hewitt 2019)

Richard described this daily encounter with the willow tree as an invitation to be in contact, even for brief moments, with his feelings about the lost baby, whom he and Christine imagined to have been a girl, Poppy. In the absence of other tangible markers such as a grave or memorial service, the tree embodied a bridge or connection to Poppy, re-inscribing a sense of her presence in a helpful way. It also became a vehicle for conversations with Christine about their baby, in a way that was meaningful for them both in jointly navigating their experience of grief.

[We] notice
[...] how everything
is reaching down into the earth
or into the water, each thing quietly

at its work, trying to bring some life
up to the surface, unharmed.
(Hewitt 2019)

Christine became pregnant again, and she and Richard continued to attend therapy for ongoing support, until the safe arrival of their son, Oliver.

Vignette 3: Caroline

Caroline (38) attended therapy, having had two ectopic pregnancies, which required the removal of both fallopian tubes at an interval of six years. In the intervening time, she had also experienced a series of miscarriages. Ectopic pregnancies often carry additional trauma, due to the need in some cases for emergency surgery. An ectopic pregnancy occurs when the embryo implants outside of the uterus. These may initially be experienced as 'normal pregnancies', but acute symptoms then develop, typically before the twelfth week, which can include abdominal pain and bleeding. The abrupt loss of the pregnancy may be compounded by a sense of threat to the mother's life. If surgery is required to remove the fallopian tube, this can also cause significant anxiety about future chances at conception.

As Caroline reflected back in therapy on her pregnancy history, she recalled her hopes for a baby 'shrinking' after her first ectopic pregnancy. She articulated a sense of not feeling able to process this at the time however, 'of not letting anything in – just doing what needed to be done'. As pregnancy after pregnancy subsequently went on to end in miscarriage, she and her partner pursued a range of investigations at private clinics to optimise their chances of a healthy pregnancy. The absence of any clear medical reason for the miscarriages was particularly difficult for Caroline. She described putting her available energy into researching various options, and described a sense of numbness or 'nothingness' in relation to the miscarriages themselves, perhaps in an attempt to protect herself from the impact of continuous loss.

Caroline described an image she held in her mind across this time, of the daughter she wanted so much, and whom she named Leah. She spoke about how she had imagined Leah trying to reach her with each successive pregnancy, and her inner sense of her body letting Leah down, each time a pregnancy ended in loss. I sensed in her description, an image of Leah waiting in another parallel place or dimension, wanting to 'cross over'. There was a poignancy and longing in Caroline's desire to be able to 'somehow cut through the layers of time and space' to access or retrieve the daughter she had imagined in her mind. Caroline's words reminded me of Philip Pullman's wonderful trilogy The Dark Materials. In the second of these books, the protagonist Will discovers 'the subtle knife': a knife imbued with special powers, which enables the owner to cut portals through the fabric of the universe, into alternative places and spaces. The second ectopic pregnancy and surgery brought with it a painful reality however, due to the implications of the removal of Caroline's second fallopian tube. She could no longer conceive naturally, and felt unable to tolerate the uncertainty and further expense of IVF. As such, there could be no further portals for Leah to travel through. This heralded an acute onset of grief and inner turmoil for Caroline, as she began to confront the real possibility of remaining childless.

Caroline described a complex relationship with her body at this time. Her scars from the more recent ectopic pregnancy and surgery were a visible reminder to her of the procedures and losses she had endured. However she also saw the scars as tangible markers of her connection with Leah – proof that she'd actually been pregnant, and that Leah had made her way to her, even transiently. The idea that in time these scars would fade was profoundly distressing to Caroline, as it seemed to carry the threat of losing Leah yet again.

In parallel with starting therapy, Caroline underwent several long sessions with a tattoo artist, in order to have a pre-existing image on her back enlarged. The tattoo depicted a pair of beautiful feathered wings extending down and across her back, delicately outlined in black ink. I wondered about the further wounding (or re-wounding) of her body in these painful tattoo sessions, each of which lasted many hours. Caroline described a sense of agency, however, in choosing to undergo this process, and in her careful selection and development of the design. This contrasted powerfully with the traumatically abrupt and unexpected nature of the two ectopic pregnancies and many miscarriages, which had left her with no sense of choice or control over what happened her body. Later in therapy, Caroline began to acknowledge that she had sought out the physically painful procedure, as a means of feeling 'something' other than the profound emotional distress that had permeated the aftermath of her second surgery. The tattoo also had symbolic significance for Caroline; she described a sense of it representing a guardian of some kind, a being who could embrace her in her distress, and contain her suffering. I was reminded of Hermes, messenger to the gods in Greek legend, and guide also to souls into the underworld. Caroline's angelic image seemed to carry the potential to moderate her own distress, as well as offering comfort too perhaps to Leah in her parallel dimension.

In discussing the meaning and importance of her physical scars and wounds, Caroline also showed me a tattoo she'd had inscribed on her lower arm, after her fifth miscarriage, and recounted the context to this. She said:

> I wanted to do something different at that point, to do something for the baby: for my baby who was really trying to join us and meet us, but kept being held back. The tattoo is a heart within a heart, with a small ribbon around it. It represents my baby's heart within my heart, as this is where she lives, even though we have not been able to meet.

These tattoos became touchstones of sorts within Caroline's therapy process, finding their way into our discourse, in various ways. As we unpacked their meaning, they seemed to allow Caroline the possibility of maintaining a sense of connection with her daughter: she could experience a sense of Leah 'written into her body', rather than Leah having to remain distant in another dimension.

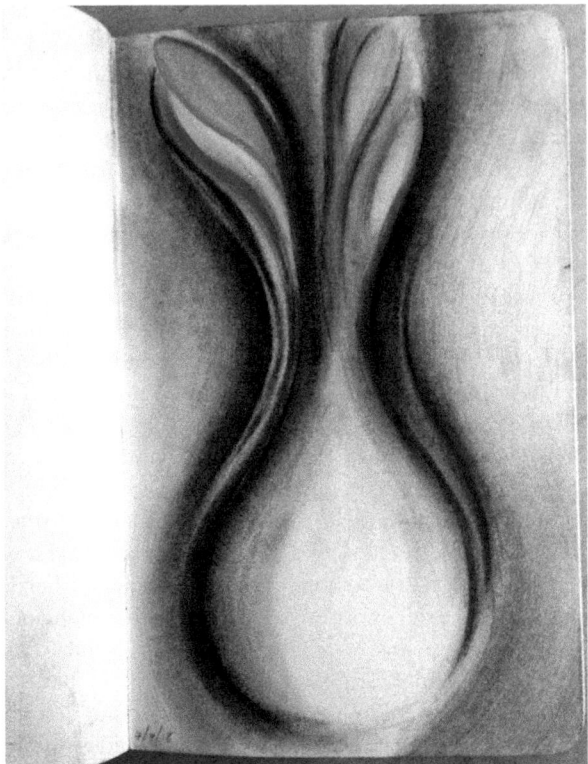

Figure 5.9 Blooming. Claire Flahavan.

There was a comfort for Caroline in the permanence of the inked drawings, given the brevity of each of her pregnancies. This became particularly important to Caroline, as her surgical scars faded. The writer Sinead Gleeson, describes powerfully in her memoir *Constellations* (2019, p. 175), the narrative impulse within the body that has been injured, describing scars as 'openings', or invitations into the stories that lie underneath or within them.

In Caroline's case, the inscription of her baby's story on her body in both tattoos carried a powerful sense of purpose: a determination to own her desire to be a mother, and a defiant intention to 'make visible' her invisible losses. Caroline used her therapy space to articulate her story around motherhood, and to mourn her losses: the loss of Leah and the likelihood too that she would remain childless. We embarked on a process of co-writing her story, so as to allow her relationship with Leah to be recorded and documented, and this in turn seemed to allow Caroline to grieve Leah more fully. Over time the beginnings of a new narrative began to emerge: a desire to no longer be defined by loss, and to shape and create a life that was meaningful and generative in other ways.

Conclusion

This chapter has explored something of the complexity of working with perinatal loss, and the myriad ways in which it can be experienced, imagined and expressed in therapy. The three concluding vignettes sketch out the uncovering of enabling metaphors in therapy: Mary's wild landscape, Richard's willow tree and Caroline's tattoos. These metaphors facilitated remembrance, place-making, bridging and connection in ways that were deeply personal and meaningful to each individual.

As Bertman (1999, p. 15) notes, grief 'captures us, but we capture it back and reshape it'. As therapists we use our imaginative capacity to lend a thinking presence to our clients (Frosch 1997, p. 93). The culmination of this kind of work can never be a return to the 'pre-grief' state, but is perhaps best defined by a reinvestment of energy into life and living (Figure 5.9). This involves 'a repositioning and revival of [what has been lost] in an inner space and time, accessible forever, whenever one needs, wants or is forced to feel the connection' (Bertman 1999, p. 15).

Acknowledgements

Lines from *The Wild Places* Copyright 2008 by Robert Macfarlane, reproduced by kind permission of Granta (UK edition) and Penguin Random House (US edition).

Lines from *Milk* Copyright 2018 by Dorothea Lasky, reproduced by kind permission of Wave Books.

Lines from *Ephemeral Art: The Art of Being Lost* Copyright 2009 by Mary O' Neill in Smith, M., Davidson, J., Cameron, L., Bondi, L. (eds) *Emotion, Place and Culture*, reproduced by kind permission of Taylor and Francis Group.

Lines from *The Fish Ladder* Copyright 2015 by Katharine Norbury, reproduced by kind permission of Bloomsbury Publishing Plc.

Lines from *Lantern* Copyright 2019 by Seán Hewitt, reproduced by kind permission of Seán Hewitt.

References

Bertman, S., ed. 1999. *Grief and the Healing Arts: Creativity as Therapy*. Oxon: Routledge.

Carey, F. 2018. *Spatiality, Dimensionality and the Visual. In The Place of the Visual in Psychoanalytic Practice: The Image in Countertransference*. Oxon: Routledge.

Cartwright, I. 2015. Why Do We Read? *The Irish Times*. Available at: www.irishtimes.com/culture/books/why-do-we-read-1.2084524 (accessed April 2020).

Cheng, J. 2019. What the Retelling of Myths Reveals of the Teller. *Literary Hub*. Available at: https://lithub.com/what-the-retelling-of-myths-reveals-of-the-teller/ (accessed April 2020).

Frosch, S. 1997. Postmodern Narratives: Or Muddles in the Mind. In R. K. Papadopoulos & J. Byng-Hall (eds), *Multiple Voices: Narratives in Systemic Psychotherapy*. London: Duckworth.

Gleeson, S. 2019. *Constellations: Reflections from Life*. London: Picador.

Hewitt, S. 2019. Kyrie/Petition. In *Lantern*. London: Offord Road Books.

Holmes, J. 2008. Mentalisation and Metaphor in Poetry and Psychotherapy. *Advances in Psychiatric Treatment, 14*: 167–171.

Lasky, D. 2018. The Miscarriage. In *Milk*. Seattle: Wave Books.

Leon, I. 1990. *When a Baby Dies*. New Haven and London: Yale University Press.

Levine, S. 2009. *Trauma, Tragedy, Therapy: The Arts and Human Suffering*. London: Jessica Kingsley Publishers.

Macfarlane, R. 2008. *The Wild Places*. London: Granta Publications.

Macfarlane, R. 2019. Speaking the Anthropocene. Available at: https://emergencemagazine.org/story/speaking-the-anthropocene/ (accessed April 2020).

McCarthy, A. 2016. Who Can Call Herself a Mother? *Psychotherapy and Counselling Journal of Australia*. Available at: https://pacja.org.au/?p=3002 (accessed April 2020).

Norbury, K. 2015. *The Fish Ladder: A Journey Upstream*. London: Bloomsbury Publishing.

O'Neill, M. 2009. Ephemeral Art: The Art of Being Lost. In M. Smith, J. Davidson, L. Cameron, & L. Bondi (eds), *Emotion, Place and Culture*. Surrey: Ashgate Publishing.

6 Reframing motherhood

Photography as a creative application to re-image mother

Amy Lockhart Chilton

Personal preface

In the final stages of fulfilling the requirements towards completion of my Master's degree of psychotherapy and spirituality, specialising in Art Therapy, I had a baby. While I expected that life would be different, I did not expect to be a fragmented version of who I thought I was. I remember thinking, *becoming a mother has brought out the worst in me.* I was angry, frustrated and impatient. I felt like I was doing something wrong. I was thinking, *a mother is not supposed to feel this way, where is the 'bliss'? If I was doing it right, he wouldn't cry and fuss this much.* I was aware of and uncomfortable with the psychological shifts taking place within me. In moments of clarity where I could zoom out from the micro-scale of breast-feeding and diapers, I would think about: my own research and writing; barriers to care for new mothers; timing conflicts with feeding and naps; the personal hurdle of physical exhaustion; and the stigma associated with maternal distress. As I fluctuated from graduate student to new mother, I could see that I was now my own case study for a thesis about the ways in which Art Therapy – and particularly the therapeutic use of photography and photos – can be an active part of re-self-identification during the ongoing period of matrescence (becoming mother). Through my own self-reflexive process, baby in one arm, laptop beneath the other, I thought deeply, critically, painfully, about the ways in which the particular version of Western culture I am most familiar with exerts untenable demands upon new mothers.[1]

I made attempts to read about mothering, or to write down ideas for an academic project worthy of a Master's degree but found myself caught between the creative process of academic work and the totality of what it means to be responsible for another being's worldly existence. In moments of presence, when the baby slept after elaborate put-down efforts requiring Cirque du Soleil-level acrobatics, after a brief shower to regain a moment of body-autonomy, I would have slivers of thoughts that became notes of my own process of matrescence. As both a new mother and graduate student, I found the responsibilities collided. Coupled with my own academic throughline of photography as a therapeutic method, I started to arrange thought fragments into what would eventually become my thesis. So, without knowing exactly where it would lead me, I began to research the ways in which Art Therapy can support this transformative and confusing time.

This chapter

reveals through personal experience, listening and working with others, researching matrescence, and applying Photo Art Therapy as an active part of

the process of becoming a mother...

And recognising

the feelings of distress and depression that are commonly experienced but uncommonly discussed, prepared for, educated about or supported in personal,

social or professional situations.

So that

my experience

and research

can be part of a growing body of resignifying the ways in which women can embrace and embody mother

with the support of art therapy.

Introduction: what is a mother today, 2019?

The image of motherhood, at least in my own feedback loop in the West, is often viewed through a monochromatic lens – a binary reduction of black or white perceptions: medical birth or natural birth, doctor or midwife,[2] hospital birth or home birth, vaginal birth or caesarean section, happy or depressed, breast or formula, crib or co-sleep, stay-at-home or working, good mother or bad mother. The subjective experience of becoming a mother is well documented in the related literature (Held & Rutherford 2012; Stitt 2012, Mauthner 1999), and in contrast to the dominant and mainstream discourse, presents a much more diverse image of experience – offering a rich and multidimensional image of mother. By giving space for deep engagement, such as when researchers are themselves experiencing matrescence, the image can become multiple and non-binary revealing rich depth, contrast and shadow, where distress, exhaustion, ambivalence, depression, anxiety, resentment and anger are part of the tonal curve. The nuanced images of mother reveal a much greater range of light and dark, soft and hard; love and hate – in short the myriad experiences that come with matrescence, the becoming of mother.

Throughout the next pages I will present an exploration of the ways we can reframe the images we hold, as individuals and as communities enmeshed within and across cultures, of mother and motherhood – conceptually, therapeutically and artistically. In this chapter I will: (a) offer an exploration of a current Western cultural discourse using the term *matrescence* (Raphael 1973); (b) elaborate on therapeutic considerations related to becoming, being, a mother, such as maternal distress and post-partum depression with the intention to educate, support and normalise a wide spectrum of emotions that are part of becoming a mother; and (c) conclude by exploring the ways photography and the use of photographs are now readily accessible tools for self-reflection and ways in which they can be used as a creative application to guide Art Therapy clients to re-imagine their own image of mother.

Reframing motherhood into matrescence

What images come to mind when we consider *becoming a mother*?

My experience and research tells me that the process is usually imagined, discussed, categorised and experienced as distinct stages – pregnancy, labour, post-partum, and the fourth trimester (Brink 2013), etc. While these terms are accurate and explanatory descriptors of time, they compartmentalise the breadth and depth of the process of becoming a mother. The focus tends to be shifted to the physical changes and physical experience and the psychological, emotional, spiritual components are often overlooked (Speier 2001). For many mothers, the process begins to reveal itself first through the physical trans-formation made evident by a growing womb. The actual birthing process affirms the metamorphosis – a woman brings forth an infant(s) from her own body. Meanwhile, unseen changes are taking place – intrapsychically, a new identity is emerging, that of 'mother'. It is a vulnerable time where physical, psychological, social and spiritual changes can take place simultaneously, over the course of months, years, a lifetime perhaps. Matrescence affirms that becoming a mother is a complex, multilevelled and transformational experience.

Matrescence[3] (Raphael 1973, 1975) is a process and is central in helping to resignify and reframe motherhood – for mothers, for families, for (art) thera-pists and health practitioners, and for a cultural conversation about mother-hood. Matrescence acts as a catalyst to approach, dialogue and experience motherhood in a holistic way. The term first appeared in 1973 when Dana Raphael used the term in her book *The Tender Gift: Breastfeeding*, where she wrote extensively about the importance of the major life transition towards mother-hood. Raphael's ethnographic approach meant that she had a micro and privileged perspective on the behaviours of mothers including breastfeeding and social relations. Her research allowed for a close and emotional knowing that granted her the opportunity to bear witness to the emergence of 'mother' (Stone & Menken 2008).

> A woman's most critical rite of passage occurs when she becomes a mother … [I]t is a major life crisis and should not be taken for granted. Childbirth brings about a series of very dramatic changes in the new mother's physical being, in her emotional life, in her status within the group, even in her own female identity. I distinguish this period of transition from others by terming it matrescence to emphasise the mother and focus on her new lifestyle…

A woman in a mastrescent state should be highlighted and this particular period is singled out as unique and important.

(Raphael, as cited in Thomas 2001, pp. 89–90)

Raphael (1975) reflects upon matrescence as a critical event of cultural and/or interpersonal importance and acknowledges that it is a subjective process within the constructs of a given cultural milieu. Raphael's work on matrescence in relation to considerations for the therapeutic context is as follows:

1   Culture varies in approach, understanding and acknowledgment of matrescence.
2   The start and length of matrescence varies subjectively and culturally.
3   It is a biological, cultural, interactional and interpersonal transition.
4   Mastrescence is experiential – a learned process.
5   First-time mothers experience a more difficult transition than with subsequent children.
6   The individuals that surround a new mother act as guides to help her assimilate a new identity of mother.
7   'Mother' is a person; an activity; a behaviour.

Trudelle Thomas (2001) expanded on Raphael, suggesting that matrescence presents a woman with an opportunity for spiritual growth or a spiritual awakening – asserting that matrescence is a powerful time in which a woman will meet a new aspect of herself, others and ultimately, God (Thomas 2001, p. 90).

More recently, matrescence has re-entered the contemporary conversation through Alexandra Sacks, a reproductive psychiatrist and researcher, in her TED-X Talk (Sacks 2018) and in her *New York Times* article 'The Birth of a Mother' (2017). Sacks' work focuses on the psychological challenges of matrescence and highlights four challenges in the process of becoming a mother: changing family dynamics, ambivalence, fantasy versus reality, and feelings of guilt and shame. Maternal psychologist Aurélie Athan suggests that matrescence can be likened to a literary hero's journey, who faces many trials and tribulations during an adventure but prevails, returning home with insight and a newfound strength (cited in Zimmerman 2018).

The importance of matrescence

Matrescence is made manifest through acknowledging that becoming a mother is a complex, multilevelled and a transformational experience. Matrescence helps to situate motherhood on a continuum rather than inside of pre-determined time periods and/or independent events. By viewing matrescence in relation to life-course, it is a continual process and offers an opportunity to gain perspective – to see it as a time of evolution – in the same way as the circuitous journey from young to old. Sacks (2017) suggests that focusing on the shifts a woman experiences in her personal identity allows for personal understanding of emotions, which in turn can have a positive effect on behaviour and healthier parenting.

For Art Therapists, matrescence offers a broader therapeutic lens. It helps to signify a major transitional life stage and serves to frame and reclaim this as a critical period in which mothers may need and would benefit from extra support. Art Therapy can nurture a re-imaging of mother while offering a safe space to explore all aspects of motherhood and be supported through matrescence (Hogan 2015; Snyder 2016).

Unhappy mother = totally normal

Cultural norms informed by various religious traditions suggest becoming a mother is a natural process; one in which women were created to do and therefore should be 'good' at (Miller 2005). While there are many layers of cultural analysis regarding motherhood, persistent motherhood ideologies have been reified and have contributed to a stereotypical image of 'the good mother' (Johnston & Swanson 2006). The good mother narrative is imagined as a full-time, stay-at-home mother who embodies and is content with maternal qualities such as protective, nurturing, caring, moral, socialising, proud and organised (Guendouzi 2005). This image of mother paints a happy, natural, love-filled, maternal, bliss-filled image. The subjective experience of becoming a mother in academic literature presents a much more diverse image. For many women, becoming a mother is actually deeply disorienting and distressing (Terry 2014; Knaak 2009; Miller 2005, 2007; Thomas 2001; Sethi 1995; Hogan 2015). The academic image of mother, echoed by personal narratives I have collected reveal a 'dark side of maternity' (Almond 2011, p. 10) where mixed feelings, distress, exhaustion, ambivalence, depression, anxiety, guilt, resentment and anger come into focus.

Unhappy mothers have long been considered abnormal; however, research suggests that maternal distress is normal (Held & Rutherford 2012; Stitt 2012, Mauthner 1999). To demonstrate this discrepancy, Held and Rutherford (2012) examined the history of post-partum distress in popular magazines and advice books from the past 50 years. Their literature analysis revealed a continual theme that maternal distress or depression is the result of a personal deficiency (psychological or biological), rather than a result from the stress of motherhood itself (p. 112). This darker side of motherhood is often branded as 'post-natal depression' where hormonal shifts, low mood, anxiety, depression, distress, etc. are lumped together (Oakley 1988, p. 115). Feminist theorists have led the way in questioning the commonly held assumption that post-partum depression is the result of a personal inadequacy. Feminist sociologist and motherhood researcher Ann Oakley outlined her thoughts of post-partum depression in *Time* magazine (1980) stating that 'the recipe for depression is to create an unrealistic myth about motherhood, offer unfeeling medical care, and then set the new mother down in a social system that offers her little support for her new child and new role' (cited in Held & Rutherford 2012, p. 115).

The point here is not the existence or pathology of post-partum depression but rather to address the binary reduction of the image of mother. As Sacks articulates 'there are two poles. There's this idealized, unrealistic myth ... not human, not nuanced in the way that human experiences are. And then there's postpartum depression' (cited in Zimmerman 2018). By acknowledging, educating, supporting and normalising a wide spectrum of emotions and experiences that are part of becoming a mother, the cultural image of mother can be reframed – where the dark is embraced and honoured along the light. In order to do so, it is essential to understand the scope of potential changes and challenges that may arise throughout the period of matrescence, which can be noted biologically, psychologically, socially, and spiritually (Bartell 2005). See Figure 6.1.

Physiological challenges might be experienced by shifts in perception of self-image (King 2014); physical pain (e.g., post-surgical, vaginal, breastfeeding) (King 2014); physical intimacy (e.g., decreased libido; painful intercourse) (Hogan 2008); breastfeeding challenges (e.g., milk supply issues, latch challenges, plugged ducts) (King 2014); fatigue (Runquist 2007), resulting in challenges to utilise 'normal' coping skills, manage negative feelings, and access wellness support (Giallo et al. 2010). All of which may involve psychological impacts such as feelings of inadequacy, depression, affect the bonding relationship and increase overall maternal stress.

Emotionally, becoming a mother can prompt a range of uncomfortable emotions including jealousy, anger, rage, envy, confusion, guilt (Thomas 2001); depression in many forms such as low mood, sadness, and diagnosable depressive disorder with post-partum onset (PPD) (Marangoni 2012); anxiety (Reck et al. 2012); ambivalence (Lupton 2000; Almond 2011); cognitive dissonance where expectations do not match reality (Miller 2005; Thomas 2005); loss and bereavement experienced through a loss of freedom, earning power, mobility, physical functions, or conceptually, as a loss of sense of self/identity (Thomas 2001; Oakley 1988).

Psychologically, the changes to a woman's self-identity in matrescence are complex and can result in a reinvention and expanded sense of self. It is

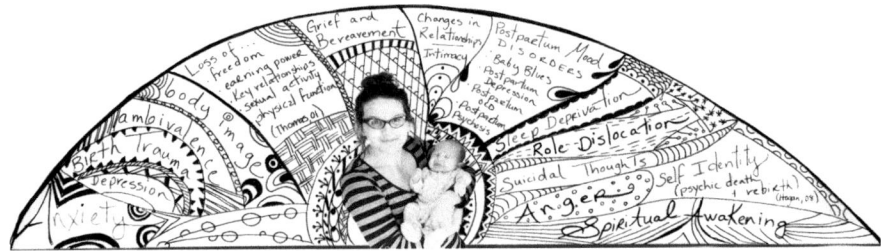

Figure 6.1 Mind-full Mama Zen Tangle. A visual summary of some therapeutic considerations that can be experienced in matrescence, which offers an example of a Photo Art Therapy directive – combining personal photo with doodle art. Amy Lockhart Chilton, 2017.

important to be aware of the continual 'mental work' (Laney et al. 2015, p. 141) taking place for a new mother. Additionally, post-partum mood disorders (PMD) are a group of mood disorders that can arise during matrescence (Curtis et al. 2007) which are understood as a spectrum of distressing emotional and mental symptoms ranging from mild depression (i.e., 'baby blues'), clinical depression (i.e., major depressive disorder with post-partum onset), obsessive-compulsive disorder, anxiety disorder, post-traumatic stress disorder and psychosis (Stone & Menken 2008).

Socially, changes to interpersonal relationships and dynamics in a multitude of ways may be experienced, such as a new division of 'labour' or lack of support from a spouse can take place, and extended family relationships can create issues of interference or a change of expectations that can cause new mothers stress (Hogan 2003).

Additionally, matrescence can be a time of spiritual transformation (Thomas 2001; Athan & Miller 2005). The intense emotional experiences of becoming a mother can nurture the opportunity for spiritual growth. For some, this may be a comfortable place and welcomed opportunity for personal growth; for others, it may bring confusing, uncomfortable feelings, or even trauma.

Photography, photographs and Art Therapy

Reframing is an essential process in photography. Framing an image is selecting what is to appear in a photograph by adjusting the camera position or lens choice (Warren 1993). Therefore, *reframing* can be a continual process as a person decides what should appear, or not appear in the photograph. The same can be achieved with photographs, the product of photography. Photographs are reframed by cropping, enlarging, matting, modifying, arranging, embellishing, elaborating, reconstructing, etc. The photographic arts lend themselves, naturally, to be a powerful tool to explore reframing.

Through my personal experience and professional training, I have come to understand the process of photography and the product of photographs to be powerful tools for self-reflection, self-discovery and personal growth. Both process and product of the photographic arts offer a catalyst for communication (Gibson 2018) including rich metaphors that conjure personal reflection and linguistic symbolism that can inspire the imaginations (i.e., shadow, focus, light, dark, seen/unseen, contrast, saturation, etc.). Today, photography has transcended its own professional boundaries and has become an accessible art form in the guise of a mobile phone (Gibson 2018).

Photography is both a visual art method and media (i.e., photographs) and can be used in therapy in active and passive ways (Moon 2010). In a therapeutic setting, clients can actively take photographs or manipulate photographs (i.e. digital manipulation, or graphic elaboration (Fryrear & Corbit 1992; Kopytin 2013) in therapy or reflect on existing photographs (Moon 2010). Photography for therapeutic purposes emerged in the 1850s shortly after the invention of the camera (Wolf 2007), when Dr H. Diamond used photographs to document and treat the mentally insane (Stewart 1979). By capturing the appearance of various stages of mania, Diamond felt this visual record would offer his patients awareness of their condition and hoped these photographs would offer them reflexive tools to separate themselves from their illness (Trifonova 2010). Today, the use of photography and photographs in therapy has evolved into various methods and practices such as PhotoTherapy (Stewart 1979; Weiser 1999), therapeutic photography (Gibson 2018), and the use of photography and photographs in Art Therapy categorised as 'Photo Art Therapy' (Fryrear & Corbit 1992; Weiser 2014; Kopytin 2010, 2018) or re-enactment phototherapy (Martin 2019). It is important to note that in practice the distinctions are not absolute and the methods are often interconnected (Loewenthal 2013).

Methods on a therapeutic spectrum

Photo Therapy

> The use of photography or photographic materials, under the guidance of a trained therapist, to reduce or relieve painful psychological symptoms and to facilitate psychological growth and therapeutic change.
>
> (Stewart 1979, p. 42)

PhotoTherapy, from a North American perspective, is recognised as a set of interactive, photo-based interventions, i.e., using personal snapshots and family albums, used in a therapeutic setting (Weiser 2014). The purpose of PhotoTherapy is to help people explore and learn about aspects of themselves by viewing and taking photographs (Blinn 1987, p. 254). While it can be used in an Art Therapy setting, PhotoTherapy techniques are considered as a system of interventions that can be used in any therapeutic setting, regardless of theoretical orientation (Weiser 2014).

Therapeutic photography

Therapeutic photography is the individual pursuit of photography and is used as a tool for self-discovery (Weiser 2017a). It encourages participants to research themselves through the art of photography, outside of a professional therapy setting, and in doing so can be an empowering process that enhances self-esteem (Gibson 2018).

Photo Art Therapy

The term has been used to classify Art Therapy that integrates the use of photography and/or photos into the art-making process, including the adaptation of PhotoTherapy techniques, as part of an Art Therapy session (Weiser 2014, 2017b; Kopytin 2018). For some, the classification of 'Photo Art Therapy' may seem redundant as photographic media are a visual art. However, as Kopytin (2018) suggests, the application of photography in Art Therapy has been limited due to; ethical considerations, technical competence (by clients and therapists), traditional focus, a favouring of tactile arts media, a lack of personal experience and a lack of theoretical training (p. 107).

Photography-based therapeutic practices represent a spectrum of forms that offer exploration for therapists and clients alike, including; to support the understanding of events and their importance (Halkola 2013); to encourage communication (Martin 2013), to support storytelling and resignification (Gibson 2018), to express feelings (Kopytin 2013); to tap into a client's unconscious (Loewenthal 2013) and to allow integration into consciousness (Kopytin 2013); to activate memory capacities, aid recognising emotions, and promote self-understanding (Halkola 2013); to improve self-esteem (Kopytin 2013); and to support exploration of self-identity (Gibson 2018). With the number of published works in these areas, and the proliferation of digital photography and the ubiquitousness of cameras in other devices, the list is sure to keep expanding rapidly.

Phototherapeutic practices to support matrescence

While Art Therapy literature suggests (Florschutz 2013; King 2014) and aligns (Hogan 2015; Snyder 2016) to confirm that Art Therapy can be a source of nurturing a re-imaging of mother while offering a safe space to explore and support all aspects of motherhood, literature using photographic interventions in Art Therapy with mothers is limited. Blinn (1987) suggested using a PhotoTherapy intervention with pregnant adolescents as a means to improve their self-concept, which was hypothesised to reduce subsequent pregnancies. Hogan (2015) listed PhotoTherapy among therapeutic practices used in group work for new mothers, but specifics on its use, efficacy or process were not given.

PhotoVoice is a branded practice that combines photography and social action (Wang & Burris 1997). PhotoVoice is not considered a therapeutic practice but has been shown to be a beneficial photographic practice for matrescent women. Nash (2014) uses PhotoVoice to explore body image during pregnancy and cultural ideals of post-partum bodies. A PhotoVoice project in Northern Ontario, Canada aimed to increase awareness of post-partum mood disorders (Postpartum Mood Disorder Project, n.d.).

The benefits of using phototherapeutic practices with mothers may include: (a) easy accessibility (Gibson 2018); (b) minimal skill required (simple/easy to use/familiar material); (c) facilitates non-verbal communication; (d) aids memory recall (Halkola 2013); (e) naturally lends itself to self-discovery and self-exploration (e.g., self-image); (f) provides an at-home self-reflective practice; and (g) activates positive change and improve personal relationships (Weiser 2017b).

Examples for creative application

A guide for using Photo Art Therapy in practice.

Art Therapy group to support matrescence

This is an Art Therapy group protocol, influenced by phototherapeutic practices, to support women through part of their matrescence. The Mama Bare Art Therapy Group is designed to give up to six new mothers (and their infants, 0–6 months) emotional support and the opportunity to creatively explore their feelings about pregnancy, birth and early motherhood in a confidential, closed group setting over the course of eight weeks.

The purpose is to:

- provide emotional support for new mothers;
- help new mother find resiliency and self-compassion;
- give space to explore and articulate a changed sense of self;
- acknowledge and provide space to explore difficult emotions such as fear, ambivalence, losses, anger, resentment, etc.;
- normalise experiences;
- foster optimal mother-infant attachment;
- create a community of support;
- provide information and resources to best support participants through their matrescence.

Weekly themes such as Connection, Birth of a Mother, Expectations versus Reality, Masks of Motherhood and Re-imaging Self offer a unified starting place for group members, and also provide structure and containment, as well as a way to connect the group members towards the common therapeutic goal (Liebmann 2004) of exploring matrescence.

Photography and photographs are incorporated into the Art Therapy process because they are accessible (Gibson 2018) and familiar mediums (Moon 2010) which are ideal for a potentially fatigued client. Here the art directives are simple, low skill level, contained (i.e. non-messy) and non-chaotic. As part of the Mama Bare Art Therapy Group, group members are invited to begin an at-home therapeutic photography practice where the purpose is twofold. This practice serves as an at-home reflective practice that can be a channel for creative expression; also, the photos taken can be used during the art making process throughout the group sessions.

Photo Art Therapy directives

Therapists may choose to familiarise themselves with one or more of the following modes of Photo Art Therapy directives that could be used to support mothers (inspired by Fryrear & Corbit 1992; Wolf 2007; Weiser 1999; Nuñez 2013).

Embellished/elaborated photographs

Photographs (printed on photo paper or photocopied) can be embellished upon with other art materials (e.g., paint, pencils, stickers, found objects,

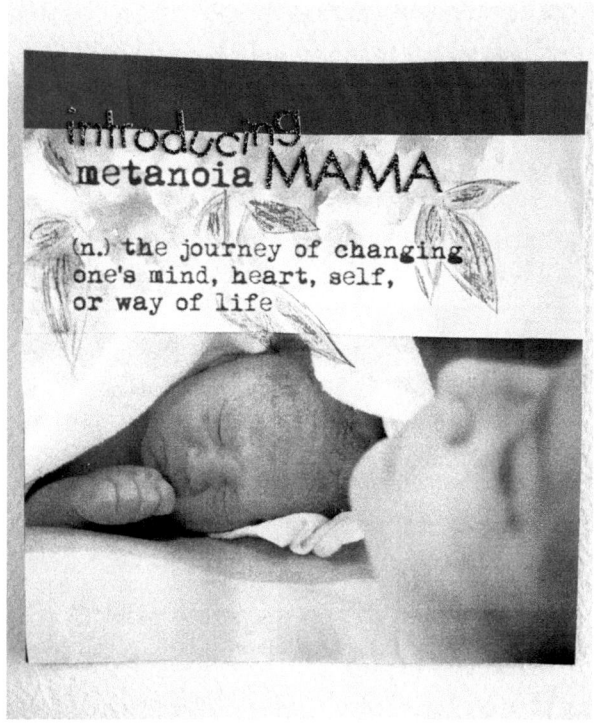

Figure 6.2 Mother Birth Announcement. Amy Lockhart Chilton, 2017.

fabric, etc.) or digitally manipulated. The photograph can be added to or the subject removed then elaborated on another piece of paper (Kopytin 2013).

Example. 'Graphic Elaboration' (Fryrear & Corbit 1992). Mother Birth Announcement – direct client(s) to create a birth announcement of themselves as mother. This can incorporate personal photographs. See Figure 6.2.

Photo collage

Collage is a common art form used in Art Therapy that serves as a non-intimidating activity that can support self-expression through images and materials while symbolically creating order (Moon 2010) in a directed or non-directed manner (Weiser 1999).

Example. Create a collage using personal photos, images and other materials that speak to my own journey of becoming a mother. See Figure 6.3.

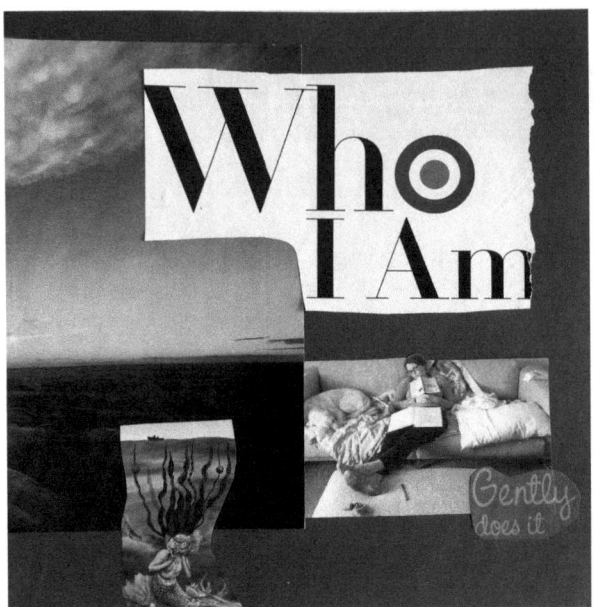

Figure 6.3 Becoming Mother Collage. Amy Lockhart Chilton, 2017.

Photo series, photo-journaling

Photographs can be arranged or reconstructed in a series that can offer opportunity for reflection from multiple perspectives, allowing images to be reframed visually and metaphorically.

Example. Using a picture frame with multiple opening or creating a digital grouping of photos, arrange the photos to narrative the journey through matrescence so far. See Figure 6.4.

Self-portraits

Self-portraits can allow for exploration of identity; Nuñez (2013) suggests the therapeutic benefit of self-portraits that convey challenging emotions as a means to 'objectify our "dark side"' (p. 102) providing distance and opportunity for a new perspective.

Example. Reality versus expectations self-portrait – create a pair of photographs that represent the reality of motherhood and one that represents your expectation of it.

Example. Take a 'self as mother' portrait. See Figure 6.5.

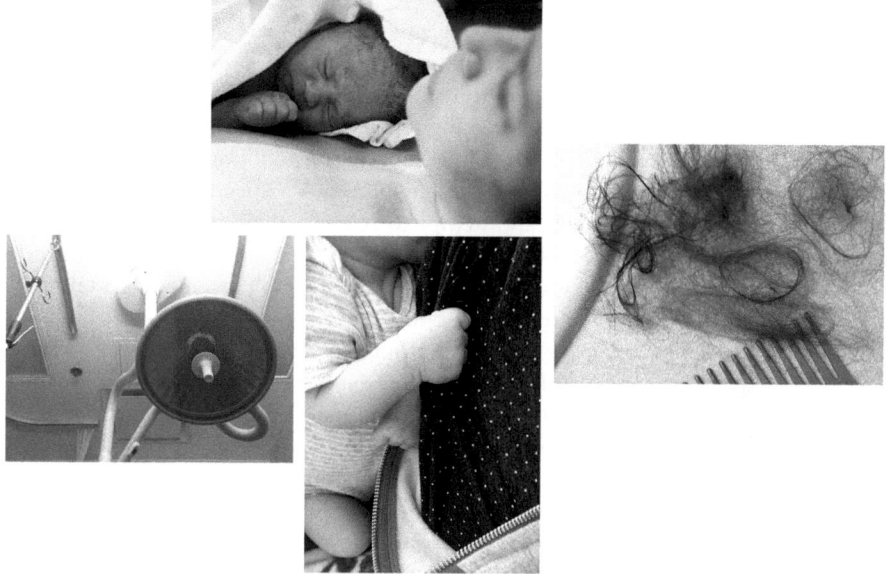

Figure 6.4 Matrescence photo series. Amy Lockhart Chilton, 2017.

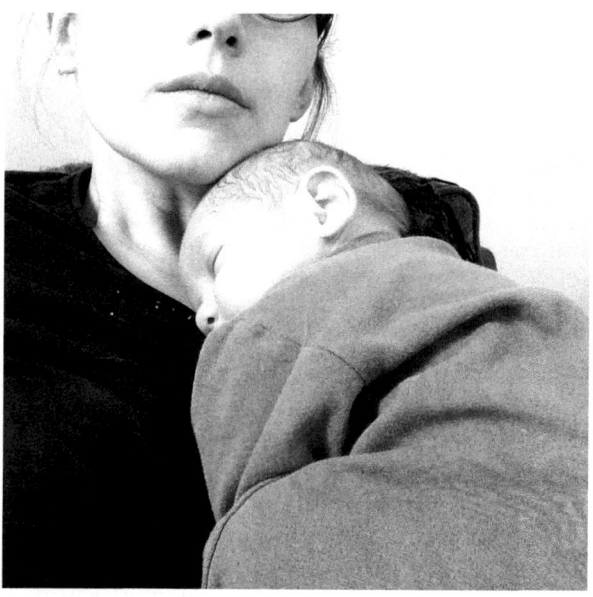

Figure 6.5 The Absence of I. Self-mother portrait. Amy Lockhart Chilton, 2015.

Concluding thoughts

To reframe is take a new perspective. It can be a physical act or psychological process of taking what is and attempting to understand it in a new way. This chapter explored the concept of matrescence to help to reframe the process of becoming a mother affirming and revering it as a subjective, continual experience that can involve physical, psychological, social and spiritual transformation. Then, perceptions of maternal distress were highlighted and a spectrum of therapeutic considerations was presented in an attempt to reframe them as a normal experience of motherhood rather than an abnormal one. Lastly, an overview of phototherapeutic practices in the context of Art Therapy were presented as a tangible means to apply these creative tools to support matrescence.

In 2020 our global cultures are undergoing a process of reframing. Many terms, concepts and categorisations are being examined and expanded beyond binary constraints. Gender is fluid; sexuality sits on a spectrum; stigmas of disability are dissolving into inclusivity; beauty ideals are being expanded and reshaped. The shift to reframe motherhood is happening. It can be *heard* on TED-X (Sacks 2018), *seen* on Instagram (breast pumping at work... #momtruths) and *felt* by mothers who simultaneously love and hate mothering.

For me, becoming a mother has been transformational – expanding my physical, mental, emotional and spiritual self. Since I was pregnant, birthed a baby and became a mother, I have encountered some of the darkest and brightest moments of my life. It was through discovering the term *matrescence* that I was able to reframe those dark times into a time of personal expansion. In considering my own self-image as mother, I see that it continues to expand and change as I grow through my mastrescence. My self-image acknowledges the shadows, embraces the contrast, and softens with highlights.

Notes

1 In this chapter I have chosen to focus the discussion of mother as the identity that I embody – a hetero-cis-gendered biological female who identifies with 'mother'. This acknowledgement is a caveat that identifies the limits of my own perspective, and does not seek to marginalise, disempower or degrade anyone else's experience or even interest in this chapter. It is simply an identification of the limits within this chapter. At the heart of this work is a fundamental belief that any individual could very well experience many of the emotional, psychological phenomenon described here, and that there may very well be a spectrum of experiences for individuals who also happen to have bodies, hormones and a physiology.

2 In Canada, maternal care and birthing support are categorised into two systems: the medical system with care through an obstetrician/gynaecologist and birthing in the hospital or with the midwifery network, which offers care with a midwife and a variety of birthing location options.

3 It is important to note that *matrescence* has been a relatively dormant term and therefore very little research has been generated about it. It does not specifically address subgroups of women/people who are experiencing various stages of matrescence such as adoptive mothers, step-mothers, same-sex mothers, trans women or childless mothers (i.e., childless through miscarriage or infant death). That said, it acknowledges and affirms that mastrescence is a subjective process and each person will have their own unique experience coming to parenthood.

References

Almond, B. 2011. *The Monster Within: The Hidden Side of Motherhood*. Berkeley, CA and London: University of California Press.

Athan, A., & Miller, L. 2005. Spiritual Awakening through the Motherhood Journey. *Journal of the Motherhood Initiative for Research and Community Involvement*, 7(1). Available at: http://jarm.journals.yorku.ca/index.php/jarm/article/view/4951 (accessed April 2020).

Bartell, S. 2005. On Becoming a Mother: The Psychological Journey. *International Journal of Childbirth Education*, 20(1): 28–30.

Blinn, L. M. 1987. Phototherapeutic Intervention to Improve Self-Concept and Prevent Repeat Pregnancies Among Adolescents. *Family Relations*, 36(3): 252.

Brink, S. 2013. *The Fourth Trimester: Understanding, Protecting, and Nurturing an Infant through the First Three Months*. Berkeley, CA: University of California Press.

Curtis, R., Robertson, P., Forst, A., & Bradford, C. 2007. Postpartum Mood Disorders: Results of an Online Survey. *Counselling & Psychotherapy Research*, 7(4): 203–210.

Florschutz, A. (2013). *The Art of Birth: Empower Yourself for Conception, Pregnancy and Birth*. London: Engage Press.

Fryrear, J. L., & Corbit, I. E. 1992. *Photo Art Therapy: A Jungian Perspective*. Illinois: Charles C. Thomas Pub Ltd.

Giallo, R., Wade, C., Cooklin, A., & Rose, N. 2010. Assessment of Maternal Fatigue and Depression in the Postpartum Period: Support for Two Separate Constructs. *Journal of Reproductive & Infant Psychology*, 29(1): 69–80.

Gibson, N. 2018. *Therapeutic Photography: Enhancing Self-Esteem, Self-Efficacy and Resilience*. London: Jessica Kingsley Publishers.

Guendouzi, J. 2005. 'I Feel Quite Organized This Morning': How mothering is Achieved Through Talk. *Sexualities, Evolution & Gender*, 7(1): 17–35.

Halkola, U. 2013. A Photograph as a Therapeutic Experience. In D. Loewentahal (ed.), *Phototherapy and Therapeutic Photography in a Digital Age*. Hove: Routledge, pp. 21–30.

Held, L., & Rutherford, A. 2012. Can't a Mother Sing the Blues? Postpartum Depression and the Construction of Motherhood in Late 20th-Century America. *History of Psychology*, 15(2): 107–123.

Hogan, S. 2003. *Gender Issues in Art Therapy*. London: Jessica Kingsley Publishers.

Hogan, S. 2008. Angry Mothers. In M. Liebmann (ed.), *Art Therapy and Anger*. London: Jessica Kingsley Publishers.

Hogan, S. 2015. Mothers Make Art: Using Participatory Art to Explore the Transition to Motherhood. *Journal of Applied Arts & Health*, 6(1): 23–32.

Johnston, D., & Swanson, D. 2006. Constructing the 'Good Mother': The Experience of Mothering Ideologies by Work Status. *Sex Roles*, 54(7–8): 509–519.

King, K. 2014. *The Authentic Mother: Creative Art Engagement to Support the New Parent*. Lancashire: Quantum Publishing Group.

Knaak, S. 2009. 'Having a Tough Time': Towards an Understanding of the Psycho-Social Causes of Postpartum Emotional *Stress*. *Journal of the Motherhood Initiative for Research and Community Involvement*, 11(1).

Kopytin, A. 2013. Photography and Art Therapy. In D. Loewentahal (ed.), *Phototherapy and Therapeutic Photography in a Digital Age*. Abingdon, Oxon: Routledge, pp.147–155.

Kopytin, A. 2018. Photo-Art Therapy. In C. Malchiodi (ed.), *The Handbook of Art Therapy and Digital Technology*. London: Jessica Kingsley Publishers, pp. 106–125.

Laney, E. K., Hall, M. E. L., Anderson, T. L., & Willingham, M. M. 2015. Becoming a Mother: The Influence of Motherhood on Women's Identity *Development. Identity*, 15(2): 126–145.

Liebmann, M. 2004. *Art Therapy for Groups: A Handbook of Themes and Exercises*. London: Psychology Press.

Loewenthal, D. 2013. *Phototherapy and Therapeutic Photography in a Digital Age*. Abingdon, Oxon: Routledge.

Lupton, D. 2000. 'A Love/Hate Relationship': The Ideals and Experiences of First-Time Mothers. *Journal of Sociology*, 36: 50–63.

Marangoni, T. 2012. What is Postpartum Depression? *Birth Issues*, Spring: 36–39.

Martin, R. 2013. Inhabiting the Image: Photography, Therapy and Re-enactment Phototherapy. In D. Loewenthal (ed.), *Phototherapy and Therapeutic Photography in a Digital Age*. Abingdon, Oxon: Routledge, pp. 69–81.

Martin, R. 2019. Look at Me! Representing Self: Representing Ageing. In S. Hogan (ed.), *Arts Therapies and Gender Issues: International Perspectives on Research*. Abingdon, Oxon: Routledge, pp. 188–210.

Mauthner, N. S. 1999. 'Feeling Low and Feeling Really Bad about Feeling Low': Women's Experiences of Motherhood and Postpartum Depression. *Canadian Psychology/ Psychologie Canadienne*, 40(2): 143–161.

Miller, T. 2005. *Making Sense of Motherhood: A Narrative Approach*. Cambridge and New York: Cambridge University Press.

Miller, T. 2007. 'Is This What Motherhood is All About?' Weaving Experiences and Discourse through Transition to First-Time Motherhood. *ResearchGate*, 21(3): 337–358.

Moon, C. H. 2010. *Materials and Media in Art Therapy: Critical Understandings of Diverse Artistic Vocabularies*. Abingdon, Oxon: Routledge.

Nash, M. 2014. Picturing Postpartum Body Image: A PhotoVoice Study. In M. Nash (ed.), *Reframing Reproduction*. London: Palgrave Macmillan, pp. 115–134.

Nuñez, C. 2013. The Self Portrait as Self-Therapy. In D. Loewentahal (ed.), *Phototherapy and Therapeutic Photography in a Digital Age*. Abingdon, Oxon: Routledge, pp. 95–106.

Oakley, A. 1988. *Women Confined: Toward a Sociology of Childbirth*. New York: Schocken Books.

Postpartum Mood Disorder Project. n.d. Available at: www.postpartumresource.com/ (accessed November 2016).

Raphael, D. 1973. *The Tender Gift: Breastfeeding*. New York: Schocken Books.

Raphael, D. 1975. *Being Female, Reproduction, Power, and Change*. Berlin and Boston: De Gruyter Mouton.

Reck, C., Noe, D., Gerstenlauer, J., & Stehle, E. 2012. Effects of Postpartum Anxiety Disorders and Depression on Maternal Self-Confidence. *Infant Behavior and Development*, 35(2): 264–272.

Runquist, J. J. 2007. A Depressive Symptoms Responsiveness Model for Differentiating Fatigue from Depression in the Postpartum Period. *Archives of Women's Mental Health*, 10(6): 267–275.

Sacks, A. 2017. The Birth of a Mother. *The New York Times*. Available at: www.nytimes.com/2017/05/08/well/family/the-birth-of-a-mother.html (accessed April 2020).

Sacks, A. 2018. *A New Way to Think about the Transition to Motherhood*. Available at: www.youtube.com/watch?v=jOsX_HnJtHU (accessed April 2020).

Sethi, S. 1995. The Dialectic in Becoming a Mother: Experiencing a Postpartum Phenomenon. *Scandinavian Journal of Caring Sciences*, 9(4): 235–244.

Snyder, K. 2016. Postpartum Imagery: Finding the 'Good' Enough. *Art Therapy Today*. Available at: http://multibriefs.com/briefs/aata/postpartum012016.pdf (accessed December 2016).

Speier, D. 2001. Becoming a Mother. *Journal of the Motherhood Initiative for Research and Community Involvement*, 3(1). Available at: http://jarm.journals.yorku.ca/index.php/jarm/article/viewFile/2079/1287 (accessed April 2020).

Stewart, D. 1979. Photo Therapy: Theory and Practice. *Art Psychotherapy*, 6(1): 41–46.

Stitt, J. 2012. Tom vs. Brooke: Or Postpartum Depression as Bad Mothering in Popular Culture. In E. Podnieks (ed.), *Mediating Moms: Mothers in Popular Culture*. Montreal: McGill-Queen's University Press, pp. 339–357.

Stone, S., & Menken, A. 2008. *Perinatal and Postpartum Mood Disorders: Perspectives and Treatment Guide for the Health Care Practitioner*. New York: Springer Publishing Co., Inc.

Terry, M. 2014. Feminism, Gender and Women's Experiences: Research Approaches to Address Postnatal Depression. *International Journal of Innovative Interdisciplinary Research*, 2(3): 19–32.

Thomas, T. 2001. Becoming a Mother: Matrescence as Spiritual Formation. *Religious Education*, 96(1): 88–105.

Thomas, T. 2005. *Spirituality in the Mother Zone: Staying Centered, Finding God*. New Jersey: Paulist Press.

Trifonova, T. 2010. Photography and the Unconscious: The Construction of Pathology at the Fin de siecle. Theory beyond the Codes. Available at: www.ctheory.net/articles (accessed December 2016).

Wang, C., & Burris, M. A. 1997. PhotoVoice: Concept, Methodology, and Use for Participatory Needs *Assessment. Health Education & Behavior*, 24(3): 369–387.

Warren, B. 1993. *Photography*. St Paul: West Publishing Company.

Weiser, J. 1999. *Phototherapy Techniques: Exploring the Secrets of Personal Snapshots and Family Albums*, 2nd ed. Vancouver: Phototherapy Centre Press.

Weiser, J. 2014. Establishing the Framework for Using Photos in Art Therapy (and Other Therapies) Practices. *Arterterapia: Papeles de arteterapia 7 educacion artistica para la inclusion social*, 9: 159–190.

Weiser, J. 2017a. Therapeutic Photography. Available at: https://phototherapy-centre.com/therapeutic-photography/ (accessed March 2017).

Weiser, J. 2017b. Related Techniques. Available at: https://phototherapy-centre.com/related-techniques/ (accessed March 2017).

Wolf, R. I. 2007. Advances in Phototherapy Training. *The Arts in Psychotherapy*, 34(2): 124–133.

Zimmerman, E. 2018. The Identity Transformation of Becoming a Mom. Available at: www.thecut.com/2018/05/the-identity-transformation-of-becoming-a-mom.html (accessed October 2019).

7 Representations of motherhood

Normative and transgressive constructions

Marián López Fdz. Cao

> The equation woman = mother does not respond to any essence but, far from it, it is a representation – or set of representations – produced by culture.
>
> (Tubert 1996, p. 7)

The patriarchal representation of the mother

> The ideal of motherhood provides a common standard for all women, which does not translate into the possible individual differences with respect to what one can be and desire. Identification with that ideal allows access to an illusory identity, which provides a falsely unitary and totalizing image that confers security in the face of uncertainties as it seems to be the definitive answer to all the questions.
>
> (Tubert 1996, p. 10)

The images surrounding motherhood have carried with them many types of significance, from the ancestral rites of divinity to the codification of motherhood through the figure of the Virgin Mary in the Catholic religion. Willendorf's Venus or the Mexican maternity figures show us a cult of fertility that is present in all civilisations – such as Ala, from Nigeria, the ruler of the Underworld, protector of the harvest and fertility of both animals and man; Arianrhod from Wales, associated with fertility, reincarnation, and beauty; Brigit from Ireland, the goddess of home, hearth, healing, and fertility; Inanna, Sumerian goddess of love, fertility, and war; Mylitta, Babylonian and Assyrian goddess of fertility and childbirth; Rhea, a Titan goddess of fertility and motherhood, among others. Maternity and childbirth are essential elements for the survival of the group and are therefore considered of crucial importance. The group appeal to the divinity in order to sustain and guarantee their continued existence.

An example of the importance given to fertility and pregnancy are the Mesoamerican figures of Cihuateotl (600–900 CE). These life-size female terracotta sculptures are a typical feature of downtown Veracruz and represent women who died in their first childbirth. When they died giving birth, they were

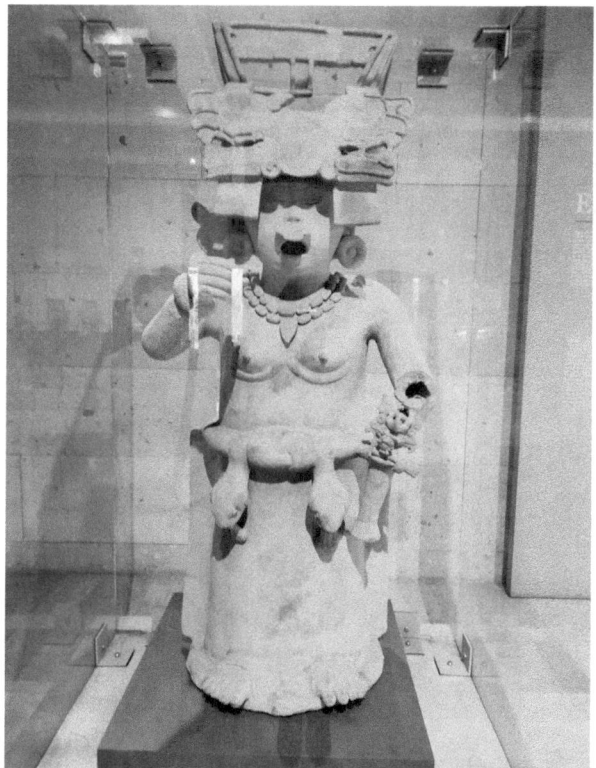

Figure 7.1 Cihuateotl. Veracruz, Late Classic 600–900 CE. Xalapa Anthropology Museum.
Photograph: Marián López Fdz. Cao.

considered warriors, thus obtaining the right to accompany the sun during its journey through the firmament. The closed eyes of the statuette reflect the last image of the earthly world, and the spirit escapes through the half-open mouth. The woman becomes divine and ascends to another plane in the universe. The snakes that they have around their waist represent fertility and the bag of copal that they carry on their left arm indicates that they are purifying their walk.

The lifeless bodies of women who died in childbirth were revered as divinities, and their bravery admired by the majority of society. After the funeral ceremony, the closest male family members were to take care of the remains, which were sought after by warriors as amulets for their worth. On the one hand, the Cihuateotl went to live for eternity in Cincalco, the dwelling of corn, to serve as guides to the Sun each sunset and became an object of worship, directly related to Cihuacōātl, mother goddess who was part of the deities known as Tonantzin, creative mothers. On the negative side, women with power are feared – it was

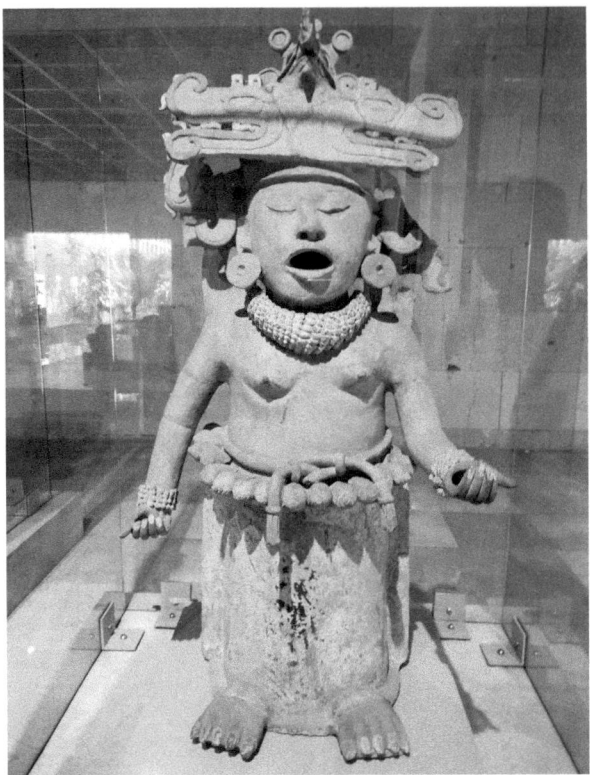

Figure 7.2 Cihuateotl. Veracruz, Late Classic 600–900 CE. Xalapa Anthropology Museum.
Photograph: Marián López Fdz. Cao.

believed that they could take away life. These entities came to earth to try to fulfil what they lost dying. As Nicholson states:

> On the five days that commenced the 13-day periods of the 260-day divinatory cycle assigned to the West, these female spirits were believed to descend to haunt the crossroads, hoping to kidnap young children since they had been deprived of their opportunity to be mothers.
>
> (Nicholson & Keber 1983, 68)

Thus, we can see an example of how female figures acquire the ambivalent character that, when they have symbolic power, they become threatening in patriarchal societies.

As a result, the representation of motherhood becomes a fundamental process for the social group, but also linked to a state to fear because of the danger it entailed.

Throughout history, and precisely because of the high level of mortality in childbirth, it becomes an object of representation, and deities that protect motherhood proliferate in all cultures. Having children (especially when infant mortality is tremendously high) is necessary for the survival of the species and a symbolic construction is needed that not only protects the act, but teaches women that this is their primary function; that childbirth is not only necessary but is desirable and something that truly makes them women, linking femininity and motherhood in an indissoluble way.

We can thus observe how a control over the inheritance of property is constructed through the control of female sexuality, enthroning, on the one hand, the virginity of women and justifying the control of conjugal fidelity as specific to the 'good woman', while urging women, on the other hand, to be mothers again and again to ensure the continuity of lineage and property. This makes the construction of sexuality and the body of women an almost impossible requirement of chastity, sexual limitation and motherhood.

The representation of motherhood, childbirth and lactation in Christian and Catholic images

The researcher Antonia Fernández Valencia (1997) highlights several representations of maternity and childbirth in European Christian iconography from the end of the Middle Ages to the seventeenth century. The births of the Virgin, Jesus and the Baptist are massively represented in medieval painting and in that of the sixteenth century and, although to a lesser extent, that of the seventeenth. In those of Mary and the Baptist, there is a common characteristic: the absence of men – except for the father, who may appear as a passive observer – and the numerous cast of female figures that surround and attend to the mother and the newborn baby.

Following Fernández Valencia, these representations coincide with the formation of a new concept of 'the state' in Europe, a fact that required population growth in order to generate resources and a civil and military workforce. Publishing in favour of the growth of the birth rate comes from civil, secular and religious authorities, from Protestantism (Luther in the sixteenth century) and Catholicism. Since the population is the main source of a country's wealth, it is not strange that iconographic themes are supported that exalt and dignify motherhood, moving it away from the idea of danger and death. On the other hand, representations abound on the theme of childbirth protection. That the act was a dangerous one could not be denied, and there are many testimonies to the high mortality rate during childbirth. In 1519, in his *Guide to Sinners*, Fray Luis de Granada recognised that many women die in childbirth (Caro Baroja 1978), and in 1792, the priest of Garganta la Olla wrote: 'Another plague walks and is always there. There are such births that at each point we go to take final Confession from the women who do not stop dying from this cause' (Fernández Vargas & López Cordón 1986, p. 21). Joseph Illick, referring to childhood in England in the seventeenth century, points out the high mortality of mothers and their infants in the first month, accusing the midwives of lack of care (Illick 1982).

This demographic role of women is very clear in the realm of Protestantism. Women can be sacrificed. 'Even if they are exhausted and die in the end of giving birth, no matter how much they die of giving birth, that is what they exist for', is Luther's thesis (King 1993, p. 15); the Catholic Church, for its part, condemns any birth control and does not accept any sexual relationship in marriage other than that which has procreation as its purpose. The Protestant reformer John Calvin accepts that the number of children be limited by continence, accepting responsibility based on the possibilities of upbringing and maintenance (Burguiere et al. 1988). Despite the very high infant mortality rate due to post-partum infections, women were still urged to fulfil their reproductive obligation. Following Fernández Valencia, it is likely that the proliferation of birth re-presentation in art, especially the birth of Jesus (in contexts where the birth of male children was prized over that of girls), showing Mary in a calm and safe situation, surrounded by a group of women who attend to her, reinforces on the one hand the message of the essential role of motherhood in women, and the importance of care and the essential role of women in it, and the promise of a smooth delivery, on the other hand.

It is important to point out how, although the maternal function is essential in the continuation of the lineage, society and the configuration of the state, the

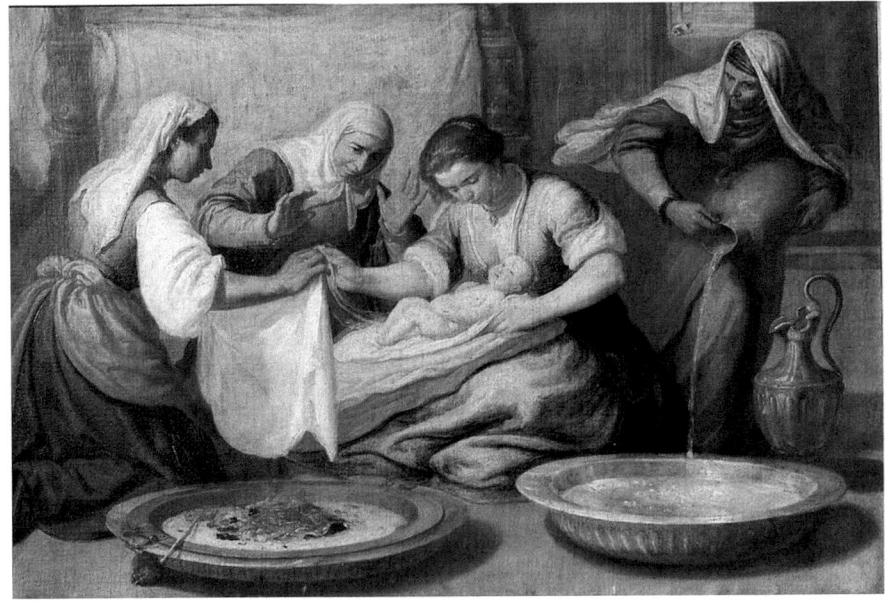

Figure 7.3 Nativity of Mary. Oil on canvas, 101 × 142cm, Spanish, seventeenth century. Reproduced by kind permission: Wikimedia Commons, https://en.wikipedia. org/wiki/Nativity_of_Mary#/media/File:Nativity_of_mary.jpg.

infant, as soon as it is born, is automatically transferred to male property, eliminating the mother's surname and filiation. Maternity thus becomes a social and political act, offering only lineage to the father dispossessing mothers of logos and authority in most societies. Mothers provide, as Celia Amorós (2004) points out, only flesh, while fathers provide logos and social and political legitimacy. That is why 'bastard' births are considered outside the law and social order, and mothers of bastards were condemned socially, legally and politically, both in private and public spheres.

The construction of lactation in Western history

As well as constructing an ideal of motherhood to be followed by women – even when this ideal is practically impossible and leads women to dissatisfaction, guilt and shame – another ideal appears linked to motherhood: the construction of lactation. We know, through paleo-archaeological research that the survival of the first human beings depended practically exclusively on their mothers through breastfeeding. Women were essential not only in reproduction but also in the care of the species, at least in the first years. Breastfeeding and lactation have therefore been the object of prescription and proscription towards women throughout human history. History is full of religious images that seem to encourage lactation by mothers, rather than the widespread use among the upper and middle classes of the wet nurse. From Fernández Valencia we can see what qualities were prized in breastfeeding women by sixteenth-century. In 1541, for example, Damián Carbón advised they should 'be of middle age, neither skinny nor fat, white and lucid, muscular, broad breasts, hard flesh, good character and neither sad nor shy' (quoted in Simon Palmer 1984, p. 58).

But Fernández Valencia (1997) points out that, at that moment of Spanish religious purity – Muslims and Jews having just been expelled from the country – the most characteristic feature of the Spanish case is the racism that is applied: the prevention against Moorish and Jewish wet nurses. Father Simón de Rojas even believed that Moorish children should be expelled from Spain because 'they have sucked the hatred they have for our Catholic religion and the infected root they have inside their entrails' (Caro Baroja 1978, p. 490). The literature in this sense is very broad. Jesuits like Pablo José de Arriaga displayed similar sentiments.

It is important to remember, on the other hand, the iconography of the symbol of the French Revolution, *La Marianne*, that often bears characteristics of the Virgin Mary, or the 'happy mothers' that appear in France from Rousseau's ideas, encouraging the women of the bourgeois and noble classes to breastfeed their own infants – which would have been frowned upon among these classes at the time. The essence of motherhood as it appears here is sacrifice, including the sacrifice of breastfeeding. As Jean-Marie Roulin (2001) states, making the mother into a symbol of the republic means doubly excluding the woman from the polis: in reducing her to either the virgin or the mother she is kept at a distance from

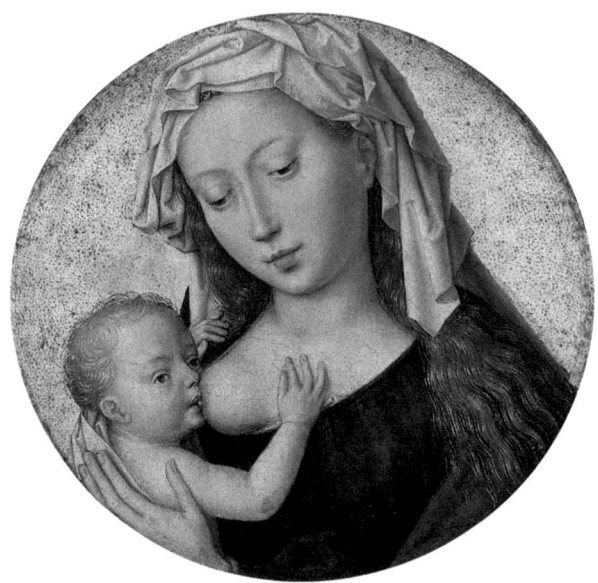

Figure 7.4 Virgin Suckling the Child. Hans Memling, c. 1433. Reproduced by kind permission: Wikimedia Commons, https://commons.wikimedia.org/wiki/File:Hans_Memling_-_Virgin_Suckling_the_Child_-_WGA14966.jpg.

the order of desire sexuality, under cover of elevation to allegory or metaphor she is refused political citizenship.

The obligation or dispensation of lactation has been, as we can see, a cultural construction. Let us not forget how advertising in the 1950s made the claim that powdered milk was better quality than breast milk, resulting in this type of product becoming popular among the more affluent classes.

The im/possible construction of the woman/mother in Catholic tradition

Kristeva associates the ideal of woman with the icon of the Virgin Mary, considered 'one of the most powerful imaginary constructs known in the history of civilizations' (1985, p. 163). Following Rodríguez Salas (2004) this prototype of woman has to be imitated by the rest according to the monolithic Christian-patriarchal model: the Virgin Mary stands for the sacrificed image, subdued to men's superiority. Later, this Marian cult of medieval times was progressively secularised until it gave way to the image of the 'Angel in the House' extended all over the Anglo Saxon world and established itself strongly within Victorian Puritanism.

Christianity, quotes Kristeva in her *Stabat Mater* (1985, p. 133) 'is no doubt the most sophisticated symbolic construct in which femininity, to the extent that it figures therein – and it does so constantly – is confined within the limits of the Maternal'. But it is an ideal no individual woman could possibly embody. The figure of the Virgin Mary is that of the unique woman. As Kristeva points out:

> Unique among women, unique among mothers, and, since she is without sin, unique also among humans of both sexes. But this recognition of the desire of uniqueness is immediately checked by the postulate that uniqueness is achieved only by way of exacerbated masochism: an actual woman worthy of the feminine ideal embodied in inaccessible perfection by the Virgin could not be anything other than a nun or a martyr; if married, she would have to lead a life that would free her from her 'earthly' condition by confining her to the uttermost sphere of sublimation, alienated from her own body.
>
> (1985, p. 149)

Alienation of herself and near immolation, the Catholic construction of mother reinforces the idea of women at the service of patriarchy, denying their individuality as women and their capacity for both pleasure and sexual freedom. As Bruzelius (1999, p. 215) states:

> It is depressing to note that the identification of motherhood with suffering and the validation of the maternal voice through that suffering, which has been so effectively fostered by the church in the case of Mary, continues almost unquestioned today.

According to Rodríguez Salas (2004, p. 102) the idea of motherhood participates in the artificiality of the 'feminine'; both maternity and femininity being patriarchal constructions with an appearance of reality, since women adopt these roles, although they are a pure fantasy that authors like Kristeva endeavour to dismantle.

Thus, trapped in the construction of femininity within a closed codification of the maternal ideal at the service of patriarchy, women tend to live the fact of having or not having children from an extreme prescription, but deeply internalised: immolation for the care of children, living-for-others, the feeling of not being truly feminine if they do not become mothers, the guilt of society and the learned self-culpability, together with the instant dispossession of children in patrilineal society through the male surname, and the taking of second place in all official documents (where the father always occupies the first place) make the experience of motherhood a personal, social and political battlefield, as the artist Barbara Kruger pointed out in her work of the 1990s.

Figures of transgression

For some decades now, feminist theory has vindicated the role of motherhood, trying to get rid of patriarchal inheritance and seeking to re-signify the act of giving life. Since Julia Kristeva, many theorists – such as Luce Irigaray and Hélène Cixous – have tried to deconstruct, on the one hand, and re-signify, on the other, the term *maternity*, trying to get women to appropriate its meaning: As Adrienne Rich points out, it is necessary for women to claim the power of their reproductive and productive capacity:

> the repossession by women of our bodies will bring far more essential change to human society than the seizing of the means of production by workers. The female body has been both territory and machine, virgin wilderness to be exploited and assembly-line turning out life. We need to imagine a World in which every woman is the presiding genius of her own body. In such a world women will truly create new life, bringing forth not only children (if and as we choose) but the visions, and the thinking, necessary to sustain, console, and alter human existence – a new relationship to the universe. Sexuality, politics, intelligence, power, motherhood, work, community, intimacy, will develop new meanings; thinking itself will be transformed. This is where we have to begin.
>
> (1976, pp. 285–286)

In *Of Woman Born*, Adrienne Rich – in common with O'Reilly – distinguishes between two meanings of motherhood, one superimposed on the other: the potential relationship of any woman to her powers of reproduction and to children; and the institution that aims at ensuring 'that that potential-and all women-shall remain under male control' (O'Reilly 2004, p. 2).

Motherhood autobiographies

> Lives do not serve as models, only stories do that. And it is a hard thing to make up stories to live by. We can only retell and live by stories we have heard. Stories have formed us all: they are what we must use to make new fictions and new stories'
>
> (Heilbrun 1988, p. 32)

In recent decades, art, through creative processes, has helped women to express, de-structure and reorganise the states resulting from difficult processes in pregnancy, childbirth and puerperium, which question their own body and its limits, identity, alterity and relationship with the other. Artists such as Käthe Kollwitz, Frida Kahlo, Mary Kelly, Rineke Dijkstra, Louise Bourgeois and Ana Casas Broda have shown how motherhood can be lived and expressed.

Paula Modersohn-Becker (1876–1907)

'This woman from Worpswede, who became famous after her death, is a huge disappointment,' wrote the Nazi censors in the exhibition catalogue.

Her artistic vision is so vulgar, so unfeminine … Her work is an insult to German women, to our peasant traditions. Where is the sensitivity, the maternal essence of the feminine spirit? An incoherent and inharmonious use of colour, deformed figures that pretend to represent farmers, distorted and degenerated children, the scum of humanity.

(in Darrieussecq 2019, paragraph 8)

Thus the transgression of the representation of pregnancy ignites the reaction to roles and models of cultural prescription about women's bodies and their functions. With this scandalous expression, images are rejected that try to re-signify and re-appropriate the discourse about motherhood by women who try to internalise their biological processes.

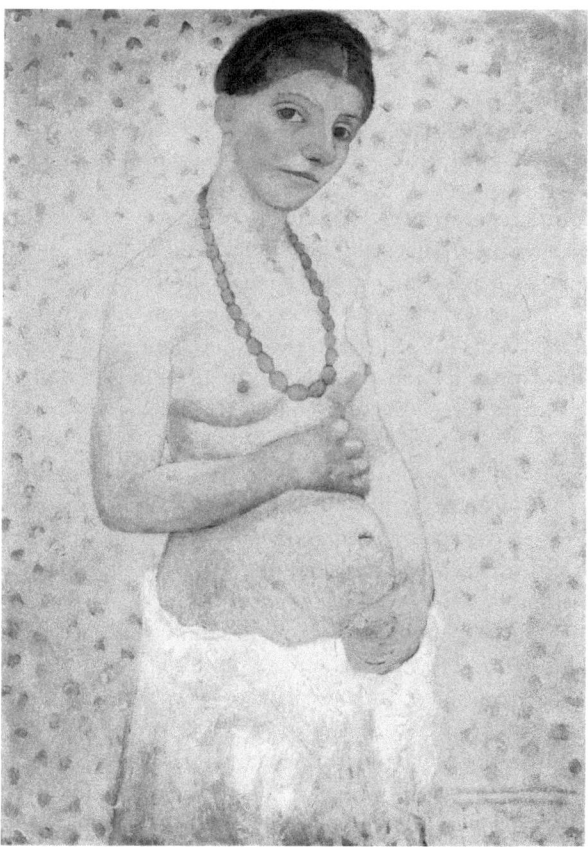

Figure 7.5 Self-Portrait on the Sixth Wedding Anniversary. Paula Modersohn-Becker, 1906. Reproduced by kind permission: Wikimedia Commons, https://commons.wikimedia.org/wiki/File:Paula_Moderson-Becker_-_Selbstbildnis_am_6_Hochzeitstag_-_1906.jpeg?uselang=fr.

Modersohn Becker was the first woman to represent herself naked and pregnant in her work 'Self-Portrait on the Sixth Wedding Anniversary' (1906). Her nudes embody, perhaps for the first time in the history of art, an introspective gaze towards herself, imagining herself as a pregnant woman. She questions, in the act of painting herself, the possible meaning of existence. Her works are not style exercises on the feminine body. They are not treatments of the body object as a motive for power, domination and dualistic conformation. Nor are they exercises of autobiography. They are rather exercises of reflection and introspective sincerity, intimate reflections of the self, which confront us with the question of existence.

It is paradoxical and overwhelming that Modersohn-Becker died of a stroke two days after the birth of her daughter. Her work becomes, with greater motive, a question about life, a question about death and the condition of women to give life at the expense of their own lives. The work seems to reflect on the difficult framework of being born, living to die and dying give birth, to give life, which often accompanies and has accompanied women in an act of self-immolation that society applauds and supports.

Käthe Kollwitz (1867–1945)

Kollwitz's women's bodies acquire the character of truth and testimony: they tire, crawl and embrace with strength the life that flees through misery and violence. They stand as a protective force against the destruction of life. Her two collections, 'Peasants' War' and 'Weavers' Uprising' symbolise how the poor classes, women and men, confront power and fight for a dignified life. In them women are a primary part of life, both sustaining it daily, preventing violence, and ultimately seeking the dead bodies of their sons on the battlefield.

They are unusual images for the gaze accustomed to the beautiful, canonical bodies of Western art. They are the bodies of people impoverished by the economic crisis, by inequality, by repeated pregnancies, by the deaths of their children due to hunger and misery. They are the image of unemployed people, taken to the extremes of misery, which draw the gaze of the spectator.

Rarely do we find the bodies of people, without idealisation, with all humanity, as in the work of Käthe Kollwitz. They are the image of those forced to go to the battlefield, to death, to disappearance. In them is recognised the injustice of a power that manipulates, condemns and orders, that prescribes and proscribes. But at the same time, Kollwitz shows us the greatest dignity in their bodies, their faces, their hands that embrace, assist, gather. The mother who embraces the dead child of misery in her arms, the group of women who close their children around them. Kollwitz said in her writings that she found much more beauty in poverty than in the refined environments of the upper classes. Kollwitz unites ethics and aesthetics, where beauty is a moral category.

Kollwitz made a commissioned poster for a campaign of the women's secretariat of the KPD (German Communist Party) against paragraph 218 in 1923.[1]

During the Weimar Republic, abortion discussion led to a reduction in the maximum penalty for abortion, and in 1926 a court's decision legalised abortion in cases of grave danger to the life of the mother.

Käthe Kollwitz draws the picture of the overstrained proletarian woman who can hardly feed two children and is pregnant again. Thus the right to abortion due to economic hardship is demanded. Already in a diary entry of the artist from 1909 it becomes clear that the numerous pregnancies of the women contribute significantly to the misery of the proletarian families. In her diary, Kollwitz writes: 'The man leaves, the woman complains. Always the old song. Illness, unemployment, drunkenness – that always goes round in circles. She has had eleven children, 5 are alive, the big ones died and little ones keep coming again and again' (30 August 1909, in Kollwitz 1984, p. 8).

Reproductive rights and improvements in women's lives

According to Pujal, after the Second World War a new rethinking of femininity and maternity arose, initiated by the North American Betty Friedman with her work *The Feminine Mystique* (1963). This work denounces the idealisation and normalisation of the role of women in terms of self-realisation based on the social construction of women as mothers, wives, kind and asexual, characteristics that according to the author mask their reality: their social isolation, their lack of life expectations and autonomy due to submission to the patriarch (Pujal 2002, p. 19).

Thanks to the emergence of the feminist movement, the 1960s and 1970s saw a profound deconstruction and reconceptualisation not only of femininity but also of maternity. The introduction of the contraceptive pill, the fight for equality in sexual rights, improvements in women's access to the labour market, the recognition of women's right to sexual pleasure and their right to choose resulted in a dramatic change in mentality. During these years, the sociology lecturer Hannah Gavron researched, among others, the lives of young mothers from middle- and working-class families in north London. Her research was published as *The Captive Wife: Conflicts of Housebound Mothers* (1966). She pointed to a domestic and maternal narrative of isolation, frustration and confinement for women (Aston 2000). Since then, women have brought to the table many of the contradictions that being a woman and mother entailed and the cultural and symbolic imperatives that accompanied them. In all parts of the world, artists and movements began to emerge that, along with feminist and self-consciousness movements, questioned the figures of motherhood from the equation of immolation and happiness. In Spain, artists such as Esther Ferrer pointed out that sexuality and productive capacity was an 'intimate and personal' issue for each woman and in the US, Mary Kelly, with her artwork 'Post-Partum Document', chronicled her personal mother–child relationship in a rigorous and subjective way for six years. In this way, first-person voices emerged documenting women's bodily changes and their consequences in a society that demands a particular behaviour from women when they become mothers, introducing the famous phrase 'the personal is political'.

The artists, through various forms, dealt with the subject of motherhood and care. Whether Barbara Kruger's social activism or Bobbi Baker's performance art, many artists focused on disclosing and denouncing the use of the female body in reproduction, the rights and restrictions on their bodies, the inconsistencies inherent in it, while using irony to spread their messages. The care of children came to be considered as not only for mothers; timidly men began to realise that equal participation in care favoured not only the father–child relationship, but that of the couple itself.

Your body is a battleground

In April 1989, Kruger designed fliers for the pro-choice rally in Washington, DC. This powerful flier was distributed during the march and the phrasing became a rallying cry for women while the *Roe v. Wade* decision was in the process of being overturned. Over 25 years later, Barbara Kruger's work, message and art remain relevant. As Kruger put it: 'I think that it's important for me to somehow, through a collection of words and images, to somehow try to picture – or objectify, or visualize – how it might feel sometimes to be alive today' (in Mitchell 1991, p. 445).

In 1992, Kruger designed another poster entitled 'How Come Only the Unborn Have the Right to Life?' At the top, Kruger asked 'Women or incubator?' And in the lower part 'Celebrate the fetus and starve the child'.

In this way, Kruger denounced a two-faced society that legislated on women's bodies and their right to reproduce while disregarding deprived children, by abandoning them to misery and helplessness.

In this sense, the artworks produced in recent years express, in one way or another, the questioning of the role imposed on women over care, at the same time that society itself takes away their rights over them. The work of the Spanish artist Cristina Llanos is exemplifying in this sense. She released in 2015, a 'Secret Agreement' where the mother must renounce to all right on the child before the society, at the same time that acquires all type of obligations for its preservation and care, all this in a social agreement that should not be explicit (Hervás Hermida 2016).

Cristina Llanos. The Secret Agreement. 2015

CONTRACT

Once the two parts have been brought together: one part, the mother and the other, the rest, made up of citizens who are not the mother, decides, without the testimony of the part we have called the mother being necessary or binding, the following:

1   Interest in the unborn always prevails. The part corresponding to the mother will have to silence any painful or traumatic episode that she suffered, whether during childbirth, the postpartum period or during the puerperium.

Any interest of the mother shall be subject to the protection of the survival of the species and its public significance.

2 Once the baby has been born, either by natural birth or by Caesarean section, and without attending to the vicissitudes that occurred during the

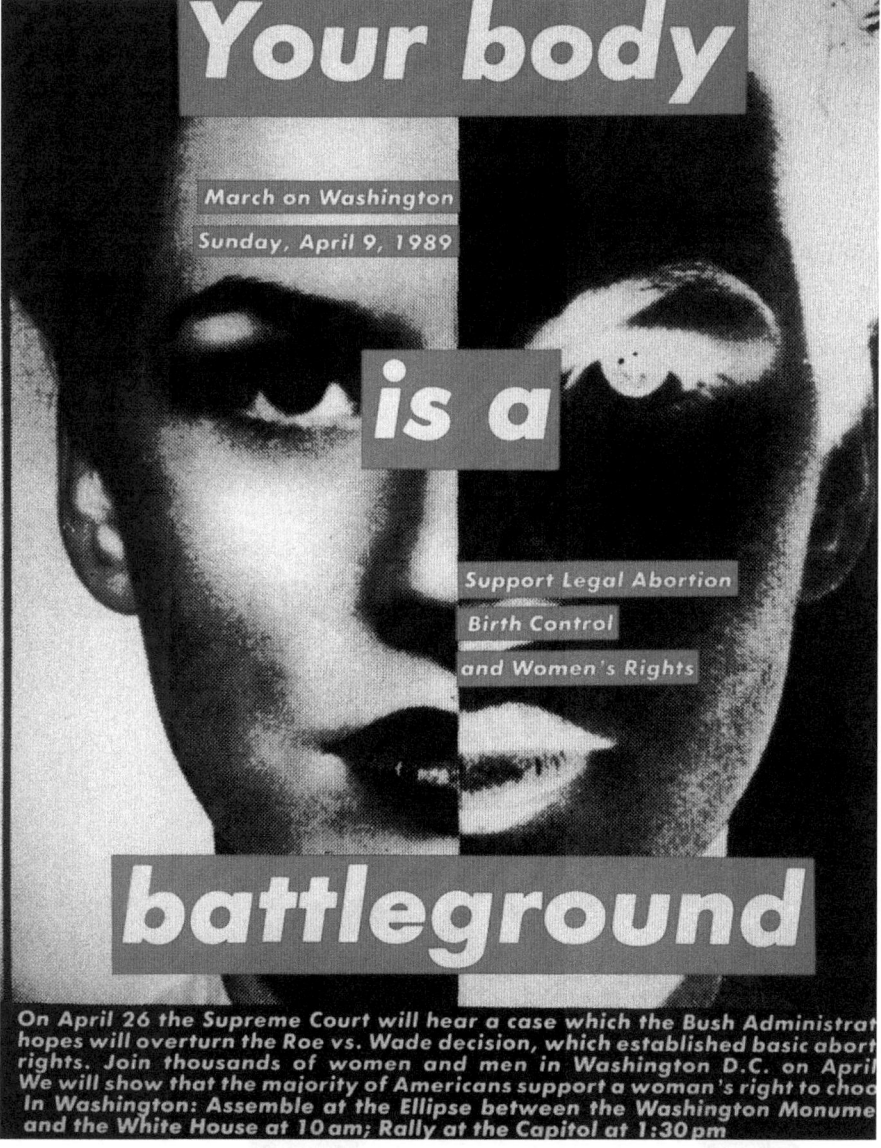

Figure 7.6 Poster distributed in Washington to defend the right to abortion. Barbara Kruger, 1989. Reproduced by kind permission: Wikimedia Commons, https://commons. wikimedia.org/wiki/File:Untitled_(Your_body_is_a_battleground).jpg.

gestation period, if any, the mother will cede moral authority over the child to the rest, thus delegating this responsibility in defense of what we can call the 'status quo'. This does not exempt the mother from her obligation as a food producer of the child.

3   This agreement is binding and obligatory for the mother and will not be subject to her consent, nor will her decision be required at the time the contract becomes effective.

4   The fulfillment of the agreement requires absolute confidentiality and therefore at no time will the obligations required by the agreement be made public. If the mother violates this confidentiality clause, the other party will obtain the necessary authority to take appropriate action to the detriment of the other party.

Finally, within the 'artivism' of recent years in relation to reproductive rights, we can observe the strength of Argentine illustrators for the right to decide on the body of women (see Figure 7.7).

Contemporary artworks can serve as mirrors or triggers for each woman's personal narratives. In the Art Therapy work that this book explores, artworks such as those we have just examined have great power to open up narratives related to the gender mandates imposed by society. Women, and especially women artists, break and make evident these mandates, expressing their suffering, but also the contradictions of family and social requirements, of the public and the private spheres, opening up the possibility of legitimising new narratives through creation.

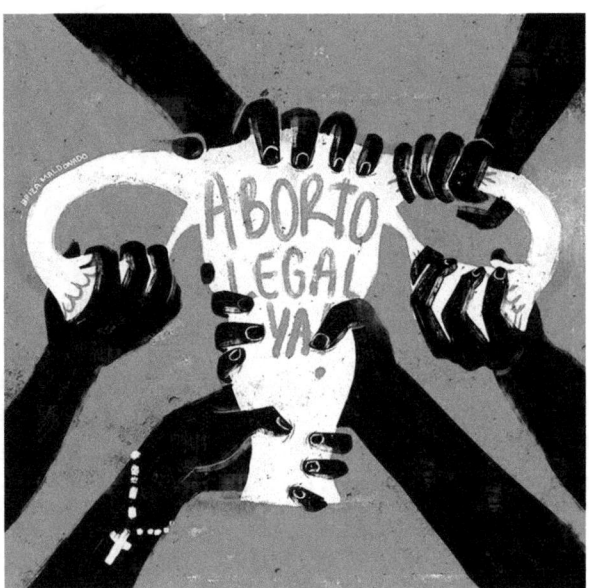

Figure 7.7 Aborto Legal Ya, Briza Maldonado, 2018. Poster for abortion rights in Argentina. Reproduced by kind permission of Briza Maldonado.[2]

A glance to today: From the mother against the woman to the commercialisation of motherhood

We are currently witnessing a dislocation of concepts around, on the one hand, the essentialism of care and, on the other, the banalisation of traditional motherhood through the merchandising of genetic inheritance.

Elisabeth Badinter in her book *The Conflict: How Modern Motherhood Undermines the Status of Women* (2012), highlights how in recent years more social mandates have emerged confining women again to the role of caring through the use of biological naturalisation arguments. Badinter explores how women find themselves subject to the 'conflict': trying to live up to the standards of a culture of 'overzealous motherhood' that can require obsessive levels of immersion and self-sacrifice, while simultaneously preserving their own 'personal pursuits' – their careers, sex lives and their identity as independent adult women. The domination of modern maternal culture by naturalist/essentialist ideology can generate extreme guilt in those who do not, or cannot, live up to its high standards: the guilt of feeling like a bad or unnatural mother.

At the same time, the irruption of surrogacy has revealed the contradiction of neo-liberal society on property, on the one hand, and the symbolic construction of maternity towards women, on the other. If the latter was linked to the body and the carnal, moralising women as life-givers, capitalist subrogation tries to deny the equation, emphasising genetic property over the corporal, splitting biology to schizoid terms. Elizabeth Kane, the first commercial surrogate in the US, now active in the National Coalition Against Surrogacy, wrote: 'A woman (surrogate mother) feels like a meat-coated test tube throughout the experience. As the fetus grows, the woman is depersonalized, becomes fragmented, losing her integrity as a person – she becomes a mere vehicle for feeding babies!' (in Allis 1997, pp. 21–22).

As Kajsa Ekis Ekman states (2014a, paragraph 5):

> surrogacy is emerging as a new form of women's oppression which has more in common with prostitution than one might think. While the sex industry commodifies women's sexuality, surrogacy commodifies women's reproduction. [...] surrogate motherhood is nothing more that the transference of pain from one woman to another. One woman is in anguish because she cannot become a mother, and another woman may suffer for the rest of her life because she cannot know the child she bore for someone else. Surrogacy also turns children into commodities and is, effectively, baby trade.

As Balza Múgica (2018) notes, the insistence on limiting the maternity and paternity of the baby born by this reproductive technique only to those who provide the genetic material – ovules and spermatozoids – means that the one who conceives and gives birth to the baby is discarded as a mother. This, in contrast to the Judeo-Christian tradition, results in a process of abstraction that divides the subject into a duality: subject/object, anima/body/flesh or person/non-person. Thus, women are valued for their productive material body, as mere work machines, rather than for their subjective spirit or soul. In this process of reification of pregnant mothers, 'a part of the I becomes "another thing" that belongs to "another person"' (Ekman 2014b, p. 191).

Some reflections

Throughout this chapter we have seen how the different constructions of motherhood have been linked to the representation of femininity and the social engendered mandates – economic and political – that this entailed. All of them are the result not of biology, but of culture. Supported by certain alibis of biology, culture has naturalised the union of the child with the mother's body, in the same way that it now disconnects it to support surrogacy. This fluctuation in the connection and disconnection of the mother's body with the child exemplifies more than ever the cultural construction of motherhood and femininity.

Through different theological, social and biological chicanery, society has made women bear the burden of immanence and care; removing them from the legal and political custody of their offspring but commanding them to the responsibility of their lives and survival.

We may no longer be able to turn those women who die in childbirth into Mexican goddesses while neo-liberal biopolitics strip pregnant women of their value, disassociating them from their connection with the life they have within. Consider the Aristotelian and Cartesian distinction of matter and shape – *res cogitans* and *res extensa* – giving supremacy to shape over matter and considering matter to be shapeless and formless – always lacking something. Capitalist biopolitics takes up again this concept – with *res extensa*/mother/matter/feminine on the one side, and *res cogitans*/form/masculine on the other – to dispossess women's body of logos and spirit, now justified in genetic rights. Through the open mouth of the dead women in a surrogate birth there is no spirit that escapes because new laws have taken that away from them.

The woman's body, the battleground, has been and continues to be the object of normativisation, prescription and proscription. The history of its representation is the history of its confinement. It is time for artists to claim, point out, denounce and transform women's desire through sharing personal experiences about their own bodies and maternity.

When working in therapeutic settings, social stereotypes and mandates around motherhood, around what society considers a 'good mother', must be present. When decoding art history and media images of motherhood and care, developing a critical eye is part of the process of deciphering the guilt that women have for being born in a sexual body. Art promotes social behaviour but at the same time, because of the inherent freedom it entails, it has the possibility of transgressing it. Art has the power, then and now, to turn the personal into the political and the intimate into social consciousness.

Notes

1 Käthe Kollwitz. Poster against Paragraph 218, 1923. Crayon lithograph (transfer of a drawing on transparent paper), Kn 198 II. See https://blogs.getty.edu/iris/haunting-images-by-master-printmaker-kathe-kollwitz-evoke-the-plight-of-working-class-women/.
2 www.bacanika.com/articulo/aborto-legal.html.

References

Allis, T. 1997. The Moral Implications of Motherhood by Hire. *Indian Journal of Medical Ethics*, 5(1): 21–22.

Amorós, C. 2004. *Salomón no era sabio*. Madrid: Fundamentos.

Aston, E. 2000. Transforming Women's Lives: Bobby Baker's Performances of 'Daily Life. *New Theatre Quarterly*, 16: 1725.

Badinter, E. 2012. *The Conflict: How Modern Motherhood Undermines the Status of Women*. New York: Metropolitan Books/Henry Holt & Company.

Balza Múgica, I. 2018 "Una biopolítica feminista de la carne: la gestación subrogada como ejemplo de los vínculos de opresión entre las mujeres y los animales no humanos". *Asparkía*, 33; 27–44 - ISSN: 1132-8231 - DOI: http://dx.doi.org/10.6035/Asparkia.2018.33.2.

Bruzelius, M. 1999. Mother's Pain, Mother's Voice: Gabriela Mistral, Julia Kristeva, and the Mater Dolorosa. *Tulsa Studies in Women's Literature*, 18(2): 220–221.

Burguiere, A. et al. 1988. *Historia de la familia*, vol. 2. Madrid: Alianza.

Caro Baroja, J. 1978. *Las formas complejas de la vida religiosa. Religión, sociedad y carácter en la España de los siglos XVI y XVII*. Madrid: Akal.

Darrieussecq, M. 2019. *Paula Moderhson-Becker: la primera mujer que se autorretrató desnuda*. Available at www.elperiodico.com/es/port/arte/20190715/paula-moderhson-becker-primer-autorretrato-mujer-desnuda (accessed April 2020).

Ekman, K. E. 2014a. Stop Surrogacy Before it is Too Late. Available at: https://medium.com/@IdeasattheHouse/stop-surrogacy-before-it-is-too-late-9910035a63f0 (accessed December 2019).

Ekman, K. E. 2014b. *El ser y la mercancía: prostitución, vientres de alquiler y disociación*. La Habana: Editorial Cenesex.

Fernández Valencia, A. 1997. *Pintura y protagonismo femenino e historia de las mujeres*. In *Arte. Individuo y Sociedad*, no. 9. Madrid: Servicio de Publicaciones. Universidad Complutense, pp. 129–157.

Fernández Vargas, V., & López Cordón, M. 1986. Mujer y régimen jurídico en el Antiguo Régimen: Una realidad disociada. In *ACTAS de las IV Jornadas sobre investigación interdisciplinaria. Ordenamiento jurídico y realidad social de las mujeres*, XVI–XX. Madrid: UAM.

Friedman, B. 1963. *The Feminine Mystique*. New York: W. W. Norton.

Gavron, H. 1966. *The Captive Wife: Conflicts of Housebound Mothers*. London: Routledge; revised edition, 1983.

Heilbrun, C. 1988 *Writing a Woman's Life*. New York: Norton.

Hervás Hermida, L. 2016. Anexo al dossier: las imágenes de las artistas y su maternidades. *Arteterapia*, 24: 209–220.

Illick, J. E. 1982. La crianza de los niños en Inglaterra y América del Norte en el siglo XVII. In L. L. Mause (ed.), *Historia de la infancia*. Madrid: Alianza.

King, M. 1993. *Mujeres renacentistas. La búsqueda de un espacio*. Madrid: Alianza.

Kollwitz, K. 1984. *Bekenntnisse*. Leipzig: Philipp Reclam Verlag.

Kristeva, J. 1985. Stabat Mater. In T. Moi (ed.) & L. S. Roudiez (trans.), *The Kristeva Reader*. Oxford: Basil Blackwell.

Mitchell, W. J. T. 1991. An Interview with Barbara Kruger. *Critical Inquiry*, 17: 434–448.

Nicholson, H. B., & Keber, K. Q. (1983) *Art of Aztec Mexico: Treasures of Tenochtitlan*. Washington, DC: National Gallery of Art.

O'Reilly, A. 2004. *From Motherhood to Mothering*. New York: State University of New York Press.

Palmer, S. 1984. La higiene y la medicina de la mujer española a través de los libros (s. XVI a XIX). In *ACTAS de las II Jornadas de investigación interdisciplinaria. Las mujer en la Historia de España*, XVI–XX. Madrid: UAM.

Pujal, M. 2002. Estudio de caso: el feminism. In M. Domemech and M. Pujal (eds.), *Psicología de los grupos y de los movimientos sociales*. Barcelona: UOC.

Rich, A. 1976. *Of Woman Born: Motherhood as Experience and Institution*. London: Virago.

Rodríguez Salas, G. 2004. Beyond Biological Maternity: Katherine Mansfield's Autobiographical Experience. *Feminismo/s*, 4: 97–108.

Roulin, J. M. 2001. Mothers in Revolution: Political Representations of Maternity in Nineteenth-Century France. *Yale French Studies*, 101: 182–200.

Tubert, S. 1996. *Figuras de la madre*. Madrid: Cátedra.

Tubert, S. 1997. *Figuras del padre*. Madrid: Cátedra.

8 Recovery stories

Transitional identities and the ambivalence of the maternal experience

Jane Hardstaff

Story: an account of past events in someone's life or in the developing of something; from Anglo-French *estoire*, from Latin *historia*, borrowed from Greek, meaning: investigation, inquiry, research, account, description, writing of history, recorded knowledge of past events.

(Anon, 2019)

How do we tell the story of who we are, even to ourselves? There are as many ways to tell a story as there are ways to interpret one. Self-narratives shift over time; perspectives and perceptions change. Storylines repeat as we circle back to significant themes, traumas or events, sifting for truths, for meaning, resolution and recovery.

This chapter weaves together two stories of recovery – one describes my experience of post-natal depression and recovery via the study of women artists and feminist art theories. The second references my work as an artist in an NHS perinatal unit, supporting the recovery of mothers experiencing mental health problems. What links them is the theme of identity, and how visual arts can influence this.

In September 1994 I was a full-time counsellor/psychotherapist, working with women survivors of sexual assault. I loved my work, it was challenging but rewarding. I was eight months pregnant, looking forward to my first child, planning to return to work after maternity leave.

In October I gave birth to a beautiful baby girl. By the following spring I knew I wouldn't be returning to work. Not then. Maybe not ever. Friends, family and colleagues were shocked – I had been so committed and passionate about my work. And what would we live on? I spoke about wanting to spend time with my daughter, of precious early years, first steps, first words. All of this was true.

What was also true was an inner terror, a sense of being utterly and completely lost, of being so far away from a clear and stable sense of 'self' that practising therapeutic work was ethically and personally impossible.

I was terrified that my daughter would be taken away from me if I revealed this deep, shameful inadequacy: I just didn't know how to be a mother.

In fact, I no longer knew how to be myself.

Over several years and many hours of therapy, I gradually began to recover, to reconstruct myself. I reconnected with my creativity and that of other women artists exploring ideas of 'the feminine', 'the maternal', and with feminist art theory. I sought out women's writing about maternal experience. I still felt alone in my maternal adequacies, but was relieved to read Rachel Cusk's assertion that, 'Birth is not merely what divides women from men, it also divides women from themselves, so that a woman's understanding of what it is to exist is profoundly changed' (Cusk 2001, p. 6).

For three years after the birth of my child I lived in a blur of what I now recognise as post-natal depression. I loved my baby, I loved being with her, but … I was lost. Why wasn't I the sparky, creative mum I thought I'd be? I was sick with guilt, with shame, a terrible example to my daughter. The world was full of women being great mothers – why wasn't I one of them? Was anyone else struggling?

Struggling to be what I thought a good mum should be, struggling to reconstruct any semblance of self-identity beyond that, I kept thinking about art. Something I'd given up years ago. Me, an artist? I could barely make a sandwich, never mind make art.

At school, I'd been the 'kid who could draw', destined for art college. But when I started an art foundation course, I lost any confidence I ever had, any sense of being an artist, or having any place in that world. What went wrong? A myriad of things, most unacknowledged, some of which I brought to the situation (unresolved childhood trauma, disrupted parental relationships), some undeniably situational. The course tutors were mostly men, either lecherously flirty or patronisingly bored. No women artists were ever referred to. The other students seemed so confident; when I visited them at home I was daunted by their big houses and professional parents – university tutors, designers, television producers. Someone's mum was actually an artist. Most of the women I knew were cleaners or cooks, working in factories, kitchens, shops and if they were really clever, in offices or the library. I had been destined for university all my life – my parents did everything they could to support that, but it was as much out of their experience as it was mine.

Somehow, I managed to pass the course and got a place to do an art degree but … I started, then transferred to an academic art history course. Maybe it was safer to study other people's art than make my own. I got a decent degree, learnt a lot about history, politics and critical theory. I became a feminist, worked in a rape crisis centre, got a grant to train as a psychotherapist. Made it: middle-class profession, middle-class life.

But now that was disintegrating. If I was unfit to return to work as a therapist, what now? I saw an advert for a free computer course: I thought I should do *something*. When I registered, the admin woman noticed I didn't seem very enthusiastic, asked if was there anything I would be enthusiastic about? Well, I said, surprising myself, I used to want to do art, but I think it's too late now.

'Why don't you go and talk to Ena who runs art foundation – see what she says?' Ena offered me a place on her course without seeing any of my work

(I didn't have any) said I didn't need to come in everyday (I couldn't) – and said if I was struggling, she could help with lifts. I was terrified but even I could see that somehow, this ridiculous idea was becoming a possibility.

On my first day, I hid in the toilet, terrified. I was a 35-year-old depressed 'housewife' – although I wasn't married. I was old enough to be the mother of most of the other students. I was stupid to even think I could do this. I looked at the rucksack on my knees – classic Nike 1996, 'Just do it' logo. I took a deep breath. Better just bloody do it then.

It wasn't easy but even I could see that I had some sort of aptitude, the 'arty kid' began to re-emerge. And this time, it was different. Most of the tutors were women – with children. Within weeks of starting, I read about an artist called Susan Hiller and her work about Freud ('From the Freud Museum', 1991–6), about her grandmothers ('Sentimental Representations: In Memory of My Grandmothers'), and her pregnancy ('10 Months'). I went to see her exhibition *Wild Talents* at Ikon, Birmingham (Hiller 1997). It was like waking up from a sleep, like the world turning from black and white to colour, from transistor radio to full orchestra. Hiller's immersive, ambiguous projections filled the vast space, the soundtrack filled the entire gallery.

This was a middle-aged-woman, an artist with an international reputation, who had come to art practice late, exploring ideas about children, power, the subconscious, film ... I was aware of boundaries shifting, realigning, disintegrating. Maybe there might be some tiny place for me in this world after all.

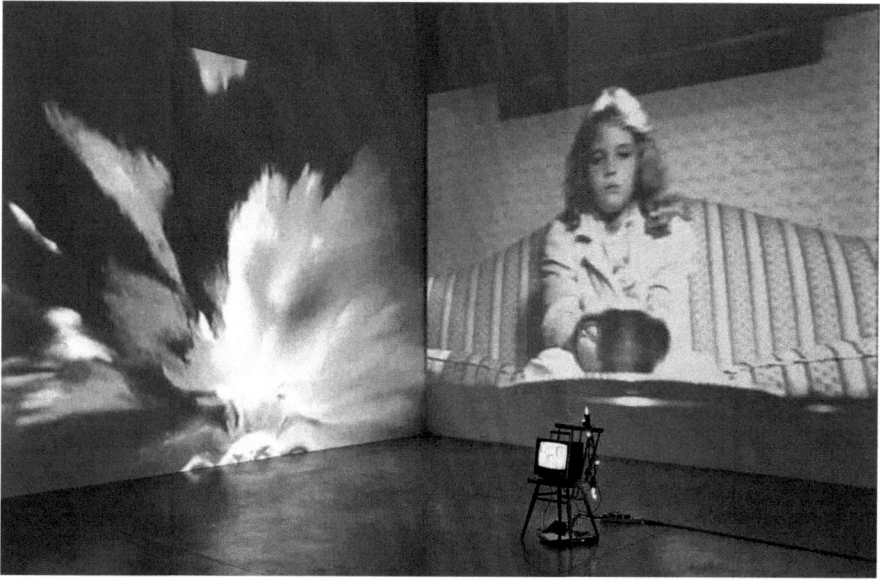

Figure 8.1 Wild Talents. Digital installation, Susan Hiller, 1997. Courtesy of the Susan Hiller Estate.

Susan Hiller led me to Mary Kelly and her groundbreaking 'Post-Partum Document', 1973–1979, a six-year exploration of the mother–child relationship. Focusing on formative moments in her son's development of language and her own sense of loss, the work moves between the voices of the mother, child and analytic observer. The installation includes Kelly's child's garments, soiled nappies, objects, texts. It brought the maternal experience, previously a private world considered of little interest or significance, into to the public domain and gave it a gravitas – the work filled a huge gallery. There was outrage at the time, with critics deriding the idea of 'dirty nappies as art' but the work is now recognised as having 'had a profound influence on the development and critique of conceptual art' (Kelly 2019).

I began to make my own work about mothers, daughters, grandmothers. I was inspired to hear an eminent female physicist say that it wasn't until she was pregnant that she could fully comprehend the wave/particle paradox – she was one/many at the same time. Interesting – motherhood bringing illumination to quantum mechanics. This became the theme of my final piece 'Superluminal Transfer'.

I was full of ideas, full of energy. I went on the college trip to London. The other students were surprised when I arrived with a three-year-old. At the Design Museum, we saw Lulu Guinness, a woman (and mother) bringing her wry humour to exquisite designs. At the Tate we saw the Turner Prize, the controversial all-women nominees of 1997: Cornelia Parker, Angela Bulloch, Christine Borland, Gillian Wearing. Apparently, the world was full of women artists.

I loved the way Cornelia Parker transforms ordinary objects – sheds, cutlery, hot water bottles, re-presenting the domestic as significant, monumental. Gillian Wearing won the prize for her 'Signs that Say What You Want Them To Say and Not Signs that Say What Someone Else Wants You To Say' (Wearing 1997). It's hard now to appreciate how shocking it was to see the image of a prosperous young city man holding a sign saying, 'I'm desperate'. Ah… I thought, not just me then.

Women artists – corporeality and the ambivalence of the maternal body

I came home inspired. Research took me to Helen Chadwick's exploration of corporeality, to Louise Bourgeois, Shirin Neshat, Cindy Sherman, Paula Rego. Women wrestling with what it means to be a woman, to be embodied within a female form that is colonised by a patriarchal society; in which arguably the most profound experience of life – birth – is conspicuously under- or misrepresented. There are endless images of women in art, but most are created by men preoccupied with women as objects of desire – all those nudes. I liked Laurie Simmons' *Underneath* series, subverting and poking sly fun at pornographic images, depicting women lifting their skirts to reveal … whole little constructed worlds (Simmons 1998).

I discovered women speaking a different 'truth' about the experience of being female, of motherhood. The 1990 US submission at the Venice biennale was

Jenny Holzer's 'Mother and Child': twelve vertical LED signs programmed with changing text, expressing conflicting and ambiguous feelings of women toward their role as mothers, and of children to their mother (Holzer 1990). 'Mother and Child' positioned the ambivalence of mothers and mothering as a bold political statement in an international arena.

Gathering momentum from the 1970s through to the 1990s, women made art about 'the feminine', about female bodies, about both the physical and internal experience of being a woman – Pipilotti Rist, playfully blurring the boundaries between internal and external, inviting the viewer to literally walk through her body in the installation 'Worry Will Vanish Horizon' (Rist 2014).

Women were not just making art; it was finally being taken seriously: the all-women Turner prize short-list of 1997 had been an acknowledgement of this. Tracey Emin's 'My Bed', Turner nominee 1999 was vilified by many critics as an 'endlessly solipsistic, self-regarding homage' (Adrian Searle cited in Cohen 2018, p. 1). Some commentators, even male ones found it to have more currency: Tate Liverpool curator Darren Pih said, 'What's interesting is that the bed is a stage for birth, depressive isolation, and death. It's a powerful symbolism found in literature and art' (cited in Cohen 2018). Emin's bed represented a specifically feminine perspective on that motif; positioned within the Turner prize at the Tate, those pillars of the canon, it 'elevates the anxieties of a woman's life to a monumental status' (Cohen 2018).

Despite the burgeoning body of work created by women in the late twentieth century, the perceived canon of art history consists almost exclusively of work by men. Feminist art historian Griselda Pollock describes art history as 'the illustrated story of man' (1999, p. 23), insisting that 'the real history of art is fundamentally and exclusively not to do with art and its histories, but with the Western masculine subject, its mythical suppressed and psychic needs' (1999, p. 29).

Man-made language

Continuing on to an MA in Fine Art, I was driven by a compulsion to understand the language of constructed art images but also the language we use to describe/define/discuss and deconstruct, moreover, the language 'we' use to define 'ourselves'. How can we understand the construction of 'the feminine' if we only have 'man-made' language to do this with: 'Language is not neutral. It is not merely a vehicle which carries ideas. It is itself a shaper of ideas' (Spender 1980, p. 183).

Through his theories of deconstruction Derrida revealed the gendering of language and cultural representation, de-universalising the masculine. Criticising the premise that language is a fundamental expression of reality, Derrida challenged the same constructs as feminism. Staying close to Freudian and Lacanian psychoanalysis he also attempts to deconstruct them, insisting that there can be no fixed signifiers: meaning is not set but shifting (Derrida 1973). Female theorists such as Irigaray, Kristeva and Cixous developed deconstructive theories further, revealing the slips, shifts and gaps between signs and their signifiers.

I became especially interested in the sign of the 'mother', which Pollock describes as 'an always sexually differentiated and always differentiating convergence of masculine and feminine interest' (1999, p. 32). She writes about mother as 'a space and a presence that structures subjectivities both masculine and feminine' but differently (1999, p. 32). In her 'Matrixial Borderspace', Bracha Lichtenberg Ettinger deconstructs psychoanalytical theory, offering a new model within which to understand the construction of self, where 'I' can be understood not in opposition to 'you', always privileging 'I', but in a shifting, constantly negotiated space (Ettinger 1993).

Pollock refers to 'the ambivalence of the maternal body' (1999, p. 24), a unique state of being where 'I' and 'we' are simultaneous, the psychic space that can hold 'male' and 'female', the lynchpin through which male and female experiences intersect and diverge. A space full of possibilities and power, a place of birth and reproduction, of creation. A space to exist as a woman, a mother and an artist. This concept informed my practice as I continued to make work about maternal experience. My final MA piece, 'Unreliable Evidence', used isolated cine-film stills to explore mother–daughter relationships; questioning the construction of identity and perceptions of memory and truth.

In 2009 I began work on a long-term project called 'Motherlines', focusing on maternal experience and its representation (Hardstaff 2019a).

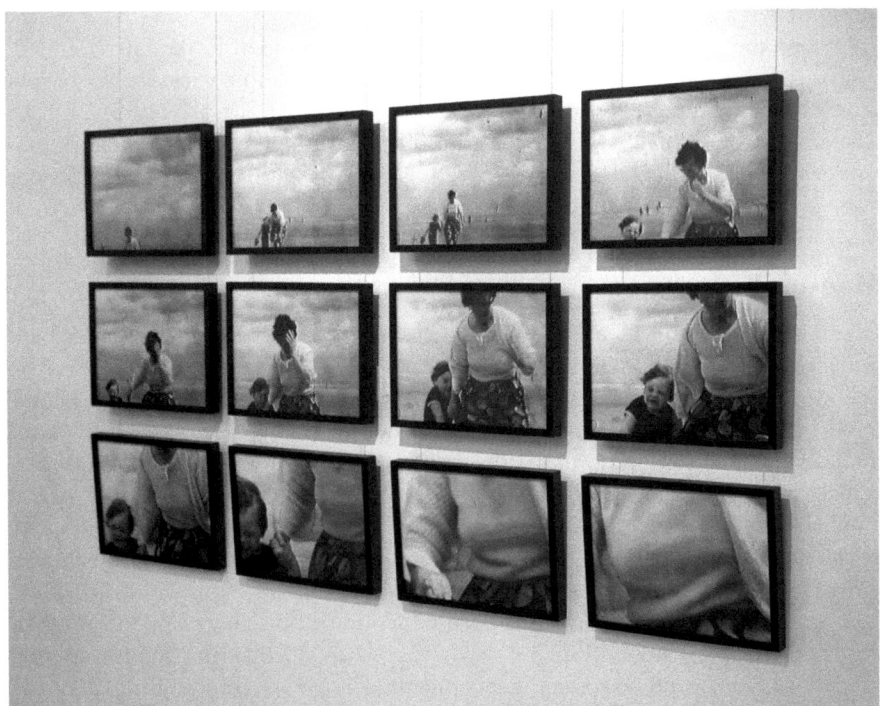

Figure 8.2 Unreliable Evidence. Digital prints, Jane Hardstaff, 2006.

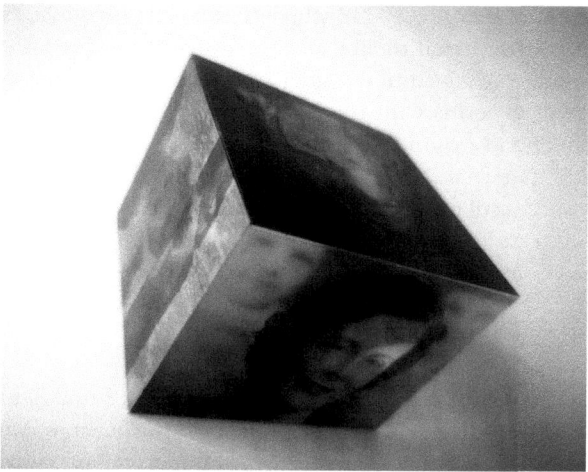

Figure 8.3 Motherlines. Self-portrait, acrylic, digital print, Jane Hardstaff, 2019.

Maternal transitions

My creative practice aims to establish a space where complex and ambivalent responses to motherhood are perceived as 'normal'. In their 2006 research, Hall and Wittkowski found that of 158 non-depressed women interviewed post-natally, all but one experienced *all* 54 negative cognitions for which they tested. 'The transition to motherhood is one of the most common life transitions experienced by women, often signifying a period of great disruption' (Nelson 2003).

Wittkowski identifies the complex process implicated in 'maternal transition' and the challenges to self-identify this can present:

1   Commitment: 'mothers are seen as giving up the concept of themselves and as "freely choosing", accepting the need for sacrifices and allowing their decisions to be formed by their new commitment to mothering' (Leonard 1993).
2   Daily life: in negotiating postpartum changes and limitations, women may use their own experience of being mothered as a guide or reject this, provoking feelings of vulnerability (Staneva & Wittkowski 2013).
3   Relationships: shifting roles within relationships with partners, friends, and family can be difficult to adjust to.
4   Work: ambivalence and anxieties can arise from decisions about work, compromising or redefining professional goals and balancing the conflicting priorities of motherhood.
5   Self: adjusting to our new identity as a mother can provoke introspection and self-evaluation. The changes we may experience within ourselves may be positive –increased patience, new understanding of love, empathy etc. – but also negative if we experience a sense of loss – of confidence, of self- esteem, of sense of self.

Becoming a mother requires us to face our past, encountering 'the ghosts in the nursery' (Fraiberg, Adelson & Shapiro 1975), which Wittkowski identifies as the major process impacting on maternal mental health. While simultaneously developing our role as a mother we need to consider our own experience of being mothered, possibly coming to terms with maternal rejection or acknowledging the reality of difficult childhood experiences.

Past experiences and maternal beliefs about motherhood/mothering orientation influence how successful our transition to motherhood will be. Those of us who struggle with that transition may need professional help to re-establish a viable identity for ourselves as mothers (Wittkowski et al. 2017).

Arts and health

When I stopped working as a therapist and returned to studying art, I couldn't have imagined that within a few years these diverging paths would re-converge into the 'arts and health' movement. Working at Derby Museums, I managed participatory arts projects, often collaborating with Derbyshire Mind and other community support organisations. In 2015 I founded Common Threads, an arts organisation which supports women living with mental health problems (Hardstaff 2019b). In 2017 I was appointed Creative Wellbeing Coordinator at Derby QUAD, an arts centre with an extensive arts and health programme. I'm currently artist-in-residence at the Beeches NHS Perinatal Unit at Derby Royal Hospital.

Creative residency at the Beeches Perinatal Unit

Inspired by QUAD's 'Listen Love Learn' programme which supports positive parenting through creative participation, the residency was developed through dialogues between QUAD and the Beeches. The project aims to:

- contribute to the recovery of residents and support improved attachment to their babies;
- provide a link between residential mental health support and the community;
- contribute to sector awareness, learning and research regarding the impact of creative participation on mental health.

Methodology

In August 2018, I began to deliver a series of 48 weekly sessions at the Beeches. Working within a person-centred psychotherapeutic framework, I set out to gently introduce creative opportunities appropriate to the vulnerability and diversity of participants. I anticipated that some residents might not be interested in creative activities or might feel they didn't have the skills or ability to participate.

Activities would need to be suitable for residents at all levels of recovery, and able to be completed in two hours. By creating an accessible, supportive and inspiring environment we hoped residents would be encouraged to participate and, as a result, feel more engaged, more connected, learn new things. Where possible, sessions would engage residents with creative opportunities beyond their stay in the unit, echoing the elements of the CHIME recovery model (Leamy et al. 2011):

Connectedness
Hope and Optimism
Identity
Meaning
Empowerment

The residency presented professional challenges: for each session, I didn't know who participants will be; how many there will be; where they will be in their recovery; how they will engage. It's difficult to build in continuity as we can't predict how long women will be resident. Flexibility and sensitivity, both in the activity and my approach has been key, responding to residents' cues, recalibrating 'success' for each individual participant.

Supporting my own wellbeing throughout this learning process has been important. In the first few weeks I experienced intense feelings of inadequacy until, with the supervisory support of a co-practitioner, I recognised the reactivated echoes of my own post-natal experience.

Supporting new mothers in recovery

The women I've worked with vary in age, socio-economic background, race, levels of recovery and wellbeing. What we all have in common is that the birth of a child has knocked us off-kilter, to a place where we lost our confidence, our self-esteem, ourselves. Most weeks I hear women saying, 'I can't do this', 'I don't know how to do this'. Themes of inadequacy, failure and fear permeate most women's stories.

I also see women beginning to recover, finding ways to be themselves *and* a mother.

One of the strengths of the Beeches is its collaborative approach and inclusive engagement of staff with residents. Shelly Brough, nurse manager, is open about her own post-natal struggles, encouraging a '#realmums' ethos. An advocate of creative intervention to support recovery, Shelley ensured that I felt welcomed into the ward and part of the staff team. I've worked closely with staff to develop the project, working collaboratively wherever possible.

The creative sessions have included simple crafts such as collage, textiles, printing, etc., often linked to the seasons, festivals and themes suggested by ward staff. Some of the most successful activities have been those with a purpose, or that enable participants to 'give' or 'share' with others.

Measuring impact

Our evaluation strategy included inviting written feedback from residents about their experience during and after sessions; formal written feedback from staff and observations by myself and staff. Some residents fed-back formally but more often evaluation was captured via spontaneous comments or observations. Some residents chose not to engage with sessions, but most have had some contact, even if only briefly, or though conversations.

Of the mothers we consulted formally:

- 100 per cent said the sessions had helped to improve their mood 'a lot';
- 100 per cent said they'd enjoyed the sessions;
- 100 per cent said what would improve the sessions was 'more'.

Based on my observations and analysis of the feedback given by residents and staff, it's possible to conclude that sessions have had a positive impact in the following ways.

Distraction/relaxation

Sessions provide calming distraction from women's anxieties and can alleviate boredom and/or focussing on negative thoughts.

> Doing this is fun and it passes the time really quickly. The days can be quite long and empty, but Wednesday afternoons fly by.
>
> (Resident feedback)

> The mums talk about the sessions as relaxing and something they can do at home when they leave.
>
> (Staff feedback)

> It helps to lift their mood, encourage motivation and enjoyment and distracts them for a short time from their worries/fears/anxieties.
>
> (Staff feedback)

Creating connections

Sessions can facilitate connections between residents, and between residents and staff. Residents who find it difficult to connect can find it easier via a shared activity: making Christmas trees from old paperbacks enabled a conversation with a dissociated resident about the books she enjoyed reading.

Sessions can also facilitate a connection with life 'beyond the ward', creating a thread to home life, or to future activities:

> I was really pleased with how my owls turned out! It's inspired me to make them at home for my son, for his sensory room. We might even be able to make them together.

I want to carry on being creative and come to your group at QUAD. I'd like to become a volunteer and do what you do.

Work by staff and residents was displayed in QUAD's *Self Portrait* exhibition project and viewed by thousands of visitors.

Expression

Sessions can offer an opportunity for women to express and articulate emotions:

> These sessions are very useful for mums who have struggled to express their emotions verbally regarding their situation through creative means. I think it has also been helpful for ladies that may have been initially sceptical to take part in crafts, to see the potential therapeutic benefit.
>
> (Staff feedback)

Self-esteem

Activities can support residents to make something of which they are proud, building self-confidence, nurturing optimism and feelings of empowerment, re-building positive self-identity.

> I've really enjoyed doing this. I like to do crafty things, but I don't ... this is good because you don't have to be able to draw or anything to do it – it's all designed for you.
>
> I've really enjoyed this – I'm not very creative but I've loved doing this, and it's turned out so well – I feel quite proud of what I've done.
>
> (Resident feedback)

> It's good to learn a new thing. Thank you.
>
> (Resident feedback)

Pride/raised aspiration

Creating work and displaying it at 'gallery' standard has had a positive impact: the ward is more visually interesting, participants feel proud of their work, new residents are inspired.

> The artworks produced and presented on our walls are beautiful – inspirational to other mums and a great talking point.
>
> (Staff feedback)

Inspiration

Sessions can motivate residents to be creative, to have more agency.

> I wasn't here for the session to make the woodland creatures, but I love them

so much, I took them off the wall to work out how they've been done, and I've made my own versions for ****'s room at home. It's really inspired me to be more creative.

Collaboration

Projects in which residents and staff worked collaboratively have been particularly successful, supporting the 'mutual recovery' model (Crawford 2018), providing ways of breaking down social barriers and helping to rebuild identities.

We worked together on a decorated Christmas ward and a sensory room 'woodland scene' collage over several months. Both projects won awards, which boosted the morale of the whole ward. The sensory room project was awarded a 'Special Commendation' in the annual national Care Coordination Association Art & Photographic Competition:

> The Woodland Scene is a brilliant collaboration. You told your own stories which together make this hopeful and cheerful image. I loved the theme of the mother and baby owl – the baby owls are ready to start their journey, with the mother owls protecting and helping them all the way.
>
> (Naomi Tipping, Judge)

Helping others

Many residents are motivated to support the recovery of other mothers. Over a period of months, I worked with mums to collect text and images for a *Welcome to the Beeches* booklet for new residents. Residents nearing discharge took part in the 'Motherlines' project, creating clay 'Birthmarks' and sharing their stories of childbirth and motherhood.

Identity

Sessions can support residents as they redefine their identity:

> Doing creative activities with you is the one time – the only time – I ever feel I am really doing something that's just for me, when I can switch off and have a break from being a mum. Even though I'm creating something for my children, or about my children it's time to just be me, and I really need that.
>
> (Resident feedback)

> My stay in the hospital had its good and bad points, but I really enjoyed the art sessions. It helped me to feel more positive about myself, about my relationships with my children and my future. It really helped to find my creative side again, thank you.
>
> (Resident feedback)

Supporting staff

Sessions support staff, bringing new ideas and inspiration to the ward. Staff are encouraged to participate in sessions when possible, with positive results:

> You give us ideas about creative things to do here and with our own children!

> I can't believe how relaxing this is!

> You always bring new ideas.

Staff feedback

In formal, anonymous staff feedback:

- 100 per cent identified 'a lot' of positive impact on residents;
- 100 per cent identified 'a lot' of positive impact on the Beeches Unit in general;
- Nine out of ten identified 'a lot' of positive impact on patient recovery;
- One out of ten identified 'some' positive impact on patient recovery.

Staff commented on the therapeutic benefits from the sessions:

> I believe craft activities have had a very positive effect on recovery. Jane has role-modelled how we can reflect and express our emotions through creative processes, whilst demonstrating the therapeutic value this may provide for ladies and their babies.

> The sessions are an outlet for emotions/creativity and can lead to therapeutic discussions.

> Jane listens to the patients' thoughts, ideas, she puts patients at the centre of the session and makes them feel valued. Several of the patients have commented on this.

Nurse manager Shelly Brough said: 'There has been a definite impact on the residents and staff from the project and we'd love to extend its duration.' Since then, Shelly has been able to secure funding to extend the project for a further year.

Working with photography

Although more than 90 per cent of residents took part in creative sessions, craft activities are not for everyone. As a way to engage with mums who expressed a lack of interest, I brought in a camera. Residents didn't want to use the camera themselves but were enthusiastic about me taking photographs of their babies. They didn't want to be photographed themselves but as the session went on and they saw the images, that changed. Together, we captured beautiful moments of intimacy between the mothers and their babies which represent the tenderness and bond the women may have been struggling to feel. A pregnant resident commented that:

> Doing this has made me feel more positive about the baby coming.

The photographs possibly showed the mums an image of themselves as they wanted to be, but felt they weren't:

> They have captured such a special time. I love them.

They also constitute a positive memento to take home, tangible proof that even during an episode of mental illness, mothers have special moments with their babies that they want to remember. Women reported displaying the photographs on their walls when they got home, and most gave permission to share their images.

> I love these! I have never liked any photograph of me before but I'm showing these to everyone. Thank you.

'Seeing is believing'

Around the same time that Winnicott published his 'good enough mother' theory of attachment, (Winnicott 1973, p. 173), Berger's *Ways of Seeing* first articulated the complex relationships between visual imagery and societal ideologies: 'A woman must continually watch herself. She is almost continually accompanied by her own image of herself ... This determines not only most relations between men and women but also the relation of women to themselves' (Berger 1972, pp. 46–47).

The Beeches has recently introduced Video Interactive Guidance (VIG) as a tool to support recovery. VIG has proved useful when working with women who have experienced a period of mental illness, when the bond between mother and baby had been ruptured and/or the mother feels she has a poor relationship with her child, questioning her ability to be 'a good mother'.

In the VIG process, the practitioner videos three or four minutes of mother–child interaction, selecting just a few seconds on which to focus, noting significant actions and responses from both mother and infant. The practitioner and mother then review the clips together, reflecting on areas where the interaction was 'attuned': 'a moment or sequence of connection where the parent has left space for and then received the child's initiative in a sensitive or joyful way' (Kennedy 2019). This process is repeated three or four times.

VIG can help mothers to recognise the signs and signals that pass between a mother and a child, enabling them to see instances of positive interaction. This can be a powerful way of countering the mother's belief that they 'can't do this' by presenting irrefutable evidence. It can be a significant moment in her recovery when a mother realises, she is 'doing it right'.

> Watching the footage back: that was just, I mean, that was huge for me [...] actually being able to see myself, like, almost step out of myself and see myself, and see my interaction – it really helps me understand and digest what was happening.
>
> (Kennedy & Underdown 2019)

The Beeches practitioner reported one mother saying that the VIG review had been the pivotal turning point in her recovery.

Shifting stories

The Beeches supports women to construct new self-narratives within which to find acceptance of themselves as mothers. This can be by bringing attention to and valuing positive achievements and attributes, but also supporting women to be less critical of their difficulties, understanding that they do not necessarily define them as 'failing' or 'bad mothers', but rather as ordinary women, having normal responses to a challenging experience.

On what are we basing our ideas/ideals of motherhood? We are exposed, consciously and unconsciously, to a million personal, societal and cultural references. Rosemary Betterton's research explores how visual art practices might offer the means of reconfiguring the maternal (Betterton 2002). But do cultural representations shape our expectations, define experiences and influence the way we construct our own identities? We are currently flooded with images of 'super-mums' – Beyoncé, Madonna, Victoria Beckham – who display no conflict, no ambivalence about maintaining their perfect woman/ perfect mother image.

In contrast, the *BirthRites Collection* brings together a collection of challenging contemporary images of birth and motherhood which represent diverse and ambivalent experiences and perspectives. Similarly, *Studies in the Maternal* online journal has created an international forum for contemporary critical debate about the maternal experience.

Through raw, honest texts, writers like Caitlin Moran (2012), Maggie Nelson (2015) and Roxanne Gay (2017) reveal ambivalence, vulnerability and inadequacies about their experience as women while maintaining their authoritative voice. *Fleabag* (Waller-Bridge 2016–2019) and *Motherland* (Horgan & Linehan 2016–2019) present transgressive representations of the female/maternal experience. In 2019 *The Testaments* (Atwood 2019) co-won the Booker Prize with *Girl Woman Other* (Evaristo 2019). Dialogues about maternal experience have never been so diverse or numerous.

Stories of motherhood are shifting. In multiple registers, both publicly and privately, women continue to create more nuanced, self-defined narratives, more self-defining spaces for our lived experiences.

Acknowledgement

Thanks to the residents and staff at the Beeches Perinatal Unit, Derby Royal Hospital.

References

Anon. 2019. *Oxford English Dictionary*. Available at: www.lexico.com/en/definition/story (accessed September 2019).

Atwood, M. 2019. *The Testaments*. New York: Vintage Publishing.

Berger, J. 1973. *Ways of Seeing*. London: Penguin Books.

Betterton, R. 2002. Prima Gravida: Reconfiguring the Maternal Body in Representation. *Feminist Theory*, 3(3): 255–270.

Crawford, P. 2018. Creative Practice – Mutual Recovery. Available at: www.mentalhealth. org.uk/news/creative-practice-mutual-recovery-connecting-communities-mental-health-and-wellbeing (accessed November 2019).

Cusk, R. 2001. *A Life's Work*. New York: Faber and Faber.

Cohen, A. 2018. Tracey Emin's 'My Bed' Ignored Society's Expectations of Women. Available at: www.artsy.net/article/artsy-editorial-tracey-emins-my-bed-ignored-societys-expectations-women (accessed August 2019).

Derrida, J. 1973, *Speech and Phenomena: And Other Essays on Husserl's Theory of Signs, trans. David B. Allinson*. Evanston: Northwestern University Press.

Ettinger, B. L. 1993. *Matrix – Borderlines*. Oxfordshire: Museum of Modern Art.

Evaristo, B. 2019. *Girl, Woman, Other*. London: Hamish Hamilton.

Fraiberg, S., Adelson, E., & Shapiro, V. 1975. Ghosts in the Nursery: A Psychoanalytic Approach to the Problems of Impaired Infant–Mother Relationships. *Journal of the American Academy of Child Psychiatry*, 14(3): 387–421.

Gay, R. 2017. *Hunger: A Memoir of a Body*. New York: HarperCollins.

Hall, P., & Wittkowski, A. 2006. An Exploration of Negative Thoughts as a Normal Phenomenon after Childbirth. *Journal of Midwifery and Mental Health*, 51(5): 321–330.

Hardstaff, J. 2019a. Motherlines. Available at: https://cargocollective.com/jane-hardstaff (accessed November 2019).

Hardstaff, J. 2019b. Common Threads. Available at: www.common-threads.org (accessed November 2019).

Hardstaff, J. 2019c. Listen Love Learn. Available at: www.derbyquad.co.uk/whats-on/get-creative-families-and-young-people/listen-love-learn (accessed November 2019).

Hiller. S. 1997. Wild Talents. Available at: www.susanhiller.org/home.html (accessed November 2019).

Horgan, S., & Linehan, G. 2016–2019. *Motherland*. BBC. Available at: www.bbc.co.uk/iplayer/episodes/p05j1jkp/motherland (accessed November 2019).

Holzer, J. 1990. Mother and Child. Available at: https://projects.jennyholzer.com/LEDs/venice-1990/gallery#3 (accessed November 2019).

Kelly, M. 2019. Post-Partum Document. Available at: www.marykellyartist.com/post_partum_document.html (accessed November 2019).

Kennedy, H. 2019. VIG in a Nutshell. Available at: https://maternalmentalhealthalliance. org/video-interaction-guidance-in-a-nutshell/ (accessed November 2019).

Kennedy, H., & Underdown, A. 2019. Video Interaction Guidance: Promoting Secure Attachment and Optimal Development for Children, Parents and Professionals. Available at https://vigknowledge.wikispaces.com (accessed August 2019).

Leamy, M., Bird, V., Le Boutillier, C., Williams, J., & Slade, M. 2011. The CHIME Framework for Personal Recovery. Available at www.therecoveryplace.co.uk/chime-framework/ (accessed November 2019).

Leonard, V. W. 1993. *Stress and Coping in the Transition to Parenthood of First-time Mothers with Career Commitments: An Interpretive Study*. San Francisco: University of California.

Moran, C. 2012. *How to Be a Woman*. London: Ebury Press.

Nelson, A. M. 2003. Transition to Motherhood. *Journal of Obstetric, Gynaecologic, & Neonatal Nursing*, 32(4): 465–477.

Nelson, M. 2015. *The Argonauts*. New York: Graywolf Press.

Pollock, G. 1999. *Differencing the Canon: Feminist Desire and the Writing of Art's Histories*. London and New York: Routledge.

Rist, P. 2014. Worry Will Vanish Horizon. Available at www.hauserwirth.com/hauser-wirth-exhibitions/5154-pipilotti-rist-worry-will-vanish?modal=media-player&mediaType=artwork&mediaId=15805 (accessed November 2019).

Simmons, L. 1998. Underneath Photographic Series. Available at www.lauriesimmons. net/photographs/underneath (accessed November 2019).

Spender, D. 1980. *Man Made Language – Language and Reality*. London and New York: Routledge.

Staneva, A., & Wittkowski, A. 2013. Exploring Beliefs and Expectations about Motherhood in Bulgarian Mothers: A Qualitative Study. *Midwifery*, 29(3): 260–267.

Waller-Bridge, P. 2016–2019. *Fleabag*. BBC. Available at www.bbc.co.uk/programmes/ p040tlqx (accessed November 2019).

Wearing, G. 1997. I'm Desperate. Available at: www.tate.org.uk/art/artworks/wearing-im-desperate-p78348 (accessed November 2019).

Winnicott, D. W. 1973. *The Child, the Family, and the Outside World*. London: Penguin.

Wittkowski, A., Garrett, C., Cooper, A., & Wieck, A. 2017. The Relationship between Postpartum Depression and Beliefs about Motherhood and Perfectionism during Pregnancy. *Journal of Woman's Reproductive Health*, 1(4).

9   Where can we make our home?

In-utero images and thinking in the running of a small therapeutic group for mothers and their young children affected by domestic abuse

Heather Tuffery

Five little ducks went swimming one day, over the hill and far away … Sad Mother duck said, 'Quack, quack, quack' and no little ducks came swimming back.

The Multi Cultural Family Base (Early Years Project) in Scotland works with parents and children aged three and under, from black, Asian and minority ethnic communities. This project includes group work and individual support for mothers and children who have experienced domestic abuse. We consider domestic abuse to be a form of gender-based abuse perpetrated by partners, ex-partners and/or family members, which can include physical abuse, sexual abuse, emotional abuse, financial abuse and coercive control. It may include forced marriages, female genital mutilation or so-called 'honour-based' abuse. Research and theory both highlight the impact of domestic abuse on individuals, including infants and unborn children, the adverse effect on parenting abilities and its implications for attachment and relationships, which can be undermined or significantly damaged.

The group

This chapter explores the work of an early years group for black, Asian and minority ethnic (BAME) women and their infants and toddlers, who have experienced domestic abuse.

The group is described as a 'Being and Playing Together Group' for women who have experience of difficult and painful relationships. In this work we consider domestic abuse to be perpetrated by partners or ex-partners and/or within the women's wider family. This can include physical, sexual, and psychological abuse. In setting up this group, we were challenged in our understanding of domestic abuse perpetrators, extending our understanding of this to include other family members (Mirza 2017). Research, with particular attention to South Asian women's experience, has supported our understanding of the perpetrator: proposing the wider family as a potential source of abuse with particular reference to affinal kin relationships (e.g., non-biological kin affiliations through marriages). Co-facilitated by myself, an Art Therapist, and Isabelle Mercadante, a social worker – both of us white women, British and French Canadian respectively – the group runs in eight-week blocks, with families able to attend continuing blocks across an academic year. The group encourages parents to think about what their infants are communicating and explores ways of re-sponding or showing curiosity. We think about ways of being together, con-taining parents' experiences and promoting sensitive responsiveness from the parent, with a view to strengthening the parent-child relationship. *Weaving the Cradle: Facilitating Groups to Promote Attunement and Bonding between Parents, Their Babies and Toddlers* (Celebi 2017) offers a comprehensive overview of Early Years groups, and it is within this cradle that we place our Being and Playing Together Group. Art making, including play, sand trays and singing, are central to the running of the group.

An introduction

This chapter looks at Rahma, her partner Yusuf and the child she was able to bring with her called Ahmad, and their time in the group. At our first meeting Rahma was in the second trimester of pregnancy and Ahmad was two years old. The family had recently arrived in the country, having been smuggled out of their home country. The family had been held captive upon arrival in the UK and had then been abandoned without any resources. In addition to the cir-cumstances of their journey and their initial weeks in the UK, Rahma and Ahmad had experienced significant physical and psychological abuse in their home country, with Rahma having to leave for her own safety, leaving behind her young daughter, Zaynab, with a family member. In our initial meeting with the family, grief and distress were clearly expressed for 'little sister' (age two) and her presence by her absence was at the forefront of everyone's thinking.

I reflect on the ways in which Rahma and Ahmad were able to use the group, with emphasis on the growing presence of Rahma's pregnancy. What space could be provided and held within the group by other families, the co-facilitators, the wider agency and linked organisations, for the expected birth of a new baby? Central to this were artworks made by Rahma and Ahmad that appear to de-scribe in-utero images. These paintings were made in relative quiet, with workers feeling highly protective. A family of salt dough ducks accompanied by singing were also central to this work.

Initial meeting

In our initial meetings with a family, the link is made between the experience of being a mother and the woman's own childhood. 'Ghosts in the nursery' (Fraiberg, Adelson & Sharoro 1975) often appear or are made reference to in this meeting. As is routine for the group, our initial meeting with the family took place in their home. Rahma welcomed us in to their temporary accommodation. We reflected on the family's experience of now living somewhere very different from the home they had left behind – the change in and loss of a known landscape, voiced and felt, as we all looked out of the window onto their new view. Papadopoulos writes on the experience of refugees, 'Homelessness is a state that not only encompasses physical and material dimensions but it contains psychological and existential characteristics, as well' (2002, p. 25). Rahma was distressed, crying as she described the pain of leaving her young daughter behind, naming this separation as the thing she was most upset about. Ahmad was watchful during this time, resting on the wall. Once Rahma stopped crying, Ahmad became distressed himself. He wailed with tears, moving between rooms, before settling with Rahma. We left the visit upset, and wanting to offer something for the family within their participation in the group. We were left wondering about Rahma's current experience of pregnancy, with little about Rahma's pregnancy acknowledged or shared in this meeting. Rahma confirmed that she would like to join the group and it was arranged that we could offer a taxi to support their attendance.

Claiming the baby

Salomonsson describes the process of *maternal-foetal attachment*, in which the pregnant woman's relationship to her growing foetus is understood (2018, p. 24). We understood that Rahma wanted to be pregnant, although the pregnancy was complicated by her relationship to the father, and the impact of the pregnancy on her, and her family life. We were also unsure of, and explored the differing cultural understanding of claiming a pregnancy and baby. We heard, anecdotally, of the ways in which a pregnancy could be marked – celebrations like the Indian tradition of Seemantham in which the mother's family marks the pregnancy at the fifth, seventh and ninth month, blessing the mother and supporting the safe delivery of a healthy baby. This put us in mind of the US idea of 'baby showers' in which gifts are 'showered' upon the new mother by friends and family. The connecting relationship in these rituals is 'the claiming of the baby' within a pregnant woman's family and wider community.

Colleagues told us that for Rahma the father's family would traditionally lay claim to the pregnancy. The pregnancy and children are understood as the father's possession. We thought about the alternative ways in which Rahma may lay claim to the pregnancy, her experience of being pregnant at this point in her life. This chapter offers ways in which this was held within the group.

Past, present and future

Eleftheriadou argues the need to see the person as a whole, 'Past, present, and future are all there, intertwined, and need to be explored sensitively. Being a refugee is part of the experience, but there are also many other components' (2010, p. 178). We thought about Rahma's experience of holding her position of mother to three children. This was her relationship to Ahmad, visible and thought about within the group, her relationship to her daughter whom she was separated from, and the growing relationship to her unborn child. The recent past, present and future of Rahma's life was held in the chronology of her children, in the holding of the group, and our wider agency and connected agencies.

Starting the group

The group was made up of four families, one of the four families not attending any of the eight-week group.

Week 1: salt dough

Ahmad is upset at the closing of the door to mark the beginning of the group, with a strong wish to leave the room. Another child, Ewa, joins Ahmad in the protest and we think about the wish or ambivalence from both adults and children in starting the group. Ahmad rejects the singing of his name in the welcome song – 'no, no, no'. Rahma offers reassurance, talking of going to school later, holding and stroking him. Rahma presents as responsive but her mood changes very little throughout the group, with a similar response to distress as to enjoyment. Rahma doesn't offer any introduction or acknowledgement of her pregnancy. We initiate the singing of the welcome song to 'the baby' focusing our attention on Rahma. Rahma sits down closely next to me, our legs touching. We stay like this while the salt-dough is made, Ahmad and Rahma work together and apart, with Rahma quick to mix the salt-dough to the right consistency. This continues with Rahma and Ahmad quick to form the dough into a family of birds, a snake, and a pestle and mortar (Figure 9.1). Ahmad squeezes the dough in his hand 'It's a crocodile!' He is quick to bring meaning to the dough. Rahma makes the birds for Ahmad at his request, while also making the pestle and mortar for her. Ahmad is joyful in his exploration of the dough, kneading and stretching it in his hands. Other women share their understanding of the pestle and mortar, their own name for the utensil, and the spices they would crush. Rahma and Ahmad go to wash their hands together, and Ahmad is upset on his return that their artwork has been moved on to the table for safety. He asks that his moulded dough is added to the collection. As the group ends Ahmad is very upset. Rahma says that he is like this every time they have to leave somewhere.

Reflecting after the group, we were concerned that addressing Rahma's pregnancy in the welcome song was the wrong thing to do, despite both workers intuitively wanting to acknowledge her pregnancy. We later read that it may be bad luck to talk of an unborn baby, and felt incompetent and clumsy in our intervention. We were unable to tell how Rahma felt about it, and neither of us felt able to ask her within the group time.

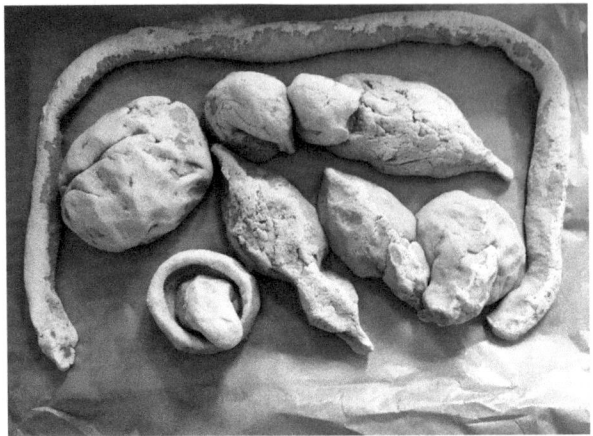

Figure 9.1 Salt dough work by Ahmad and Rahma.

Despite the difference in therapeutic setting, Raphael-Leff, professor of psychoanalysis, describes something of our feelings at this time:

> the analyst is unwittingly drawn into the powerful pull of the psychic reality dramatized within the growing belly, or evident in interaction between mother and baby. She may be thrust into the a situation of feeling contradictory responsibilities towards two clients – expectant mother and foetus – or caught between divided loyalties to two babies, teasing out confusion between her patient's baby-self and the baby visibly growing within the body or arms of the woman on the couch.
>
> (Raphael-Leff & Perelberg 1997, p. 125)

Week 2: painting

Ahmad is more settled on arrival, able to hear his name sung. The singing is extended at the start of the group; Rahma sings the song of Sad Mother duck. 'Five little ducks went swimming one day, over the hill and far away... Sad mother duck said quack, quack, quack ... and [no/the?] little ducks came swimming back.' We reflect later that that it sounded like Rahma's voice was breaking as she sang. We find it difficult to hear the end of the song as Rahma sings, but we are taken with the huge sadness of the sad mother duck separated from, and missing her ducklings. Our inability to hear whether the ducklings are reunited with their mother is important for us to stay with. The song describes the mother duck's ducklings out of her physical and visual contact.

Rahma finds the space to make her own painting, using brushes and printing from sponges (Figures 9.2 and 9.3). She is quiet while making them, showing the same physical confidence with which she mixed the dough in the first week. Workers again feel protective in defending the physical and creative space Rahma makes around her. After the first painting Ahmad becomes interested in joining Rahma, by the third painting they are working together with fish sitting both in and out of the water (Figure 9.4). While painting, Ahmad says 'Baby'. I ask where the baby is, and Ahmad points to Rahma's belly.

Rahma shares that she has to make sure she gets home in time for the delivery of the baby box (government initiative) Another member of the group called Hanna is excited when Rahma shares the due date of her baby and that the baby will be a boy. In this exchange, there is a real sense of preparing for the future and of the place that is being made in the group, for claiming the baby.

Looking together at the collection of paintings afterwards, we were taken by the way in which the children and octopuses are suspended above the ground, separated from their environment. The connection is lost they are 'fish out of water'. We counted the three printed children and thought of Rahma as a mother to three children. In consultation, the disconnect that we experienced in the paintings was thought about as in-utero images. Life is being held within the bubble in the sea. We held on to both thoughts simultaneously, also aware that Rahma had not shared her own views on the painting, but has voiced her interest in the opportunity to paint.

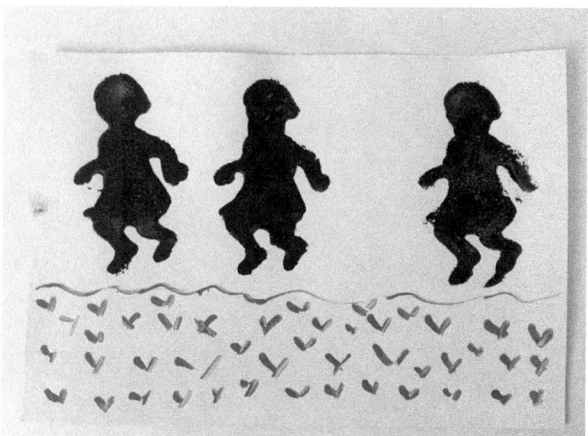

Figure 9.2 Untitled. Rahma's artwork.

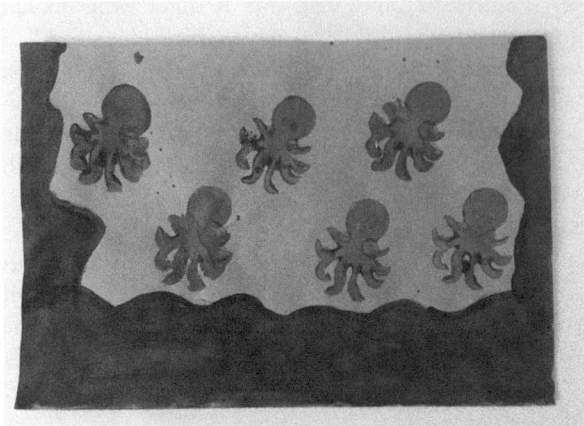

Figure 9.3 Untitled. Rahma's artwork.

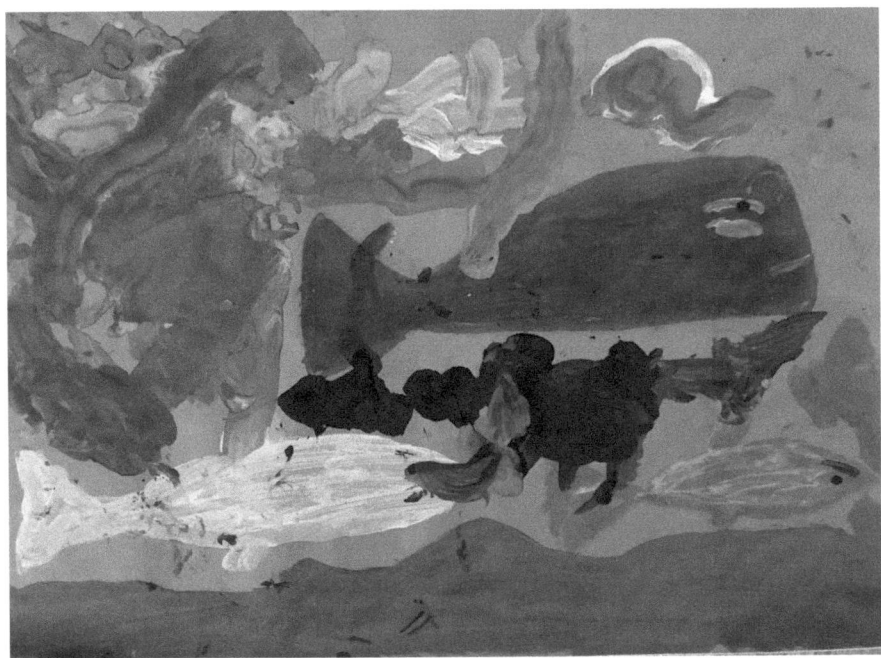

Figure 9.4 Fish by Ahmad and Rahma.

Week 3: collage

Rahma is quiet in the session today. Ahmad has brought three toy fishes with him from home and I make the link to last week's paintings. He is pleased to hear his and Rahma's names being sung in the welcome song. Hanna 'remembers' with warmth that Rahma is pregnant; at the same time Ahmad is curious about my belly. Rahma is 'flat' in response to questions about the baby box, this flatness is in contrast to the anticipation we felt last week. Hanna is tired and her daughter Ewa is unsettled, wanting to eat the glue and paint Hanna. Hanna is unable to explore the art materials, appearing embarrassed and shy. Ahmad and Rahma explore the tissue paper, shredding and cutting it up. Personal geographies are discussed with reference to the world map displayed in the room. Rahma shares the colonial history of her home country, including reference to the geographical logistics of the slave trade. This reminds us again that we, the facilitators, are representing two of the main languages of colonial rule. It is hard for Rahma to make an artwork of her own. She sets out to draw a house, using a graphite pencil and ruler, but is interrupted by Ahmad who paints on the house. Rahma is upset by this, and then, resigned to starting again, draws and paints another house with a landscape that feels unfamiliar to us but also intriguing and drawing our interest. As in previous images, the animal life in the art work hover above the ground. Her son Ahmad begins a game with the salt-dough ducks from the first session. He has a Mummy Quack Quack and Sister Quack Quack. Sister Quack Quack gets broken and Ahmad becomes upset. Rahma tries to glue the pieces back together, but the glue isn't strong enough. We feel at a loss of what to do. Rahma takes the Mummy duck and Ahmad takes one for him and one for 'baby'. Sister duck is now 'far away', 'broken', 'hurt'. We are taken back to the singing of the Mother Duck song, and feel just how far away the Mother Duck is from her ducklings. I wonder aloud, 'You have a baby sister Ahmad?' Rahma answers first, 'yes I do' and then Ahmad answers, 'yes' too. As the group comes to a close, Rahma, now heavily pregnant struggles to get her shoes on. Without being asked, both Isabelle and I move to help her, taking one shoe each and sitting at her feet to fasten her shoelaces.

After the group, we remembered fondly being helped by our own partners to put our socks and shoes on in the last weeks of pregnancy. In turn this highlighted the absence Rahma had in being alone as a parent in this pregnancy. In consultation we wondered about being in-service and extended this to the experience of being enslaved. We stayed with the fact that we belong to and represent a history of white colonial rule. I later wondered about our feelings of guilt, while also thinking about the ambivalence the pregnancy holds for Rahma.

The themes of the un/contained, captivity, holding and enslavement were expressed within the group; they were, felt, depicted and named in a range of ways. In the first session our wish to make a containing space, closing the door, was experienced with distress. There is a dichotomy in the routine, dynamic administration of group work, the protecting of a therapeutic space, mirroring the dynamics of captivity, a locked door. This dichotomy can also be seen to be held within the experience and conceptualising of pregnancy and the idea of an in-utero experience. In *Bun or Bump? The Metaphysics of Pregnancy*, Finn (2017, pp. 1–5) presents these two views, the growing foetus as part of the mother, or the baby contained within the mother. Hogan (2003, pp. 148–171) writes of four ways in which a pregnancy may be thought of, offering maternal–foetal unity. Within the politics of abortion rights, Allotey-Reidpath, Allotey and Reidpath (2018, pp. 57–60) argue that to deny a woman an abortion is to place her in involuntary servitude within a framework of international human rights law. In writing this chapter I move between the terms *pregnancy*, *foetus* and *baby*, never quite sure that the chosen term fits. The experience of pregnancy is complex, extremely personal, and held within overlapping, contradicting and colliding social-political frameworks. In thinking of Rahma during her pregnancy, it felt that the offer within the group of a liminal space, and a container for fantasies accruing during pregnancy was taken and used with quiet consideration. The group was able to be with and tolerate the experience of this during that time.

Our urge to protect Rahma's physical space while she created her artworks was felt as a powerful tug by both Isabelle and myself. At times this meant sitting close by or playing with Ahmad so that Rahma could work. Several times both Rahma and Ahmad initiated an experience of physical closeness with either Isabelle or me. We were protective of Rahma's opportunity to make art but this also felt like an offer of protection for Rahma in her pregnancy and the thought of her unborn baby, also 'being made' and developing within her and in relationship to her. Ownership of her daughter, Zaynab, marked this session, as she and Ahmad tried and failed to fix a broken sister/daughter duck. Rahma felt able to stay with and be in relationship to her three children at this point, however painful, unknown or intrusive she experienced each relationship to be.

Week 4: sand trays

Rahma and Ahmad are the only family attending the group today. Rahma is tired; she had a busy day yesterday and tells us about a friendship she has made with another single parent from her community. Ahmad hasn't brought anything with him today, he stays in close contact with the floor, rolling about and making physical contact with Isabelle and me. Ahmad and Isabelle act out a sibling group interaction with soft toys.

We confirm the break in the group next week and make plans to visit Rahma at home if the baby is born over the next two weeks.

We all play in the sand tray, the adults are assistants to Ahmad's play. Dinosaurs are at the centre of the play with Ahmad wanting everyone to hold at least one dinosaur. Ahmad is upset if anyone lets go, or isn't playing, but at the same time, he's not initiating or developing the game. There is a feeling of stuck-ness, we feel frozen in the act of holding the dinosaurs but not knowing where to go. Ahmad is not talking but making grunts, roars and cries of upset. Three ducks are also left in the sand as the play comes to an end.

We are still stuck in not knowing what is to come. There is an ending of one kind, alongside the possibilities that the break will also mark the birth of Rahma's expected baby and a new sibling for Ahmad. As the session ends we wish Rahma well, voicing our own wish to hear any news from Rahma, or from our colleague who is providing individual support to Rahma.

In notes from the group, pregnancy is named 'the baby' and I wonder again about the group's claiming of the pregnancy. The weeks before a baby is due to be born, holding fast-moving contradictory feeling and fantasies, the wish to stay pregnant and full of life, a fear of being pregnant forever, excitement, trepidation for the baby you are going to be able to look at, out of your own body but still attached (Raphael-Leff 2001, pp. 45–59).

Week 5: musical instruments

Before the group starts our colleague shares news of Rahma having given birth. Rahma and her baby are doing well, Rahma phoned from the hospital to share her news. We are tearful and there is a sense of relief.

One family is attending the group today, Hanna and her daughter Ewa. They are excited about the taxi journey, singing our welcoming hello song to the taxi, when it came to pick them up. It feels like they have been able to keep the group alive in the two weeks they were away. Hanna cradles one of the toys, rejoicing as we share news of Rahma having given birth. Ewa takes care of the soft toys laying them on their bellies and rubbing their back, Hanna shares that this is how Ewa likes to go to sleep, and that her own Mum did the same for her when she was little.

Hanna and Ewa explore the musical instruments, finding moments of attunement. We are invited to join them.

At snack time Hanna says they both like our kitchen, 'It's a good kitchen'. Hanna shares photos on her phone, telling us of a half-sister that died age one, having spent most of her short life in hospital. She shares photos of her sister at the end of her life. The fragility of life, especially that of a new-born infant, is at the centre of the group today. New life, care, death, grief and loss are all named in photos.

In reflection we are moved by the tension that the group has held over the past two months. The intensity of pregnancy, sustaining and containing new life, always holds the possibility of death, at both a medical and psychological level. The actual death of Hanna's sister makes this a reality. We see that there has been grief for both Hanna and Ahmad's sister held in the matrix of the group.

The taxi service

Hanna and Ewa both shared their excitement and enjoyment in being able to travel in a taxi to the group. This is a service the group is able to offer and is often experienced with significant meaning. For many families, it is the difference between feeling able to attend or not. Mothers spoke of how saying the taxi was coming initiated the singing of the group's songs from their children, taxis would be spotted elsewhere by children attending the group, and linked to the group and us. The taxi service belongs to the dynamic administration of the group; it supports the boundaries and holding that the group can offer. It offers a liminal space between home and the group. In reference to this group and our wider Early Years context, I began to see it as connected to images of in-utero too – the families being inside of and part of the taxi, driven and cared for, by the taxi driver.

Ending of the group

With three weeks to go till the end of the group block, we were yet to realise that Week 5 would be our last week together as a group. Rahma voiced her wish to return, but the reality of her caring for both her baby, named Yusuf after her husband, and Ahmad while in the middle of an immigration appeal, meant that they were not able to attend. Hanna and Ewa moved home and Hanna changed her working pattern. We visited families at home as is routine at the end of a group, offering both an ending and opportunity for evaluation.

Our engagement with Rahma, Ahmad, and Yusuf continued over two more home visits, and it is the ending of the work, and our place within a community of supports that is now described. Being subject to immigration procedures, Rahma, Ahmad and Yusuf were required to move to another unknown city, so that their asylum application could be processed. Feelings of loss and insecurity and the search for stability during pregnancy and birth were mirrored in the family's need to adhere to the wider social care and administrative systems. Once again this meant huge upheaval for the family, who were beginning to establish a sense of home and connection. Rahma was explicit that, should she have any say in the decision, she wouldn't want to move. We felt, as workers, both angry and upset that this was happening at such a point in their lives. A collective appeal raised from all agencies supporting the family was unsuccessful. We made relevant referrals to agencies that could potentially support Rahma after the family moved. The thought of this impending upheaval and sudden ending brought us to recognise the level to which we had, alongside other agencies, offered therapeutic care. We had a strong sense of not wanting to let go of the family, in our thinking and in their attendance at the group. In the absence of a family and/or wider community that could/may take interest in and attachment to Rahma's pregnancy, growing foetus, and the birth of Yusuf, Rahma and her family were thought of in the work of the group, and other connected agencies.

Providing a space in which mourning for separation from 'baby sister' Zaynab could be literally and symbolically played out, experienced and named within the group appeared to enable thoughts for the future and space within the family, into which Yusuf could be and was born. Volkan thoughtfully describes a state of perennial mourning that he has experienced in his work with immigrants and refugees (2017, pp. 13–25). For Rahma, her understanding of her loss was not final (her daughter not having died) but separated, and living a huge distance from Rahma, and in a situation Rahma felt was unsafe. Rahma hoped that one day she would be able to be reunited with her daughter, but when this would happen was unknown. In our first meetings with Rahma, the pain of her loss felt close to intolerable. Volkan writes (2017, p. 9),

> If the individual acknowledges the pain (Kleinians call this 'depressive guilt'), the individual may exhibit sadness, sorrow or nostalgia but will still be able to retain reparative tendencies and responsibility and discriminate between past and present.

It is something of this 'reparative tendencies and responsibility' that we felt and observed Rahma was able to provide in her experience of motherhood to three children, as our work came to an end.

In our last home visit to the family, Rahma spoke again of the friend she had made. She breastfed Yusuf, whom she held with care and protection, while getting Ahmad ready for nursery. The family were due to move but at an unknown date. We joined them part way in the walk to the nursery, Rahma pushing Yusuf in his pram and Ahmad walking at their side. This ending was difficult. We felt awkward and unsure if Rahma wanted us there, feeling like we might be an embarrassment, at the same time holding what endings Rahma and Ahmad had experienced in just the last year. As they walked away, we held on to the respect and care we had for Rahma and for her capacity to care for her children.

Rahma did have to move shortly after this ending. Since then Rahma has received confirmation of settled status and has returned to the place where she continues to make her home, both for her and her children. She has applied for her daughter Zaynab to be able to join her and her sons. We are grateful to Rahma for her permission to share this work.

In my last contact with Rahma, phoning to arrange the specific publishing consent for photos, I heard Yusuf's voice in the background. We both laughed at the sound of him enjoying his voice and Rahma shared that it was his first birthday. It felt significant that our contact was on this day.

Acknowledgements

To Isabelle Mercadante, my co-facilitator for sharing all that the group has been and will be.

To Marise Gowenlock for the space and encouragement to establish and write about the work.

To Graham Shulman and Margaret Temple for the space to think about it.

To Olly, Edith and Ida for the time to write.

References

Allotey-Reidpath, K. D., Allotey, P., & Reidpath, D. D. 2018. Nine Months a Slave: When Pregnancy is Involuntary Servitude to a Foetus. *Reproductive Health Matters*, 26(52): 57–61.

Baradon, T., ed. 2016. *The Practice of Psychoanalytic Parent-Infant Psychotherapy Claiming the Baby*, 2nd ed. Abingdon, Oxon: Routledge.

Bion, W. R. 1962. *Learning from Experience*. London: Heinemann.

Campbell, J., Campbell, C. W. J., Liebmann, M., & Brooks, F. 1999. *Art Therapy, Race and Culture*. London: Jessica Kingsley.

Campbell, P., & Thomson-Salo, F., eds. 2014. *The Baby as Subject Clinical Studies in Infant–Parent Therapy*. London: Karnac.

Celebi, M. 2017. *Weaving the Cradle: Facilitating Groups to Promote Attunement and Bonding between Parents, Their Babies and Toddlers*. London: Singing Dragon.

Dyer, R. 2017. *White*, 20th anniversary ed. London: Routledge.

Eleftheriadou, Z. 2006. Creating a Safe Space: Psychotherapeutic Support for Refugee Parents and Babies. In S. Acquarone (ed.), *Surviving the Early Years: The Importance of Early Intervention with Babies at Risk*. London: Karnac, pp. 87–99.

Eleftheriadou, Z. 2010. *Psychotherapy and Culture: Weaving Inner and Outer Worlds*. London: Karnac.

Ellis, L. 1997. *The Meaning of Difference: Race, Culture and Context in Infant Observation*. London: Routledge.

Finn, S. 2017. Bun or Bump? The Metaphysics of Pregnancy. Available at: www.academia.edu/34164778/Bun_or_Bump_The_Metaphysics_of_Pregnancy (accessed April 2020).

Fraiberg, S., Adelson, E., & Sharoro, V. 1975. Ghosts in the Nursery: A Psychoanalytic Approach to the Problems of Impaired Infant-mother Relationships. *Journal of the American Academy of Child & Adolescent Psychiatry*, 14(3): 387–421.

Garland, C., ed. 2002. *Understanding Trauma: A Psychoanalytical Approach*. London: Karnac.

Hogan, S., ed. 2003. *Gender Issues in Art Therapy*. London: Jessica Kingsley Publishers.

Jansen, C. 2019. Foetus 18 Weeks: The Greatest Photograph of the 20th Century? *The Guardian*, 18 November. Available at: www.theguardian.com/artanddesign/2019/nov/18/foetus-images-lennart-nilsson-photojournalist (accessed April 2020).

Kalmanowitz, D., & Lloyd, B., eds. 2005. *Art Therapy and Political Violence with Art, Without Illusion*. Abingdon, Oxon: Routledge.

Meyerowitz-Katz, J., & Reddick, D., eds. 2017. *Art Therapy in the Early Years: Therapeutics Interventions with Infants, Toddlers and Their Families*. Abingdon, Oxon: Routledge.

Mirza, N. 2017. South Asian Women's Experience of Abuse by Female Affinal Kin: A Critique of Mainstream Conceptualisations of 'Domestic Abuse'. *Families, Relationships and Societies*, 6(3): 393–409.

Papadopoulos, R. K. 2002. *Therapeutic Care for Refugees: No Place Like Home*. London: Karnac.

Raphael-Leff, J. 2001. *Psychological Processes of Childbearing*. London: Chapman & Hall.

Raphael-Leff, J. 2006. The Emotional Dialogue: Womb to Walking. In S. Acquarone (ed.), *Surviving the Early Years: The Importance of Early Intervention with Babies at Risk*. London: Karnac, pp. 3–17.

Raphael-Leff, J., & Perelberg, R. J., eds. 1997. *Female Experience: Three Generations of British Women Psychoanalysts on Work with Women*. London: Routledge.

Salomonsson, B. 2018. *Psychodynamic Interventions in Pregnancy and Infancy Clinical and Theoretical Perspectives*. Abingdon, Oxon: Routledge.

Selin, H., & Stone, P. K., eds. 2009. *Childbirth across Cultures Ideas and Practices of Pregnancy, Childbirth and the Postpartum*. London: Springer.

Volkan, V. D. 2017. *Immigrants and Refugees Trauma, Perennial Mourning, Prejudice, and Border Psychology*. London: Karnac.

Winnicott, D. W. 1971. *Playing and Reality*. London: Tavistock.

Whitaker, D. S. 2001 *Using Groups to Help People*, 2nd ed. Hove: Brunner-Routledge.

10 'Myself as a Tree'

The enabling power of an Art Therapy intervention in clinical work with postnatally distressed women-mothers

Sophia Xeros-Constantinides

Being constantly attentive to the needs of someone else for whom one has total responsibility at all times is a daunting task. In addition to broken nights, dream deprivation and exhaustion, a biological mother also contends with hormonal fluctuations, recovery from labour exertions and possible birth damage (and) painful engorgement or mastitis ... In the West perinatal breakdown is common, and postnatal disturbance is experienced by almost half of all new mothers and a quarter of fathers.

(Raphael-Leff 2010, p. 63)

Introduction

This chapter reflects on the experiences of procreative women, and on pregnancy, birth and early motherhood as life-changing events that challenge the status quo for women. The chapter reports on what distressed mothers have said, in words and in pictures, about their experiences of maternity, within the safe confines of a creative therapy group, the CONNECT Group Art Therapy Program[1] (Xeros-Constantinides, Boland & Bishop 2017). Using the 'Myself as a Tree' art-expression exercise, women are encouraged to represent and share their lived-motherhood experiences, using metaphor and paint. Through the combination of tree-imagery and women's words, enabling opportunities arise to normalise feelings, to redefine maternity and to empower participants in authoring their own motherhood journeys.

Lived maternity – bliss and loss: shifting between the imaginary baby and the baby of the 'here-and-now'

... in Man the survival of the young is dependent on the exertions of the mother[2].

(Bowlby 1958, p. 367)

In the context of his work on human attachment, Bowlby has articulated the inescapable fact that new-born human babies are immature at birth and are unable to survive alone in the world without the care of the mother or other primary caregiver. The maternal–infant relationship is an *unequal* one, and the burden of care falls to the mother (or primary caregiver). This responsibility, for keeping baby in mind and for attending to baby's physiological and psycho-emotional needs, places onerous demands on the mother. Many women find themselves unprepared for the nature and extent of the 'exertions' that maternity commands.

Impregnation marks the time from which the woman becomes responsible for another life, growing within the bounds of her own body. As Raphael-Leff has observed, this has consequences for a woman's sense of self:

> … being impregnated stirs up in even the most assured woman a flurry of uncertainties, which necessarily entail revision of her feminine identity, relating to her fecunded body, its unseen processes and the physical, emotional and relational changes it brings about.
>
> (Raphael-Leff 1991, p. 48)

During pregnancy, with the foetus growing in her womb, the woman-mother contemplates the future, and develops an internal *imaginative* relationship with her foetus; 'every mother infuses [the pregnancy] with her personal feelings, hopes, memories, and powerful unconscious mythologies. An imaginary baby is juxtaposed on the embryo implanting in her fertile womb' (Raphael-Leff 1995, p.8).

With the birth, the woman meets her baby face-to-face for the first time. The 'real baby' of the here-and-now comes to dominate the mother's world:

> Matching up the real baby who has come out of her with the imaginary baby who has been inside her for so long demands an effort of integration by no means spontaneous. Many mothers peer at the infant unbelievingly – where is the little girl she anticipated? … who is this 'bony frog-like baby'?
>
> (Raphael-Leff 1991, p. 52)

While pregnancy and birth are often celebrated, it is not unusual for women to find themselves also mourning their losses – the loss of control, loss of self, loss of former life, of freedom, of paid work/career and friendships. In her autobiographical book *A Life's Work: On Becoming a Mother*, Rachel Cusk eloquently describes her sense of struggle emanating from an internal rupture or division to her sense of self:

> Birth is not merely that which divides women from men: it also divides women from themselves, so that a woman's understanding of what it is to exist is profoundly changed. Another person has existed in her, and after their birth they live within the jurisdiction of her consciousness. When she is with them she is not herself; when she is without them she is not herself; and so it is as difficult to leave your children as it is to stay with them. To discover this is to feel that your life has become irretrievably mired in conflict, or caught in some mythic snare in which you will perpetually, vainly struggle.
>
> (Cusk 2003, p. 7)

There are many adjustments and challenges facing prospective parents. These include feeling unprepared for parenthood, dealing with potential loss of the pregnancy or medical complications, managing psychological/mental health problems, traumatic birth, feeding difficulties, sleep deprivation, ambivalence, anger and relationship problems. The dreamed-of motherhood journey may be confounded by any combination of these bio-psycho-social factors.

In addition, not all women respond positively to finding themselves pregnant, or to meeting baby face-to-face with the birth. Karin Vandervoort has observed that 'mother-readiness' is not a given. Rather, it is the result of sustained hard work on the part of each woman to achieve personal growth and extend identity to encompass an-Other in her life.

> Pregnancy, childbirth and bringing a baby home from the hospital do not instantly create a maternal subjectivity … as real women attempt to define for themselves an emerging maternal subjectivity, they often find that the space is already filled by ghosts and unattainable, mythical fantasies of perfection that include the Virgin Mary.
>
> (Vandervoort 2009, p. 1)

Maternity as a 'journeying to connect'

In CONNECT we appreciate the critical importance of the maternal–infant relationship, that relational 'space' where, through 'trial-and-error', mothers and babies each learn about the other, about themselves and about relationships and trust.[3]

It is important to recognise maternity as a relational, dynamic, experiential process, captured in the term 'journeying to connect'. The journey involves a steep learning curve of engagement with baby over time in which the mother endeavours to keep baby in mind – to reach out, hold, soothe and talk with baby, to try to understand and offer over time what this particular baby seems to need, in Winnicott's 'good enough' mothering way (Winnicott 2005).

The CONNECT programme functions as a safety-net for those mothers and babies who find first-line government-funded perinatal support insufficient for their needs. By providing a therapeutic space for women-mothers, we support women and foster conversations about what their lived-motherhood journeys have really entailed.

In the first week of the group, through the process of enquiry and open sharing, we examine society's 'motherhood myths' (Maushart 2000; Motherhood Myths 2001) with a critical eye, based on participants' own experiences. Examples of motherhood myths that the group has examined and challenged include: 'Mothers always know why their babies cry', 'All mothers automatically "love" their babies the first time they see them', 'All babies co-operate with their mothers, if the mother is doing everything right.' The challenging of myths allows participants to find common ground and acceptance, and to bond as a group. Importantly, this exercise catalyses a fundamental shift in the definition of motherhood, through its reframing of maternity beyond society's ideals, to encompass those 'other' experiences of lived-maternity that have been articulated by group members. We then take time to encourage women to revisit their pregnancy and birthing journeys, first in collage and then in words.

In consecutive weeks, we reach beyond words into each participant's creative and emotional depths through the use of paint, canvas and metaphor, in the art-expression exercise called 'Myself as a Tree.' Mothers are asked to imagine or envision themselves as a tree, and to give visual form to their feelings and experiences in paint. We encourage this imaginative process by asking the group a series of questions: Were you a tree, what sort of tree would you be? What would be the form of your trunk and roots and branches? Where would you be situated? What sort of environment and terrain would you find yourself in? Would you be alone, or with others in a copse or forest? What weather and climate surrounds you? Would there be any water nearby, or would it be dry like a desert? Would you have leaves and fruit, or other life living in your canopy?

> Art can be said to be – and can be used as – the externalized map of our interior self.
>
> (London 1989)

After having each painted themselves as a tree, the women are asked in turn to share their art making with the group, and to talk about their tree. Participants are also asked to write a paragraph about their tree-work – words supplement the form and colour of the pictorial image, enriching the communication. Together, the picture and the words create a uniquely personal and powerful statement made in the course of revisiting motherhood experiences.

We do not use art projective activities for *diagnostic* purposes as was done in the past. In his preface to Susan Hogan's *Healing Arts: The History of Art Therapy* (Hogan 2001, p. 16), David Lomas argues that 'to eschew altogether some process of reflection upon the visual material would be to throw the baby out with the bathwater, a step backwards to the days when the making of art by patients was a mere diversionary pastime'. In CONNECT we prioritise sharing and reflecting on the creative output. In fact, *the combination of creative imagery and words* is central to the therapeutic thrust of CONNECT – it forms the basis of redefining maternity within the group (to include women's real-life experiences) and it empowers women through the visual traces they make in the process of authoring their motherhood journeys.

'Myself as a Tree' outcomes and what they reveal about 'lived maternity'

> But see, every tree, thoughtfully considered, is a tree of knowledge.
>
> (Hermann Hiltbrunner cited in Koch 1952, p. 7)

'Myself as a Tree' offers a blank canvas for the introduction of the woman's impressions, thoughts and feelings around motherhood. Each woman's motherhood journey is particular to her, and each tree-work is likewise a unique embodiment of her experience and learning.

Themes commonly emerge in the tree-paintings. Often women represent their journeying or progression along the path of motherhood, or their *desire* to progress to a more satisfying, replenished or provisioned state. One mother painted a diptych showing a bare-branched tree in survival mode, embedded in a winter scene. Her second image depicted hope through seasonal change to spring, with the emergence of 'fluffy, pink blossom' lighting up the whole tree.

Revival, regrowth and regeneration are common themes. One mother (Figure 10.1) used birdlife to represent the flourishing of her relationships as her tree strengthened.

> My tree is a bush that almost died from frost. We almost dug it out of the yard, but decided to give it a chance. From one tiny branch right at the end of the bush, some green leaves and flowers began to grow. From this, the whole bush came back to life and flourished. When the bush was vibrant, birds like the blue wren would come and jump around, feed and delight in the flowers and bush. When the leaves and flowers were gone, the birds went away. When the bush regrew, the same birds came back, and other birds came. This represents relationships. That when there was nothing to give, no one came … I feel like I am this bush, slowly starting to regrow.
>
> (Kalyca Baker)

Recovery and functioning are frequently represented in both the productivity of the tree, and in the surrounding seasonal/weather patterns. In some images the

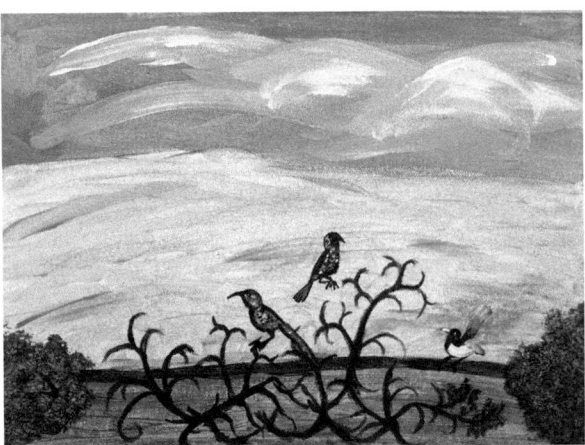

Figure 10.1 My Tree is a Bush that Almost Died from Frost. Kalyca Baker.

tree transitions from bare branch on the left, representing early motherhood, through to the present state of bearing produce (apples) on the right.

For another mother, recovery from emotional trauma is represented by re-growth in a tree that has endured a bush-fire (Figure 10.2).

> Through my experience I have been so personally distracted and have suffered deep emotional trauma … I represent myself as a tree which has stood through a bushfire. My tree has survived the fire and new sprouts are emerging. The nest and bird symbolise the future, hope and the new life, my rainbow baby. A strong, healthy tree stands beside me, my husband. People who have let me down and distanced themselves from me are symbolised by the broken limbs of my tree.
>
> (Nerida)

For some women the metaphor of light is central to the self-representation of the motherhood journey. Light can be used to represent a new day, hope, warmth, happiness.

The metaphor of Nature, and her enduring, cyclical ebb and flow, seem to offer reassurance to women in the context of their perinatal disturbance, even whilst they experience fragility and 'un-doingness'.

One mother depicted herself as a tree with slender, upward-reaching branches carrying pink dots of blossom. She wrote:

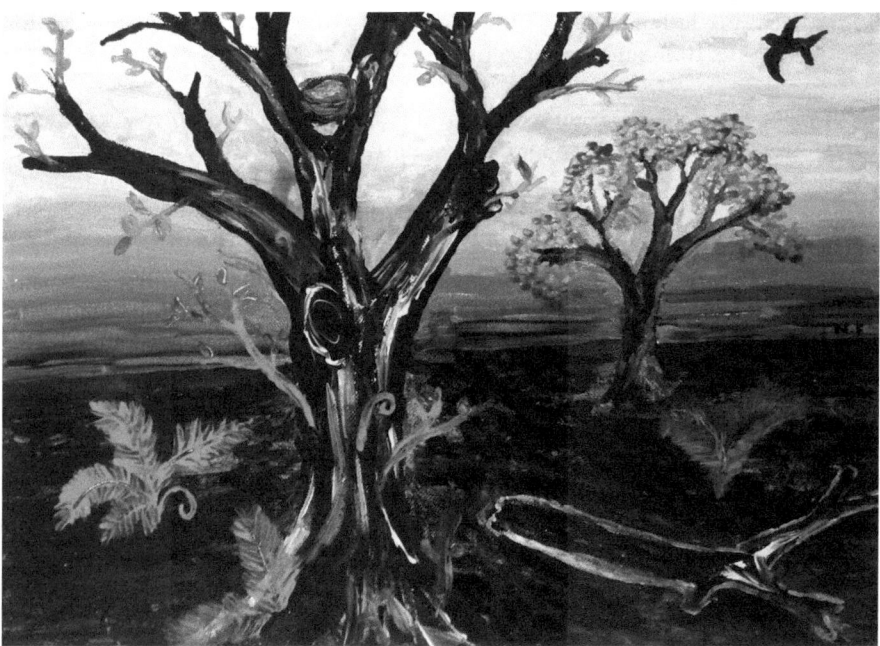

Figure 10.2 My Tree has Survived Fire. Nerida.

I walk out of the house, feeling trapped, anxious, alone, lost and over-whelmed. Breathe in the fresh air and feel better. Ah … there is a world out here after all. It's OK, everything is as it was, how it should be. Look, the sky is blue, I can feel a gentle breeze and see the trees blowing in the wind. Again, I breathe in and out. It's OK, there's a world out here. I focus on my feet on the ground, connected to the earth. I hear the birds singing. I feel the breeze on my face. I touch the trunk on the tree and wonder how long this tree has been standing here. Who planted it? How many women have stood before this tree in the past? How many will stand here after me? The wind picks up and blows all of the petals to the ground. So pretty and so fragile.

Women-mothers depict their varied struggles and losses through words and imagery pertaining to their tree-works. One mother felt that through having a baby she had suffered the loss of her identity as a 'confident, strong and young' person. She depicted this loss by separating herself into *two* very different trees, her slender young green tree on the left (see paperback cover image by Zoe Murdoch). Zoe Murdoch wrote: 'Green tree – before baby – confident and strong and young. Brown tree – after baby – old, confused, stressed, disappointed, unsure, lost. Large contrast between the two stages of my life.'

Sometimes it is through the process of depiction that realisation dawns. One mother looked closely at her tree after finishing and saw that she had alluded to her loss of freedom: 'The tree looks like it can move – I hate to be trapped.'

A bereaved mother painted a bird flying up towards her branches – she wrote: 'Little spirit, my little lost one.' Other losses for women-mothers include loss of support (Figure 10.3) and loss of control.

I painted myself as a gum tree. Strong, dependable, supportive, constant. However, I am alone – separated from my support network (family, etc., the forest behind). I feel that I stand alone and find it difficult to ask for help – I am the one who is used to helping and being the supportive one. Asking for help is the hardest thing I've ever had to do – *but* once I have – I feel like a weight has been lifted. The gum tree has a cut off branch signifying my past relationships and life in a different state – that I was very happy to leave behind … I am just struggling to do it all alone.

(Leanne Hancock)

Ambivalence sometimes manifests in the tree-works. One mother depicted her tree in a landscape setting representing mood and emotions – peaks and valleys of the hills representing the 'ups and downs'. Her ambivalence took the form of a 'small white butterfly, the hope of transformation, or the dream to be free again'.

For another mother, there is an acute awareness of internal conflict and of loss in the form of 'death but also new life' (Figure 10.4). Through her words, we glimpse the impact that thinking and talking in the group had on her psychological and creative processes. Through Art Therapy, she was able to

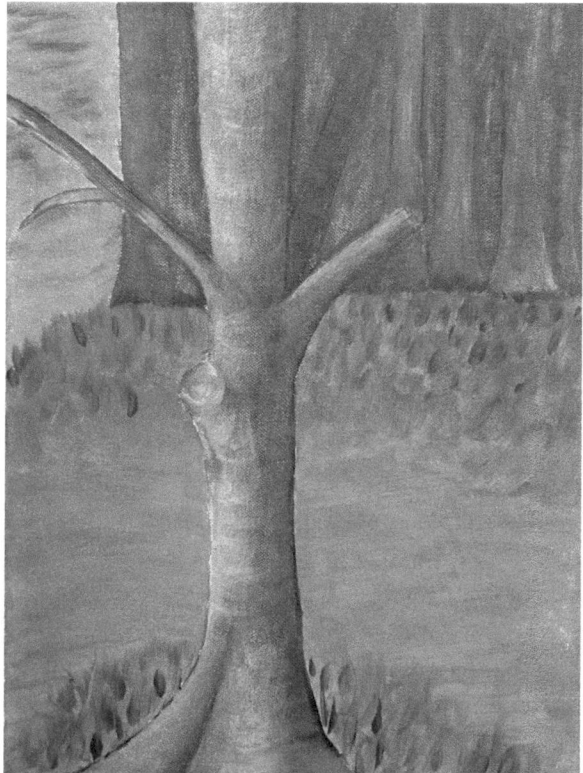

Figure 10.3 Gum Tree. Leanne Hancock.

acknowledge her loss accompanying maternity, and to find some renewal and reparation, represented by her transformation of her 'dead and grey' tree into her 'autumn tree'.

> Initially my tree was dead and grey but as I continued working on it and thinking/talking, it became an autumn tree – with death but also new life … The green ground in the foreground represents hope, but it's still covered in ice and dirt … the old life creeping in, the old self suffocating or co-existing? (not sure) with the new ground. The flowers, initially, were weeds and vines twisted around the tree and representative of my children. They are a noose around my neck, but they bring so much brightness and love to my life. Thus, I've represented them as bright flowers that break up the starkness of the landscape and bringing new life to the space around the tree. The fence is the bridge between the old and the new … it will never be an unbroken space again. Sure, you can take the fence down, but it won't be the same – I would still see the fence. Likewise, the time before the fence will never be

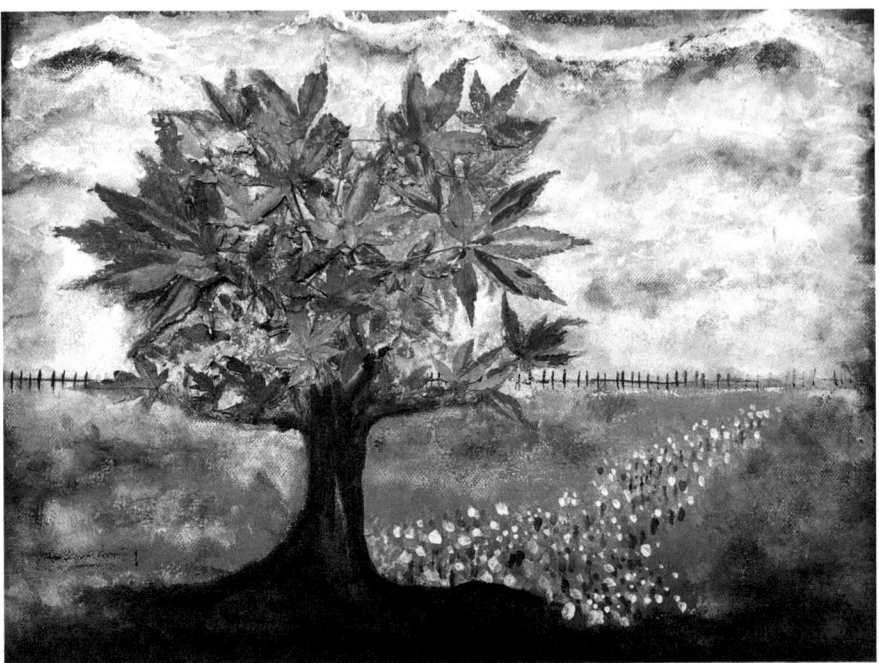

Figure 10.4 Autumn Tree. Sarah-Jane Wentzki.

again. There's a lot of conflict in the detail of this painting hidden by the façade of order and symmetry. This is how I feel about my life.

(Sarah-Jane Wentzki)

Some women depict an absent mother, or a bad or abusive past. One mother painted a tree with curly branches and a heart in the trunk and a birds' nest with two little bird-heads peeking out. She wrote:

> My tree has thorns that are spiky and tough. But I have blood running through the trunk and branches … I do have a heart capable of love. There is some growth and seeds forming but they have a long way to go. My little birds need help to grow but the mother bird is absent… Hopefully something will grow and change soon. Perhaps a new season.

The pain and scaring of having been emotionally abused as a child remains for many mothers. One such mother reflected:

> [M]y tree represents from darkness to light. I think that's what it means. Trees can grow bad, rotten fruit and I have had people surround me through my life who were bad and rotten and tried to make me believe

I'm the same. For a long time they succeeded... gosh knows, bit by bit I've been fighting to believe that I'm not a bad person who should be and feel guilty for things I've said and done in my life, but someone who chooses to have colourful, positive thoughts. Warm bright colours make me feel happy. Edward, my son, represents unconditional love represented by the bright red colourful side (of my tree). I think the dark side might always be there, but I'm learning to accept it, and be stronger than those dark thoughts.

Another mother with a history of childhood abuse showed her two children as branches reaching up to the sun.

Sometimes mothers pretend, hiding their true self/feelings from the world:

Occasionally I hide behind a mask, not showing my real feelings. I do this for many reasons, such as not wanting to hurt others, anger them or upset them. But mostly so I don't get hurt, (or) judged or have conflict with anyone.

One participant said of her tree image:

My tree is full of fruit growing healthy and strong in the beautiful sunny weather. This represents the façade I put on a daily basis, always pretending I am doing really well and strong on the outside, but underneath the surface I am trying to push through the hard-dark black soil. The connecting roots from Eli's tree he is helping me grow lots of strong, thick roots and because of him I push through the soil.

Another said:

I'm a ghost gum. My canopy is lush and green and full of life. I feel this represents the way I present myself to others – that everything is as it should be. Below the canopy is leafless branches and barrenness that represents how I really feel. Tears crying from the branches, red river of anger and frustration, purple tent where I want to hide when I'm afraid of being a Mum.

Sometimes women are overtaken with darkness, isolation, frustration/anger and/or hopelessness/despair. For other mothers there is the added layer of mental illness to deal with (recurrent or arising de novo), along with adjustments to maternity. One participant painted a pregnant looking tree with a colourful canopy. She said of the image:

My painting represents my pregnancy. It's a large tree as I got quite big. I loved being pregnant hence the bright colours used but I always had anxiety about Hari which is represented by the storm clouds and the lightning. The storm clouds blight what would otherwise be an idyllic summer day which is how I feel about my anxiety.

Another participant said of her tree, 'I painted myself as a tree, bare, isolated, empty and vulnerable to reflect the feelings I have felt as I battle my way through the quagmire of post-natal psychosis'.

Sometimes a mother's distress follows life-threatening illness in her baby.

> Starting with the joy and peacefulness after Hayley was born and our family had grown. Things stating to become more difficult. Hayley's hospital admission to ICU. The return of OCD traits, anxiety and depression. When I was admitted to hospital and the weeks leading up to it, my world was black. I saw no hope, no future and didn't think I wanted to be here … recovery process has had many ups and downs but is slowly improving and my world is lighter. I can see the future … with my husband and two girls.

Many women-mothers feel subsumed and eclipsed by maternity and its demands. One mother described her wished-for tree:

> A Willow tree. Strong and survives no matter what's thrown at it, it's still standing. I chose this because that's how I want to be. I want to be strong. I want to be able to stand and handle everything that's thrown at me. I just want to feel strong even when I'm not in control.

Another mother wrote:

> … feeling lost and dark, still a few sparks of light. Feel like Melissa the woman is gone and Mummy is 100%. Needing to get back to where I would like to be. Need to start meditating, doing tai chi and relaxing more. Not sure if this is selfish. I feel like it is though. Don't handle stress well. I had made a stress-free life for myself before my family … Set in my own ways. Hard to break (my habits) having had kids (when) older.

Women frequently give expression to their wished-for brighter future: 'Tree trunk starts dark for my struggle at the start when Brooklyn was born. Travelling up the tree to lighter days ahead and a brighter future. I love nature.'

In her motherhood journey, each woman is faced with the task of understanding and re-defining herself in relation to both her past and her new baby. One mother painted the crown of her tree in two halves 'the old me dying off and the new me sprouting slowly'.

In conclusion

In this chapter I have touched on the demands and vulnerabilities that women-mothers face once colonised by a fertilised ovum. Through the CONNECT Art

Therapy Group Program, post-partum mothers have been invited to share aspects of their lived-maternity and to give expression to their motherhood experiences, in both imagery and in words.

The 'Myself as a Tree' painting exercise has posed a challenge to participants to think in metaphor whilst revisiting often fraught and painful territory. Use of the tree-metaphor requires each mother to place her personal experiences, thoughts and feelings onto another living thing outside of herself, and then to give those projections a visual form. Trees are living organisms – they come from seeds, and have the potential under the right conditions to germinate and grow, and in turn to produce new life. In a sense, like the tree, each woman has herself participated in Nature's cyclical ebb-and-flow in creating her baby.

We have found that women generally embrace the exercise of envisioning themselves in tree-form, giving visual expression to their challenging motherhood experiences. Through 'Myself as a Tree', a 'botanical garden' assortment of powerful tree imagery has been generated reflecting women's collective wisdom pertaining to maternity. I have offered a sample of these precious icons of maternity here for contemplation, so that we may better understand the experiences and needs of procreative women, and provide the therapeutic support that is essential for them, their infants and families.

One mother shares how she was enabled by CONNECT:

> I feel this group is the only space where I feel normal, not unusual. It has changed the way I respond to social images/pressures around being a mother.
>
> (Xeros-Constantinides et al. 2017, p. 10)

A historical postscript: background to the use of projective depictions of trees in psychiatric practice in Melbourne

There is a history of patients making tree imagery in Melbourne Psychiatric Hospitals. Between 1959 and 1967 at least 600 patients at Royal Park Psychiatric Hospital in Melbourne were administered the 'Tree Test' by doctors, in addition to undergoing more conventional mental state assessment, such as psychiatric interview (Spinks, Greenway & Hanson 2008, pp. 1–2). 'The Tree Test' (Koch 1952) is a projective test devised by Charles Koch, used to aid psycho-diagnosis, to gain a greater understanding of the creator's inner world. Koch published tables to aid in the interpretation of the tree drawings. Today, the validity and reliability of the test has been called into question (Spinks et al. 2008, p.2), but nonetheless the test provides some insight into past use of projective visual imagery in a clinical setting, to assess patients' presentations and mental illnesses. The Cunningham Dax Collection in Melbourne has approximately 1,800 of these tree-works drawn by psychiatric patients.

The use of the Tree Test in Melbourne coincided with the time that British Psychiatrist Dr Eric Cunningham Dax (1908–2008) was chairman of the Mental Hygiene Authority in Victoria from 1952 to 1969 (Cunningham Dax 1998). In this role Cunningham Dax encouraged art expression as an integral part of clinical services for mental patients' diagnosis and treatment, as well as for public education.[4]

Acknowledgements

The author wishes to thank, first and foremost, all the infants and their mothers who have bravely shared aspects of their motherhood journeys in the CONNECT programme. Without you there would be no group. To my colleagues, Lynne Bishop and Bernice Boland, I offer my sincere gratitude for being invited to collaborate in shaping a special programme for distressed mothers that distinguishes itself by placing art making at its heart. Particular thanks to Viv Miller for her wizardry in capturing the tree-work imagery and to the Yarra Ranges Council for funding CONNECT. I am indebted to Julia Young, curator and collections Manager at the Dax Centre, for bringing Koch's 'Tree Test' to my attention.

Notes

1 The CONNECT Group Art Therapy Program, currently in its twelfth year, is co-conducted by Dr Sophia Xeros-Constantinides, enhanced maternal and child health nurses Bernice Boland and Lynne Bishop, and the team, in the outer-eastern suburbs of Melbourne, Australia.
2 Bowlby, in a footnote to his 1958 paper, states: 'Although in this paper I shall usually refer to mothers and not mother-figures, it is to be understood that in every case I am concerned with the person who mothers the child and to whom he becomes attached rather than to the natural mother.'
3 Smith, Xeros-Constantinides and Cumming (2010, pp. 72–77). Case study of mother and ten-month-old daughter with impaired maternal–infant relationship and marked gaze-avoidance, referred to PAIRS mother-infant Group Therapy. Mother wrote creatively about her feelings/past as part of her group experience.
4 The Dax Centre houses Dr Dax's legacy, the Cunningham Dax Collection of Psychiatric Art, comprising more than 9,000 artworks made by psychiatric hospital patients in the UK and Melbourne. The Dax Centre in all contains over 16,000 artworks, with more recent acquisitions pertaining to mental illness and/or psychological trauma. See www.daxcentre.org.

References

Bowlby, J. 1958. The Nature of the Child's Tie to his Mother. *The International Journal of Psycho-Analysis*, 39: 350–373.
Cunningham Dax, E. C. 1998. *The Cunningham Dax Collection: Selected Works of Psychiatric Art*. Melbourne: Melbourne University Press.
Cusk, R. 2003. *A Life's Work: On Becoming a Mother*. New York: Picador.
Hogan, S. 2001. *Healing Arts: The History of Art Therapy*. London: Jessica Kingsley Publishers.
Koch, C. 1952. *The Tree Test: The Tree-Drawing Test as an Aid in Psycho-Diagnosis*. Berne: Verlag Hans Huber.

London, P. 1989. *No More Secondhand Art*. Boston: Shambhala.

Maushart, S. 2000. *The Mask of Motherhood: How Becoming a Mother Changes Our Lives and Why We Never Talk about it*. London: Penguin.

Motherhood Myths. 2001. NCAST-AVENUW Publications. Adapted from *Promoting Maternal Mental Health During Pregnancy, Theory, Practice & Intervention*.

Raphael-Leff, J. 1991. *Psychological Processes of Childbearing*. London: Chapman & Hall.

Raphael-Leff, J. 1995. *Pregnancy: The Inside Story*. Northvale, New Jersey: Jason Aronson.

Raphael-Leff, J. 2010. Healthy Maternal Ambivalence. *Psycho-Analytic Psychotherapy in South Africa*, 18(2): 57–73.

Smith, J. C., Xeros-Constantinides, S., and Cumming, A. 2010. A Decade of Parent and Infant Relationship Support Group Therapy Programs. *International Journal of Group Psychotherapy*, 60(1): 59–89.

Spinks, T., Greenway, P., & Hanson, J. 2008. *Beyond the Three Trees*. Exhibition catalogue, exhibited 13 November 2008–9 April 2009 at the Cunningham Dax Collection. Melbourne: The Cunningham Dax Collection Publication.

Vandervoort, K. 2009. *Standing in Unstable Spaces: The Emergence of Maternal Subjectivity in First-Time Mothers*. PsyD dissertation, California Institute of Integral Studies.

Winnicott, D. W. 2005. *Playing and Reality*. Abingdon, Oxon: Routledge.

Xeros-Constantinides, S., Boland, B., & Bishop, L. 2017. Journeying to Connect: Promoting Post-Natal Healing and Relationship Formation through the CONNECT Group Art-Therapy Program for Distressed Mothers and Infants – a Clinical Practice Article. *Australian Journal of Child and Family Health Nursing*, 14(2): 4–11.

11 Obstetric violence

Silenced issues

Daniela Besa Torrealba
Translated by Frédérique Champagne

Introduction

This chapter focuses on obstetric violence shown through images produced by Chilean women who work in the health sector. The objective of this chapter is to increase awareness regarding obstetric violence and reflect upon the question *how do women and healthcare professionals feel about these practices of a violent nature?* The social acceptance of obstetric violence practised in medical procedures makes it invisible. There is no law that protects against the physical and psychological damage caused by obstetric violence suffered by women and their children that may cause trauma and eventually lead to death. There are, however, health experts who show the sensitivity and capacity to perceive these violent practices and whose aim is to seek changes and ensure experiences lived are different.

The women who participated in this project work in health-related fields. They shared experiences and images of obstetric violence, which served as a trigger to initiate discussions regarding this issue, which is currently normalised and witnessed daily in Chile despite efforts by organisations and professionals for its eradication. Medical and health institutions impede women from enjoying their right that should grant them freedom of choice, safe and necessary healthcare that their children and themselves should benefit from while giving birth.

Talks were organised to highlight what is silenced using images and creative processes. These resources showed the fear and the pain suffered. Additionally, the images shown reveal contents and elements that speak for themselves and reflect aspects that no words can describe. The woman and her body remain invisible in dominating discourses, images or practices in our culture.

Obstetric violence: images produced by chilean women in the health sector

Methodology

Women who suffered obstetric violence were convened as well as partners and health experts to group discussions. The OVO (Observatory for Obstetric Violence in Chile, https://ovochile.cl/) collaborated by mailing the invitation.

It was decided to work with experts in the field of health to avoid any further trauma possibly suffered by female victims of obstetric violence. One of the women interviewed works in the health sector and also suffered violence during childbirth. She was undergoing therapy at the time and was offered to participate in other discussions to record and work on the images.

All the participants asked for the publication of their names in this chapter:

• Andrea Gómez. Nurse.
• Giorgia Pezzoli. Artist and Art Therapist.
• Karin Carrasco. Psychologist and Art Therapist.

The conception of images used was guided and supported by the author of this text using two qualitative methodology techniques: group and individual interviews, which were recorded and transcribed. Images were photographed for subsequent analysis. The role of the Art Therapist was to promote unguided free artistic creation and to offer support throughout the process. Subsequent discussions over the images produced involved greater guidance.

Giorgia Pezzoli produced a personal piece of work inspired from the image of a patient robbed of her freedom with whom she worked when practising in a women's prison under the supervision of the CEANIM institute (a research centre focused on children's and women's needs, www.resiliencia.cl/). CEANIM and the person concerned allowed the use and the publication of the image by the Art Therapist in this chapter.

Participants all signed an authorisation form to record and photograph interview results and their subsequent publication.

Obstetric violence in Chile

• 'What does obstetric violence entail?' Many individuals asked this question during the selection process of participants. Some women even questioned their own experiences:
• 'How will I know if I suffered obstetric violence?' To which the following questions were then asked:
• 'What did you feel? Did you feel subjected to some form of violence?'

This first question shows how invisible and normalised obstetric violence seems to be even for women themselves. It is essential to acknowledge and value each woman's experiences without questioning or imposing external definitions or criteria to decide what is violent or not during gynaecological and obstetric processes. On this basis, the focus was placed on the creation of images and analysis of interviews relating to obstetric violence.

The current legal void regarding obstetric violence also shows that it is an issue that has no visibility. The Chilean legislation covers other aspects of maternity such as in the professional sphere in the case of maternity leaves before or after the birth of the child. Meanwhile, the bill regarding gynaecological and obstetric violence (published in the State Bulletin 12148-11) still has not been approved. This proposal outlines the rights of women with regards to procreation and would put an end to the normalisation of obstetric violence. It declares the following: 'Violence towards women must be eradicated in all its forms, its invisibility and normalisation are not acceptable even less during such crucial and key moments of women's lives' (Bulletin 12148-11 2018, p. 1).

This proposed law not only establishes the rights of pregnant women during labour, when giving birth and post-partum but also challenges gynaecological and obstetric violence, which is defined as, stated below:

> Type of gender-based violence against the body and reproduction processes which dehumanizes the individual and which also entails the abusive use of medication and the pathologizing of reproduction processes. In other terms, this violence covers the ill-treatment of women during labour, when giving birth to her child or children. It mainly entails verbal abuse from assisting staff (doctors, midwives, assistants and so forth), the subjection of the mother to unnecessary stress, the use of violent and highly unrecommended maneuvers that go against protocols in place with regards to labour such as the 'Kristeller maneuver' or resourcing to caesareans to hasten the birth when not duly necessary.
>
> (Carvajal & Hernando 2015, p. 2)

This definition covers violent practices either physical (interventions and procedures) or psychological (insults, judgemental comments, mockeries and shouting). Here are some of the testimonies collected from Chilean women who suffered obstetric violence extracted from audio-visual records kept at the Obstetric Violence Observatory (https://ovochile.cl/testimonios/):

> They would say 'shut up'. They would manipulate any part of my body. Together with the midwife, they started mocking me. I thought I had to keep my mouth shut and not say anything – as my mum used to tell me – otherwise they would mistreat me.
> The doctor pointed the finger to me and said 'you, shut up'. They told me to stop crying, that I looked like a little girl.
> The doctor and the midwife took off. He was going to the beach so that's why they did a caesarean.

The bill emphasises the need to eradicate obstetric violence. It states alarming local figures delivered by the Obstetric Violence Observatory: '1 out of 4 women handled in the public sector suffered some form of physical violence inside the hospital and 56.4% indicate that they suffered mocking or reprimanding when voicing their pain and emotions during birth' (Bulletin 12148-11 2018, p. 1). Giving birth in Chile implies a high risk of suffering violence.

Obstetric violence occurs in paradoxical settings whether inside health institutions or else verbalised by health professionals who have vowed to care for others and restore the health of patients but who act against women by mistreating them, harming or even by terminating their lives and that of their children.

Oakley (1992) provides a deep analysis of social support with regards to maternity concluding that it is fundamental for the health of the mother and that of her children. It also mentions the fact that mothers usually lack this support. Relatives and the surrounding community can generate anxiety, stress and violence. Nor do women benefit from social support within healthcare institutions. It should be reminded that healthy pregnancies and births do not require medical attention. Giving birth is not an illness, however

> pregnancy continues to be viewed as a medical condition and is handled as such in the same facilities by the same medical professionals dedicated to curing diseases. Giving birth ... remains – more than ever – a surgical operation over which women have no control.
>
> (Ehrenreich & English 1984, p.77)

The majority of births in Chile occur in clinics and hospitals and involve mainly healthy women. Nevertheless, the physical and/or psychological condition of these women upon leaving after giving birth proves unguaranteed due to possible aggressions experienced in these healthcare institutions.

Analysis of images involving healthcare professionals

Is obstetric violence a concern for these workers? Those involved in this project are indeed preoccupied by this issue and are affected by obstetric violence.

Based on this context, four images were selected and analysed. Each one was initially observed in detail. The phenomenological method of Art Therapy of Betensky (2001) was used a reference in the subsequent review of the art pieces, but not during the process of Art Therapy focusing on phase 2 which deals with the 'What-do-you-see?' procedure regarding phenomenological evidence. All that can be *seen* is seen in the art expression itself, not surmised or thought out from a pre-established theory. 'This is achieved by guiding... and noticing specific structural components in the artwork and the feelings they convey' (Betenksy 2001, pp. 127–128). This concept allows concentration on the importance of the image that was therefore described, interpreted and analysed using the testimonies of the authors of these images. Below is the analysis of each image divided into different sections that reflects the practice of obstetric violence in its various forms.

Description: Rectangular box made of cardboard. 22 × 14.5 × 5cm. The inner edges are covered with paper of a velvety texture and dark blue colour. Bits of crumpled adhesive are stuck to some of the edges of the box. The bottom of the box shows watercolour abstract forms. Blue, green, red and yellow are the colours that dominate in the centre. The only figurative image in this piece is a red heart. Black and dark blue abstract forms surround this central image. The contour of a pregnant woman whose hand is resting on her baby inside her womb is highlighted using transparent silicone traced over the watercolour shapes.

The image shows the body of a pregnant woman and her baby made of invisible material (transparent silicone). The bodies are present, they exist as they are made of material – their texture can be felt – but they cannot be seen easily as they lose themselves in the white space of the box surrounding the colour tones that appear at the bottom of the box. The image of the female body and the material used is a key element in this piece of work as it reflects its presence as well as its absence. What is there – this central element – cannot be observed easily.

The artist, who is also a healthcare professional, reveals that a patient of hers was her inspiration. She was due to give birth in a public hospital in Chile. Her partner was not allowed to accompany her in the delivery room. After giving birth, she was left alone and was not in contact with her baby. The woman felt that she spent hours in solitude. They did not take any notice of her nor did they give her any information. She asked for her partner and for her baby to a nurse who replied: 'Didn't they tell you that your baby was born dead?' Later, she succumbed to a deep depression of a delusional nature (she would hear her baby cry and see him at home). She was unable to understand the link between her symptoms, the trauma lived and the death of her baby.

These are the words of the artist:

> My work shows how the woman is made invisible and how giving birth is seen as a productive process. She was going to have a baby but did not give birth to her baby alive. Nothing more. What happens with this woman, her emotions, this mother who was going to have a baby? In the end, in institutional terms no responsibility was taken nor interest shown to look after this person after the delivery. There was no intention to provide a follow-up of this person, to contact her. She was left drifting alone, in complete solitude. There is no structure, no space to care for her emotions. It was a failure in the line of production, something that went wrong. Let's just get on with it. I worked in the public sector for various years and I see the public sector as highly industrialised in the sense that even us, professionals who work in it, are just part of the machinery. If we are mere objects, then the patients are too. There is no space for emotions or for grief. The turmoil generated by the system leads to a lack of humanity and sensitivity. Taking in charge the emotions of a mother grieving implies getting involved in the entire process. Workers do not want to take this responsibility. They are not trained. Many of them are not trained to deal with crisis situations or extreme emotions. These mothers are left to drift away, they are left to deal with this emotional knot that leads to depressions and anxiety.
>
> (Karin Carrasco, psychologist and Art Therapist)

Description: Paper format. 27 × 37.5cm. The centre shows a rectangle shape made of black cardboard placed diagonally, outlined using a wax-based yellow pencil. A human figure with tied open legs and arms is drawn on it. Bits of red tape cover the hands, feet and the bottom part of the face. A strip of deep red velvety paper was used to cover the abdomen from one side to the other of the rectangle and is then extended using a red wax-based pencil. At the bottom of the image, we can see a group of human figures drawn using black crayon and charcoal. Wax-based pencil and black charcoal was used for the outline. In the upper part, four fingers drawn using wax-based pencil and black charcoal can be seen close to the cardboard rectangle. In the background, we can see tenuous and irregular traces of black charcoal.

What is striking in this image is the fact that the bodies are not differentiated, making it impossible to determine genders. The white body contrasts with the black background and the rest of the human figures. It represents a woman. The author states that she does not show female features. Is this a situation that reflects the exclusion of female attributes? The limbs are blurred and disappear into the black background.

The image gives the impression that the hand dominates the scene depicted for its bigger shape, the scale of the rest of the elements and the orientation of the fingers. The extremities of the character positioned over the black surface are tied. The mouth is covered. It seems the person has been immobilised and silenced. Something is happening to the abdomen of the character covered with a red element that extends to both sides. Below, we can see a group of faceless human figures witnessing the scene passive and motionless.

The worker explains she depicted a picture of her giving birth. She suffered obstetric violence. She was expecting a normal and happy delivery. She did not feel any fear and felt confident. Nevertheless, she happened to experience violence and ill-treatment in the clinic in which she had selected to give birth.

She refers to the elements of her work as follows:

> The lower part represents the people present during the delivery. I totally trusted the staff involved. I am a nurse and I worked for a long time in maternity wards. I witnessed many of these techniques and processed them as normal. I wasn't aware of the pain experienced by women and saw procedures regularly followed. I did not see that these were forms of violence. A series of interventions made me feel very vulnerable. This is why I started drawing them first (human figures at the bottom) because they were the protagonists during delivery. Here I drew myself and this is how I felt (human figure onto black background). I felt tied and silenced. They did everything that they shouldn't do. I didn't have any voice. I felt I could not talk and that I could not oppose myself to anything. They injected oxytocin without asking me. A lot of people started coming in. They were watching what was happening to me. They completed an emergency caesarean. The midwife had to press against my daughter. I felt the cut of the caesarean. I had the feeling that I could not talk and that I did not have a voice.

The last thing that I drew was this hand and this red line. I felt they confined me to this bed voiceless and devoid of any power. I find it extraordinary that this type of violence occurs in an institution with trained personnel. I ask myself when, we, workers lost this sensitivity and empathy. The system is producing thoughtless machines that serve to produce and not think about what the other one is doing. How many times have I seen myself acting like this, how many times have I generated violence, how many times have I not shown all the respect owed and denied people of their rights without realising just because of the power over others when dressed in blue or white?

(Andrea Gómez, nurse and mother)

Representations in Figures 11.1 and 11.2 depict details of bodies that prove invisible, that show no female attributes and lose themselves in the background. In both images, the bodies of women are situated either on or within rectangular structures thus referring to the use of stretchers that prove the medicalisation of childbirth.

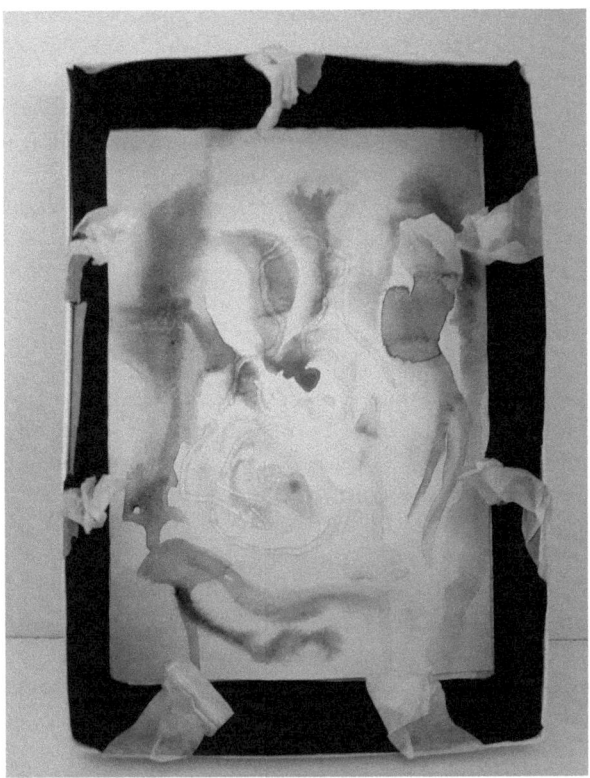

Figure 11.1 Making the Woman Invisible and Abandoning Her in the Realm of Reproduction. Karin Carrasco, psychologist, Art Therapist and mother.

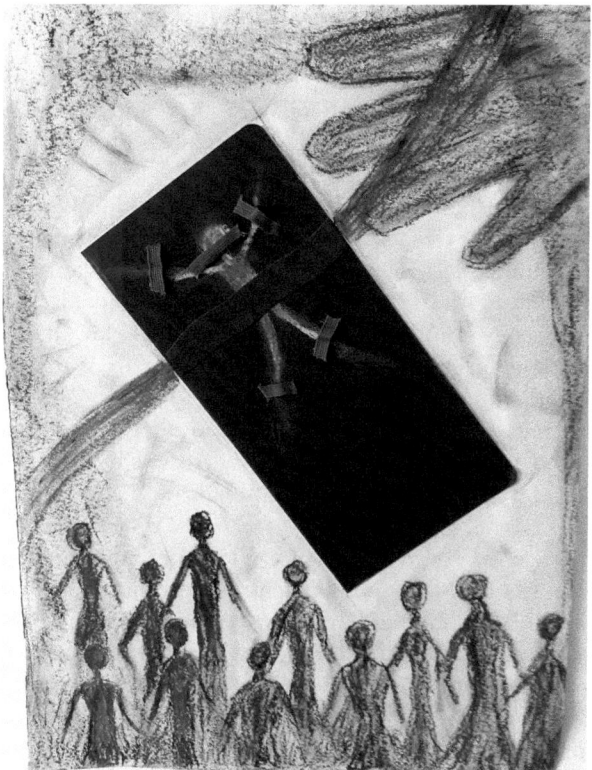

Figure 11.2 Woman Object: One More Element of the Machinery. Andrea Gómez, nurse
 and mother.

These are creations produced in reaction to obstetric violence and which describe giving birth as a mechanical process. References are made to the industrialisation of the sector, loss of human contact and denial of emotions. The woman, her body and her emotions ceased to exist and to matter. They became transparent or turned into objects or things. The body became one with the bed and the other is flattened and tied up. They could not move nor talk or give their opinion. Their objectification and silencing contributed to their oblivion and abandonment in a process of production in which each professional plays a role and the woman is just a number or a thing within this machinery.

Emily Martin (1987) researched about the imagery of the female body in women's narratives and highlighted the existence of an industrial productive process: 'to understand the medicalisation of childbirth, we must understand that the development of western thinking and medicine entails the idea that the body is considered a machine. This concept was adopted throughout the 17th and 18th centuries' (p. 54) It still remains valid today given the inhumane and emotionless treatment devoid of empathy observed and procedures ruled by current protocols whereby the woman is objectified and is part of the productive and reproductive process. Any subjectivity and human dimension are therefore left aside which is exactly what the woman introduces through her presence and her own process. The machine and mechanisms in place reject these aspects. The process must be fully controlled and production ensured and standardised. There are no bridges between the needs and experiences of women and healthcare personnel on the matter of childbirth.

Description: Paper support. 27 × 37.5cm. Drawings produced with coloured pencils. In the upper left part, black handcuffs and below an orange circle. Inside two fuchsia straight lines and a zigzag line across them, an orange dot in the middle. Below these lines, four red drops. In the upper right side, a drawing of a light or spotlight with six eyes underneath. Two rectangles below, a big one and a smaller one. Each contains a heart. An arrow pointing from the bigger rectangle to the smaller one.

This piece shows different icons that represent the idea of immobilisation (handcuffs), cuts, tears and blood drops (parallel lines crossed by zigzag lines with drops below). Eyes are watching below the spotlight and love is present (two hearts).

The creator of these images has been working for a long period of time in Art Therapy involving female victims of obstetric violence in various contexts. The main reason that pushed her to take part in this experience was the drawing (Figure 11.4) produced during an Art Therapy workshop by an incarcerated patient who had suffered obstetric violence. This image meant a total turning point for her.

The Art Therapist describes her creation (Figure 11.3) as follows:

> Here is the scar and the blood. Chile is one of the countries with the highest number of unjustified caesareans summoned by doctors. These are

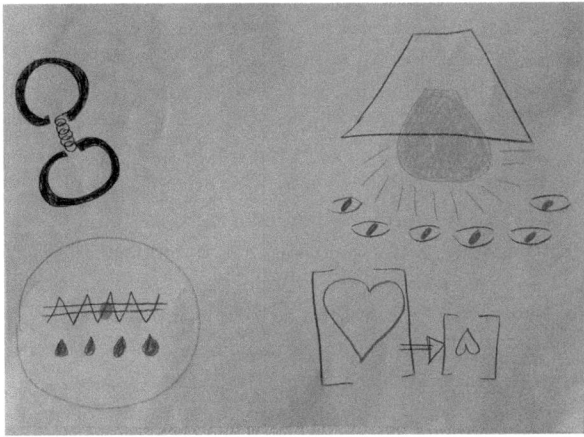

Figure 11.3 Here is the Scar and the Blood. Giorgia Pezzoli, artist and Art Therapist.

programmed for the Monday or Tuesday, as the doctor is unable to perform at the weekend. This proves natural processes are denied, especially those of women. The other image represents the actual birth. The amount of eyes, the light … the uncomfortable room is intimidating and impersonal … The two hearts that have been beating as one in warm surroundings since the conception of the baby are now separated. There is so little respect for such a grand occasion that I feel that we are dealing with some form of violence.

(Giorgia Pezzoli, Art Therapist)

The handcuffs are a relevant symbol in this piece of work. The image is more elaborate than the rest of the remaining elements with regards to its shape and the details. The colouring is also more intense. Giorgia worked together with a partner in CEANIM organising Art Therapy workshops aimed at ten female inmates. Among them there was a 36-year-old woman who had given birth to her ninth child six months before. She participated actively, showed talent and motivation when drawing. She enjoyed the workshop: 'it was the opportunity for her to express what she could not say', says the therapist. Her work was detailed and depicted daily life in a prison. In one of the sessions, she drew herself giving birth while handcuffed (Figure 11.4).

Description: Paper format. 27 × 37.5cm. The author used graphite pencil and colours. The walls and the white and blue flooring are clearly marked.

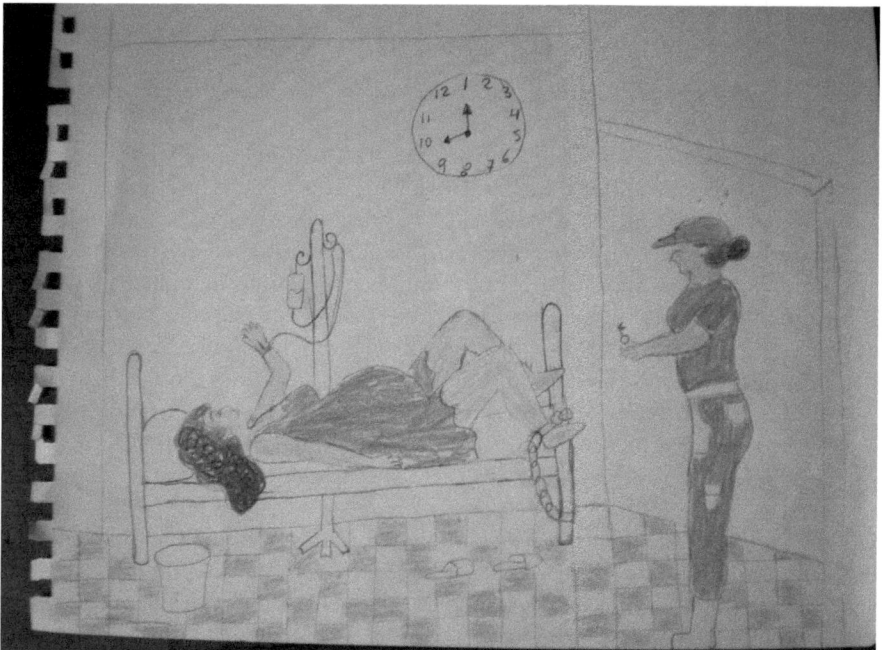

Figure 11.4 Work produced by female inmate, patient of Giorgia Pezzoli.

Another part of the room has been drawn that could represent a wall or a door. A bed and a pillow can be seen on the left which occupy a large proportion of the drawing. There is a bin and a pair of slippers at the bottom of the bed. On top of the bed, one can observe a pregnant woman with brown hair and an orange dress. She is lying down. Her legs are open and she is giving birth. One of her ankles is chained to the bed. The opposite wrist is connected to a drip. The clock above the bed indicates a precise time. A woman dressed in a police uniform holding the key to the chain or the handcuffs is standing close by.

The therapist aimed at condemning the violation of the rights of her patients. She received the support of the CEANIM:

> She had drawn herself giving birth while shackled, a police woman to her side and the door closed. Moreover, it is illegal to handcuff the mother during the delivery. This act of power is unjustified and as violating as the rest. It goes against the baby itself. I managed to talk to her after this: 'If this causes an impact, it will have been worth it then.' Together with CEANIM, I took the case to the government to show the images where supposedly those in power are literate and cultured. The only thing they said to me was 'this isn't real', 'what you've got in your drawing does not happen. What the participant drew does not occur.' The meeting was over. Together with CEANIM, we will return to the government. We want this to be publicised.
>
> (Giorgia Pezzoli, Art Therapist)

This experience led her to question her role as Art Therapist in a prison context:

> I questioned my work because I was unsure I was helping or harming. The use of power in a country such as Chile where the military uses it as it pleases is what I felt from the very first day I started working. They would open doors whenever, the police decided the ones who could participate. They would lose our equipment. There should be regulations in a place like this to oversee your work. It is a right. They restrict your actions. Materials and work produced would disappear. A lot of harm was done. Art Therapy is precious, it means freedom and openness. But wherever these concepts are oppressed, regrettably, it generates war. It's a fine line and I think it would prove beneficial to work on both sides, the inmate and the police officer.
>
> (Giorgia Pezzoli, Art Therapist)

Upon filing the complaint, the police retaliated against the inmate and excluded her from the workshop, they also separated her from her baby before the date legally stipulated. Giorgia insists on the existing legal framework to support the work of the therapists who work in closed institutions since these are not as clearly regulated and more inclined to committing forms of abuse against therapists and inmates. The image produced by the prisoner served to condemn violence and the violation of rights suffered. The reality of the image was not acknowledged by the authorities but its mere existence proves the fact that there is ongoing violence that needs to be dealt with. Justice needs to be done.

Discussion regarding the image, the body, the concept of violence and that of maternity

Our surrounding culture as well as public and private healthcare institutions show images of childbirth (in the form of advertising) that differ greatly from the existing violence suffered by a high percentage of pregnant women. Adverts visible in medical centres (web pages, leaflets or magazines) show calm and smiling women. Their partner is generally shown next to them. The professional seems friendly and caring. These images respond to the emotional state of the women and to what they would expect at such an important moment of their lives and that of their babies. Moreover, they expect and are certain that this will be the case since the centres are specialised in healthcare. This raises the following issue in institutions dedicated supposedly to providing care at childbirth. Indeed, the majority of mothers concerned are actually healthy individuals who will likely suffer some form of aggression or another.

The images sent out by our culture regarding childbirth are not real. They are idealised and do not warn of the high risk that women may suffer obstetric violence. Sometimes, close friends or relatives may tell women that this might happen. Our culture has excluded all aspects of violence and suffering experienced during pregnancy and at birth.

The workers interviewed showed existing forms of submission, manipulation, use and abuse of women at childbirth. They tackled the issue as women and as professionals specialising in this field of work, who feel healthcare personnel can be cold, unwelcoming and show limited empathy and patience. They think these personnel do not relate to the psychological and emotional dimensions of women. They consider they do not listen to them, see them or value them. Women are things not individuals: 'I worked in the public and private health care systems and both focus on production. Everything is about numbers, forcing to reach objectives meaning a decrease of empathy and communication. It's about quantity and not quality' (Andrea Gómez, nurse).

These professionals condemn the use of violence and the violation of the rights of women through the images they produce. They insist in fighting urgently for a change towards the eradication of these practices, in changing the mindsets responsible for what is really happening in Chile with regards to childbirth. They want to raise awareness among the personnel involved and wish for a greater humanisation of the staff concerned that has become part of the machinery. As Andrea Gómez witnessed in her position as nurse before and after having given birth: 'As healthcare practitioners, we have to make decisions and use our own judgement. We need to consider individuals as a whole. We are not trained to do that. We never deal with a more personal approach of our work'.

References

Betensky, M. 2001. Phenomenological Art Therapy. In J. A. Rubin (ed.), *Approaches to Art Therapy*. New York: Brunner-Routledge.

Bulletin 12148-11. 2018. *Bill that Establishes the Individual's Rights with Regards to Pregnancy, before Childbirth, during Childbirth, Postpartum, Abortion, Sexual and Gynaecological Issues*. Chamber of Deputies of Chile.

Carvajal, L., & Hernando, M. 2015. *Bill that Establishes the Rights of Women during Childbirth and Post Giving Birth as Well as Sanctions against Gynecological and Obstetric Violence*. Chamber of Deputies of Chile.

Ehrenreich, B., & English, D. 1984. *Brujas, comadronas y enfermeras. Historia de las sanadoras*. Barcelona: Ediciones La Sal.

Martin, E. 1987. *The Woman in the Body: A Cultural Analysis of Reproduction*. Boston: Beacon Press.

Oakley, A. 1992. *Social Support and Motherhood*. Oxford: Blackwell.

12 Artful trans-itions and the queering of pregnancy, birth and (m)othering

Sheridan Linnell and Asha Zappa

The material and cultural conditions of being pregnant and/or becoming-(m) other (at once self and other) swell our bodies and subjectivities beyond the persistent myth of a bounded individual identity, exceeding modernist definitions of what it means to be human. Despite being a dominant cultural expectation for women, the embodied and cultural experience of becoming-mother is, we suggest, trans-formative and intrinsically strange – even queer.[1]

At the same time, pregnancy, birth and early parenting are among the most regulated and psychologised of human experiences. This medicalisation of birthing has made some forms of agency possible while producing birthing bodies as what Rachel Chadwick describes as 'clockwork bodies' (Chadwick 2018, p. 50).

> [B]iomedical power does not just reside 'out there' … it is also an emergent, intersection, relational and ontological form of power produced by and entangled with local norms, cultural narratives, modes of technology, material institutions, sociocultural oppression and the materiality of birthing bodies.
>
> (Chadwick 2018, p. 51)

Biomedical power is materialised in equally complex and problematic ways in the discourses and practices of gender transition, where chemical and surgical intervention enables certain forms of agency but 'at a price'. This, we suggest, results not just in a doubling, but in an exponential increase in the operations of power in the lives, embodied experiences and sense of self of those trans people who wish to birth children. Paradoxically subjected to 'erasure' (Bauer et al. 2009) as (im)possible birthing subjects and yet regulated and produced as 'risky' birthing bodies, or categorised as 'unnatural individuals' when birth is rarely if ever 'natural' and never the work of one body alone, trans and other gender-non-conforming people who give birth are caught in an almost impossible contradictory ontological position.

Asha's story

Pregnancy forces mother *and* other, parent and growing child to exist in a liminal space – neither yet whole, yet both encompassing a vast potentiality. Who will we/they be? The question is not answered at birth, it takes a lifetime to unravel, yet we are so quick to ignore, and actively erase, parents whose narratives disrupt the accepted linearity.

When I became pregnant, I became a magician – the Great Disappearing Mother! I was still there, but I was no longer me. I was (m)other – a weird body open to public scrutiny, invasive questions. My living narrative not as important as my ability to fit an autobiographical trope of 'motherhood'. My strange, strained relationship with my body could only exist insofar as it fit with what was expected of a mother.

As a mother who isn't a woman, how can I exist? How can I be real in a world which still valorises binary genders, binary relationships and the hierarchies that enforce erasure?

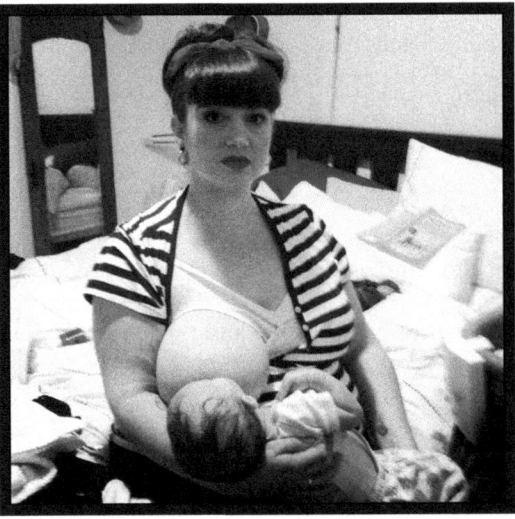

Figure 12.1 Self Portrait as (M)Other. Asha Zappa, digital photo, 2013.

Decentring tropes; queering narratives

Such contradictions are regularly erased or smoothed over in the growing number of personal and professional accounts of gender transition. There is a story we expect to read in trans bodies, a journey map of trouble, discomfort, exploration and eventual relief and liberation in 'the truth'. What McGregor (2014) terms 'trans autobiographical demand' (p. 3) is projected onto the bodies and minds of trans, non-binary, gender-independent (Pyne 2014) and gender fluid people. This linear narrative smooths over and threatens to erase the complexities and contradictions of non-conformity and queerness, restoring normative order to what might otherwise disrupt the time and place of 'our' lives.

Social norms require trans and gender-independent people to perform their narrative on-demand – to justify their existence through a lens of linear transition 'in order to explain away their difference from traditional conceptions of the stable, unalterable relationship between sex and gender' (McGregor 2014, p. 6). In our efforts to understand the journey of transition within dominant narrative tropes, we erase differences that could be more broadly transformative.

The notion of a stable, autonomous individual bounded by their own skin and bound to a linear narrative of individual progress is also radically de-centred by the experience of pregnancy itself. In what is otherwise a compelling but largely linear narrative of coming to accept and be transformed by her son's transition, Mimi Lemay captures something of this profound shock when she brings to life the embodied and emotional changes that seemed to rob her of her self as she knew it: 'I found that the heart that beat inside my chest was no longer my own … in a word, I'd been *hacked*' (Lemay 2019, pp. 1–2). For Lemay this 'loss of self' (p. 2) is prelude to a greater and more unexpected change in her 'middle child'. Indeed, Lemay is so entranced, with both the story of maternal attunement and the linear narrative trajectory of gender transition, that she expresses amazement that she missed 'the moment itself' (p. 3) when it all began – as if there were a singular point in time when she lost her daughter and very slowly began to discover her (trans) son. Nevertheless, that word 'hacked' speaks to us, as authors, of something radically decentring and queer about pregnancy itself, a sense of being 'thrown' that is further intensified when the pregnant body is not gendered female.

(Un)winding pathways to trans-parenthood

It is safe to say that trans and/or gender-independent people's experiences with the health system tend to be, at best, a minefield to be carefully navigated. Bauer et al. (2009) discuss the embedded, systemic nature of discrimination faced by trans people accessing healthcare, and the problematic, harmful outcomes this produces. Embedded discrimination takes many forms, but for trans people seeking to become parents, systemic, legislative barriers can provide a traumatic context through which people must navigate.

Although stories of trans and/or gender-independent parents are becoming more common, it is important to note that in many places across the world, sterilisation is a requirement for gender affirmation (Lee 2015), and in places where surgical affirmation is required for legal gender recognition, forced ster-ilisation is part of the process (Allen 2019). More than 30 European countries are reported to legally require forced sterilisation, and/or other practices such compulsory divorce of a partner, prior to granting legal recognition of a change of gender (Vale 2016). A client's path to parenthood may have been made all the more difficult and potentially traumatic, by the legal, as well as the social, context in which they live.

As for cisgendered people, there also exist many potential paths to parenthood for trans people, including 'natural' conception, fertility preservation (that is, the cryopreservation of gametes for future use), in-vitro fertilisation (IVF) and other assisted reproduction options, surrogacy, adoption, co-parenting and others. However, as with access to other parts of the health system, access for trans people to these options is severely limited.

It is extremely difficult, indeed often impossible, for trans people wishing to have a child to gain access to assistive technologies (Pyne 2013) or to adopt children (Pyne, Bauer & Bradley 2015). Moreover, 20 per cent of transitioning people who are already parents subsequently lose custody and/or are denied access to their children, often through the courts. Yet studies consistently suggest that it is parental conflict rather than transition itself that can have negative consequences for children of transitioning parents. Children of trans and queer parents are as healthy and happy as children of cisgender parents and (should it be of any concern, which of course we would question) are also no more likely than other children to be trans or queer (Pyne et al. 2015).

As more people are becoming aware of the benefits of allowing young people to live as their gender (Durwood, McLaughlin & Olson 2017), there is an increased need for knowledge around fertility preservation options, both in paediatrics generally, and specifically for those working with young trans people (Nahata, Curci & Quinn 2018, p. 123). Fertility preservation may also be a consideration for people who initiate medical gender affirmation in adulthood. However, it is important to note that there are access barriers faced by trans people wanting to access fertility preservation, including cost and the desire to not further delay medical transition (Riggs & Bartholomaeus 2018).

For trans men who wish to have children, pregnancy is an option. However, for those who have been taking testosterone to affirm their gender, becoming fertile requires cessation of testosterone. Considering the aforementioned difficulties in accessing medical care, and, for some, the hugely positive impact testosterone can have, the decision to cease hormones in order to conceive is not one taken lightly. In the documentary *Seahorse* (Finlay 2019), Freddy McConnell describes the difficulty of relating to his body in the absence of testosterone: 'Every time I think about it, I think, "What the fuck am I doing?" I feel like a fucking alien.'

Pregnant bodies are often experienced as both 'self and other'. Beyond this, trans pregnant bodies may, in fact, be experienced as 'other and other' through the profound discomfort and contradiction of temporarily reversing the trans-formation of the body you have fought to reclaim yours. To be dis-embodied and made other; and then for that alienated body to be inhabited by an-other who is nevertheless so desperately wanted, so intentionally created.

Asha's story

When we are pregnant, we give the developing child everything it needs to become itself – it is us, and it is other – we do not grow clones. Our entire body commits itself to the growing of a being. There's an old saying 'for each child, a tooth' – our bodies leech the calcium from our bones and teeth in order to provide enough for the growing foetus. Once they are no longer reliant on our bodies for everything, they are reliant on us to provide a safe place for them to be themselves.

If for cis pregnancies each child is a tooth, what cost to the trans male parent in becoming pregnant? And just as many cis parents would gleefully pull every tooth from their skull for their children, so, too, do many trans male parents gleefully make changes to their bodies. Difficulty does not equal resentment.

Though trans women do not experience pregnancy, they still become parents, and providing options for – and increasing the accessibility of – fertility preservation ensures that as many as possible paths to parenthood are open. And although there is less visibility around trans women who become parents, the challenges are still very real, including delaying or ceasing hormones and other medical treatments in order to produce and preserve sperm. This can impact not only emotional wellbeing but can have a genuine impact on safety. Trans women, particularly trans women of colour, disproportionately experience violence (Human Rights Campaign 2019), and trans women report their appearance – particularly with regards to whether or not they are read by the public as trans – has an impact on the way people interact with them (Blanchard 2019). Being able to 'pass' is in some contexts a prerequisite for trans women being allowed to live safely or even at all, and this capacity may be jeopardised by suspending chemical transition.

For people who are gender-independent, gender-queer, non-binary and other identities that do not 'conform' to binary notions of gender, the issues meld into complexity – in some instances pathways are clearer, in others far more difficult to traverse. The lack of representation and acknowledgement, and the constant reinforcement of binary gender – especially within the context of health systems, which are practically impossible to avoid in the pursuit of pregnancy and parenthood – serve as a constant erasure, a reminder of what is considered 'legitimate'. Having an understanding of the paths to parenthood – the difficulties, the discrimination – allows us as therapists to ensure that the burden of educating us is not placed on our clients.

Labour/labouring

Labour – perhaps a pregnant body experiences it, safe to say that most do, although not all. An intense physical experience we are, generally speaking, expected to endure. Labour denotes work, and as we emerge from the experience, covered in sweat and blood, exhausted, the work we have done is made visible – our work, our labour, plain to see.

But what of the invisible labour: those labours, which may not cause us to lose physical blood, but those which cause pain and exhaustion just the same? Emotional labour – as originally defined – is when an individual has to 'induce or suppress feeling in order to sustain the outward countenance that produces the proper state of mind in others' (Hochschild 2012, p. 7). In expecting the client to educate the therapist (or perhaps even satisfy some curiosity), the burden of emotional labour is placed on the client – contributing to the client's experience of both erasure and microaggressions.

Blumer, Gavriel Ansara and Watson (2013) discuss how therapists' underlying gender-based assumptions can influence their perception of family dynamics – how sometimes the framework of our practice is inadequate; attempting to fit a trans client into a binaristic, cis-centred framework may render invisible the client's truth. (This isn't to say that such frameworks are never useful, but they are at best incomplete.) This 'invisibilising' reinforces a narrative of normative versus non-normative, and forces 'non-normative' families into 'practicing visibility management' (Blumer et al. 2013, p. 273).

Zappa (2016) suggests that, through understanding the socio-cultural context of our work, we can reduce the burden of labour and education for our clients and 'make space for families far removed from "the norm" without pathologising them' (p. 53). And this, perhaps, is the key – that we allow our clients to bring whatever they bring, without placing a burden of self-justification on them. That we bring, instead, an awareness of our own bias, up*bring*ing, (mis)understandings, and consciously hold them so that our clients do not have to. Knowing what oppression we may replicate through our own cultural lens is challenging but essential to our work (Zappa 2017).

Sheridan's story

Looking back at my own responses over 30 years ago to my first transgender client, I'm sorry to say that I at first confused sexuality and gender. I initially asked insensitive questions about whether he might possibly be lesbian (if only he had access to the inner-city bars and clubs of Oxford Street, Sydney as I did). It 'did my head in' when he stepped forward to open the therapy room door for me, when I was uncomfortable with any man doing so. Yet this client opened the door for me in more ways than one. He was generous and patient with my misunderstandings – and indeed he had little choice about whom to see in that particular time and location. When I saw how my misrecognitions and assumptions pained him, I began to self-correct, but I wish I had not put him in that position in the first place.

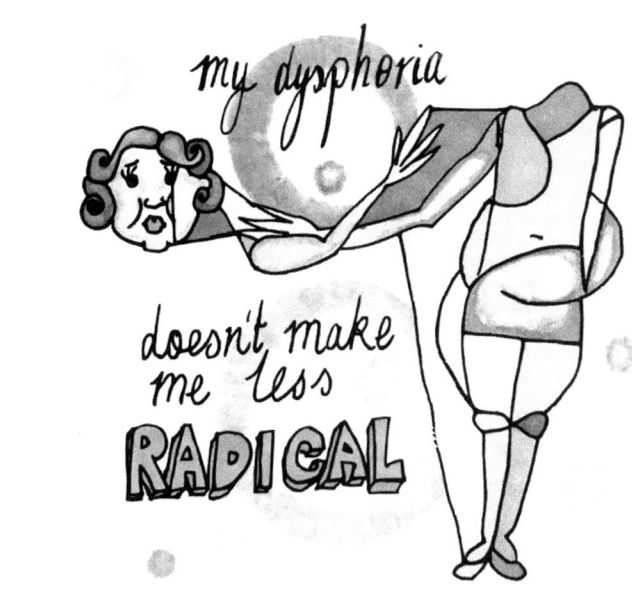

Figure 12.2 Dysphoria. Asha Zappa, copic marker on cardstock, 2017.

Linearity/Liminality

Queering the notions of pregnancy, childbirth and early parenting so as to ever-so-slightly loosen the knot that binds 'reproduction' to the reproduction of the normative world is potentially transformative. Shifting 'mother' from noun to verb, we suggest that a female body and identity is not necessarily intrinsic to the project of mothering. As people who have a commitment to the legacy of feminism in our lives, we also acknowledge the tensions in de-gendering the experience of birth, given women's historical and ongoing attempts to regain control of birthing from conservative elements of the medical establishment. Gender is complicated and requires complex theorisations – thinking that does not elide one category simply because another is more marginalised. Theories of intersectionality (e.g., Talwar 2018) go some way toward addressing these tensions, and it may be that the new materialisms (Barad 2007) can take us even further. In the latter view, birth itself is not the isolated work of one woman but rather an assemblage of every*body* and every*thing* (Chadwick 2018) that makes birthing imaginable and possible. The places, materials and processes of birth are its agents alongside birthing bodies. As a therapeutic and material practice in which relationships with place, making, materials (see Fenner 2017) and visualities are as crucial as relationships between human participants, Art Therapy can become a helpful agent in extending the conceptualisation of such birthing assemblages.

This isn't 'us versus them' – it isn't, and has never been, 'the queers versus the straights' – it's an invitation for all of us to deconstruct the systems which, in a thousand ways, big and small, restrict and erase us all. We don't need to be trans, gender-independent or queer to queer Art Therapy. Art Therapists are particularly well positioned to find *artful* ways to challenge conventional notions and complex intersections of gender, sexuality, pregnancy, birth and mothering.

Given that 'experiences of queer reproduction particularly lack visual schema' (Holland 2019, p. 5), there is a clear role for Art Therapy in making the pregnancy, birth and parenting experiences of queer and trans people visible, recognisable and negotiable for themselves and others. Art Therapy, like other visually oriented methods can 'challenge expectations of how gendered bodies should move through space, interact with one another, and present themselves in relation to gendered, familial, and reproductive discourses that are also racialized, classed, and embodied' (Holland 2019, p. 7).

Furthermore, Art Therapists' unique expertise in *therapeutic* engagement through the arts can enable queer and trans people to experience strong and sustained support as they come face to face with the pain of what dominant discourses of gender and sexuality have attempted to erase in their lives and sense of identity. Art Therapy potentially already 'queers' the medical model of therapy – it removes the hierarchy of 'expert therapist and sick client' by bringing the art, the process, the creativity to the work. It re-centres clients as experts. This kind of practice has an inherent (theoretical) queerness and can help to 'deconstruct heteronormativity and binaries that constrict what is considered normal and healthy expressions of being human' (McDowell, Emerick & Garcia 2014, p. 100).

Making unexpected critical and creative connections between embodied experiences of pregnancy and motherhood and the experiences of trans and queer bodies continues the practice of questioning of hetero and gender normativity in Art Therapy (Hogan 2002, 2019; Ellis 2007; Zappa 2016) and can be understood as part of a wider radical tradition of troubling the patriarchal, Western discourse of the autonomous, self-sufficient individual (Linnell 2010).

As Art Therapists we can continually put the hetero and gender normative assumptions of our profession 'under erasure' so as not to inadvertently erase the lived experiences and narratives of those who consult us. This includes examining our favoured and implicit theories. While the position of psychoanalysis as the theoretical antecedent of Art Therapy has been effectively disputed (Hogan 2001), it remains crucial to challenge how the residue of normative psychoanalytic accounts reconstructs the normative time and place of the nuclear family as universally true, and as the model for early infant development and parenting. A similar critique can be made of the ubiquitous use of attachment theory (Linnell 2010) and Western developmental theories (Moss 2019).

Sheridan's story

Part of my Art Therapy training in the early 1990s was foundational studies in psychotherapy, with an emphasis on Klein, object relations and the British Independent School. Much emphasis was put on early maternal/mother–infant relations. I had come from being the clinical coordinator of a feminist service for survivors of childhood sexual assault into a territory where Mother was sometimes capitalised (upon) and usually to blame. One of my first jolts into awareness of the strange planet upon which I had landed was reading: 'Each one of us has sat on mother's knee to smile at father and been held over father's shoulder to make eyes at mother' (Padel 1986 p. 172).

'But that's meant symbolically, Sheridan', protested the instructor, whom I really liked, and who until that moment had regarded me as promising. Adept at translating this patriarchal gook into something digestible, she seemed disappointed that I had turned out to be such a concrete thinker.

But then there was *this*, relegated to a footnote that sought to erase my own recognisability and viability as a same-sex attracted mother:

> The symbolic equation (in Freud's sense of the phrase) of self with parental genital is one of the regular identifications made in child-hood. Perhaps the difficulty in making such an identification should be a strong reason against the bringing up of a child by a lesbian couple.
>
> (Padel 1986, p. 169)

Surely, I pleaded, this showed that the supposedly 'symbolic' has a direct implication for clinical and social practice?

Just a few years later, Noreen O'Connor and Joanna Ryan drew similar attention to Padel's and others' 'dire warnings' (O'Connor & Ryan 1994, p. 237) against lesbian parenting, framing them as empirically baseless (see also Dempsey 2013), clinically compromising and driven by a gendered, binary opposition that marks the dominant psychoanalytic understanding of identification and sexuality.

This seductive image of the nuclear, heteronormative and cisgender family continues to have purchase in both obvious and unexpected ways. As Lauren Berlant suggests:

> Even though the shapes desire takes can be infinite, one plot dominates scenes of proper fantasy and expectation. It is a plot in which the patterns of infantile desire develop into a love plot that will be sutured by the institutions of intimacy and the fantasy of familial continuity that links historical pasts to futures through kinship chains worked out in smooth ongoing relations.
>
> (Berlant 2012, p. 55)

Such 'smooth stories' and constraining plotlines can also come to dominate apparently progressive accounts of queer and trans lives and relationships. In view of this, Ulrika Dahl argues "we must move beyond addressing hetero-normativity and begin studying how gender, sexuality, race and class get re-produced in queer kinship stories" (Dahl 2018, p. 1030). Dahl's study shows how the extraordinary social progress, whereby highly educated white, cisgendered middle-class Swedish women have moved in less than a decade from being considered sexual deviants to being exemplars of healthy, progressive mother-hood, has in itself become normative and minimising of other forms of difference, through the rise of a discourse of lesbian motherhood that she names 'becoming fertile'. This is embodied in the expression and enactment of desires by queer and trans subjects to become 'real' biologically reproductive women, and exemplified in an award-winning Swedish commercial where a Swedish skiing champion, her wife and their infant child star in a pastoral fable of progress that celebrates able-bodied white women, feminism, fertility and organic milk (Herthoni 2015).

Respectability, and the notion of the normal on which it depends, may be upheld by a middle-class logic of reproductive temporality. Judith Jack Halberstam proposes that a 'queer adjustment in the way we think about time, in fact requires and produces new conceptions of space' (Halberstam 2005, p. 6). The apparently innocuous formula of 'family time' takes on a regulatory aspect in Halberstam's account of heteronormativity. With pregnancy, birth and early parenting already subject to multiple developmental, psychological and medical discourses that work to regulate the time and place of normative reproduction, the queering of time and interruption of smooth, linear narratives of human development may be crucial in creating a space for difference.

It would be unwise, however, to entirely disavow the value of 'stories about who one is and what one wants, stories to which one clings so as to be able to re-encounter oneself as solid' (Berlant 2012, p. 76). For many people who come to therapy, restoring 'the self as narrative coherence' (Williams & Linnell 2006) and as recognisable by self and others may be the necessary antidote to a symbolic, or even actual, death. Halberstam themself (2005) suggests that identity politics are problematic yet to a degree necessary. S/he makes a strong case for a queer space and time between and beyond postmodern fluidity and modern fixity, and between and beyond academic scholarship on gender and the lived experiences of queer communities and individuals. Even gender fluidity can become another smooth, white story, and prescribing it might in some instances be no better than other more obviously normative prescriptions. The plotlines of therapy, too, can inadvertently reproduce milky-smooth, linear stories, othering the lives of clients, even in the attempt to disrupt normative discourses.

Stories from our communities

J and his father A are dear friends of one of the authors of this chapter who live in an outer suburb of a major Australian city. J and A (who asked to be known by their initials) told us many stories of how J's 'transition' had been transformative for them both. It is significant in retelling excerpts of these stories that the intimacy of friendship has cut through the professional distance that usually organises the time and space of our work as clinicians and researchers. It is also significant that while many aspects of their lives are unconventional, J and A are not especially interested or engaged with queer scholarship.

When Sheridan asked J what might assist parents of very young children to be open around the possibilities of gender, he thought deeply.

J's story

While I don't want to tell anyone they can't call their baby 'he' or 'she' or a gendered name, I wish we could drop the gendered words and products. Instead of having boys' toys and girls' toys we could let kids be kids. There are so many ways to go about your life that are not about being cisgender and white. But there is a lot of weight put on birth sex and a lot of expectations put on you from the beginning to conform with that, whether you like it or not. It's not easy or good for any kid to have those [normative] expectations about gender put on them, but it is especially hard for transgender kids...

When I went to see a therapist in my late teens, I already knew I wanted to medically transition. We didn't have much money so I saw this guy locally through the public system. He seemed nice but then asked me really invasive, upsetting and specific questions about sex, masturbation and genitals at a time that I could not even bear to think about my body. I thought I had to answer his questions or I would not be allowed to transition. I think he was trying to get at something about how bad experiences with men might have made me want to be one so I didn't have to have sex with them, or something...? Then my parents paid for me to see an expert in the city through the private health system but surprisingly he was just as bad – he insisted on calling me by my cisgender name and recording me in his records as female. I had to put up with him and answer his questions, because he had the power to refer me on for hormone therapy, as he eventually did.

My advice to Art Therapists would be – basic respect goes a long way. Get yourself educated about queer and trans people and also remember we are not all the same. Ask us what it is OK to ask about, and what we would like to be called.

Meanwhile, J's father told a story that organised his son's and his own transformation into linear time and gender binaries but also questioned the production of meaning this involves.

A's story

To be really honest, when [my wife] fronted me with the fact that J wanted to transition, at first I was aghast. I thought, but I'm fine with 'her' being gay. But then I did my research and realised this wasn't a passing fashion and it wasn't about sexuality – it was about gender. And as soon as we really believed and supported J and accepted his ideas, things changed. We went from having a kid who was depressed and very suicidal, who we were frightened we might lose at any moment, to having a kid who was really happy and 100 per cent, well, 'normal'. So I have done a 100 per cent turnaround. As the father of a trans kid I want to say to other parents – be open from the very beginning to who your kids are. Always and unconditionally. Put your kids' health and safety and happiness first, not some bigoted fundamentalist religion – that's sick, it puts transgender kids at risk of suicide and makes me so angry.

   When they are born you are just happy that they are them, and you want them to grow fully into who they are, even if you don't yet know what that is. Of course I would have been completely content with two daughters, and at the same time I'm delighted to get to know the son that I did not expect to have.

While therapists would have far less work to do if all parents of trans and gender-independent kids were as open as A, for this family too, lack of social recognition and the social embeddedness of gender regulation was so annihilating that J came close to annihilating himself. Part of what sustained J through his child-hood and adolescence was rendered in vivid visual description – wearing cord jeans and Lynx deodorant, imagining himself as a boy and the ambivalent pain and joy of being (mis)recognised as such by his peers, well before the category of trans male became discursively available to him. But the apparently linear stories of gender in the accounts of J and A were not entirely smooth. A, for instance, pondered the difficulty of ascribing a gender based on normative notions of what is 'natural' for boys and girls and wondered aloud if he had reordered events into an explanatory, linear sequence. He articulated with irony and wonder the notion that gender transition has transformed his child into someone 'normal', a word that remains under erasure in A's story. Meanwhile, J's story embraced the available cultural signifiers of masculinity; at the same time as he would prefer a world where children are not ascribed an essentialised gender at all.

That advice we were not going to give...

The complexities and contradictions in the stories we have told in this chapter suggest that there can be no prescription for how to conduct Art Therapy with trans and/or gender-independent people, and that we need to support their desires and practices around pregnancy, birth and parenting, while resisting approaches that would regulate trans lives into the normative times and spaces of reproduction. In order not to invert – and thereby reproduce – the shape of normalising power, we as Art Therapists need to both respect the longing on the part of some of those who consult us for respectability and normalcy, and to support clients in the making of images and narratives that challenge norms and radically widen that which is recognised and respected.

These seem such simple and basic requirements – respect, recognition; images and narratives with which to identify; being seen for whom one is and can become. But J's stories of the therapy available to him show that these basic relational elements are not routinely afforded to trans people who seek professional help. Meanwhile the inherently queer processes of pregnancy, birth and parenting remain among the most closely medicalised, regulated and ordered of human experiences. When these domains converge into the lives of queer and especially trans subjects there is an amplified possibility for at best insensitive, at worse abusive therapy practices that, we would argue, it is both a responsibility and an opportunity as Art Therapists to refuse.

Both authors of this chapter are Art Therapists and birth mothers who in different ways have incidentally and/or intentionally resisted the linearity of 'repro-time' (Halberstam 2005). As such we do not assume that other Art Therapists are necessarily coming from a heteronormative or cisnormative positioning. Both of us are and/or have known other people who have raised children in same sex or gender diverse relationships with or without an identified known 'father'; and indeed this has in many respects become part of the 'new normal'. At the more radical edge of our understanding there are trans men in our personal and professional lives who have suspended their hormone therapy in order to become pregnant – who give birth to and breastfeed a child who may subsequently know them as Dad.

None of this experience gives us licence to advise others how to live or tell other Art Therapists how to work. Our intention in this chapter is not, predominantly, to make recommendations for how Art Therapists could best support queer people through pregnancy, childbirth and parenting, and elsewhere we have attempted to disrupt the ubiquity of the individual case study in Art Therapy literature (Linnell 2019). Nevertheless we know, as Art Therapy educators and clinicians, how frustrating it can be when looking for practice guidelines and there are none to be found. In some ways practice recommendations can be summed up in the word 'respect' – but what are the specific practices of respect in this context? So, we will not only refuse the linearity of the story of gender transformation – although we acknowledge and honour those whose stories follow a linear narrative; we also double back on our own intentions and offer some tentative suggestions for practice that we have found useful, alongside our more theoretical and autoethnographic exploration. (Contradiction, in a queer methodological approach, is, we suggest, not a contra-indication but rather a strategy).

- Use gender-inclusive or gender-neutral language in written information, intake forms, reports, referrals and notes and encourage the institutions you work for to do the same.
- Don't assume that someone isn't – or is – queer or trans.
- Don't assume that all queer and trans people want to be known as queer and/

or trans. If someone wants or needs to 'pass' that's their decision. Please don't label it as 'denial'. If you are cisgender or heterosexual (or white, or able-bodied…), are you obliged to declare that to everyone at every opportunity?

- Ask how someone prefers to be named, known and described. Where possible and/or preferred, use the pronoun 'they'.
- Acknowledge the social and economic difficulties and profoundly negative social and psychological effects of 'erasure' for queer and especially for trans people (Bauer et. al. 2009) and how this can create issues that bring them to therapy, rather than seeing their gender or sexuality as the problem.
- Relocate and externalise 'gender dysphoria' as a problem of the 'social body' rather than of trans bodies. (Perhaps dysphoria is consequent to living in a dystopia?)
- Mediate between a non-directive stance that allows people 'free expression' and the possibility that expression is always-already bound to the available discursive and visual repertoires.
- Expand the discursive and visual repertoire of Art Therapy practice by offering collage materials with queer-friendly, gender-inclusive, gender-diverse and gender non-specific imagery and text. (If you live in a major city of some countries you could wander up the equivalent of Oxford or King Streets in Sydney, Australia and collect free newspapers, handouts and flyers. You can wander through internet sites and download images. You need to remember though that queer lives are diverse and that not everyone identifies with Western inner-city queer cultures and their signifiers. You could offer alternatives from within diverse traditional and alternative cultures of ethnicity, class sexuality and gender. You can assist people to research their preferred images and language. If you or they live and work in a place where being so explicit is dangerous, you can offer ways to work symbolically and can acknowledge the danger of doing otherwise…).
- Allow for the possibility that young trans people may or may not want to be (birth) parents one day and be prepared to discuss how technology could assist them not to foreclose on that possibility.
- However well-informed you are, and whatever your own experience with sexuality and gender, *prepare to be surprised*.

Asha's story

I can't remember a time when I wasn't fascinated by masks and makeup. I remember attempting to make commedia dell'arte masks from papier-mâché; staying up until the early hours as a teen with my drag queen friends doing each other's' makeup. It felt right, it felt true. After becoming a mother, masks came back into my therapeutic art practice – trying, desperately, to find some truth in representation. To be seen, by myself, by others. To liberate myself from feminine notions of beautiful/beatific motherhood – lies that for me caused pain and exhaustion – and to embrace the delicious grotesquery of my (m)otherness. At the same time engaging in a kind of self-destruction and reconstruction. Becoming mother, but also mothering myself in a way I never could have been as a child. Nurturing my capacity to nurture, making space where my little self could safely explore, and destroy, and remake, a complicated gender. There is an awful/awe-full power in actively rejecting a system which assures you that you don't exist.

The experience of my gender can no more be removed from my body than my experience of becoming a (m)other – the feelings embedded in my body, my muscles and bones straining to break out. I plunge my hands into paint, clay, sand, let them rip through as though I were able to tear off my own skin, to be free. This is not new, or unique. How many times have I sat with clients – cisgendered and not – and sat with them through those same feelings. Holding space for their other-ness. In allowing our clients the safety to be "other" without being 'othered', are we not actively mothering them? Replicating the deepest attachment of child and mother.

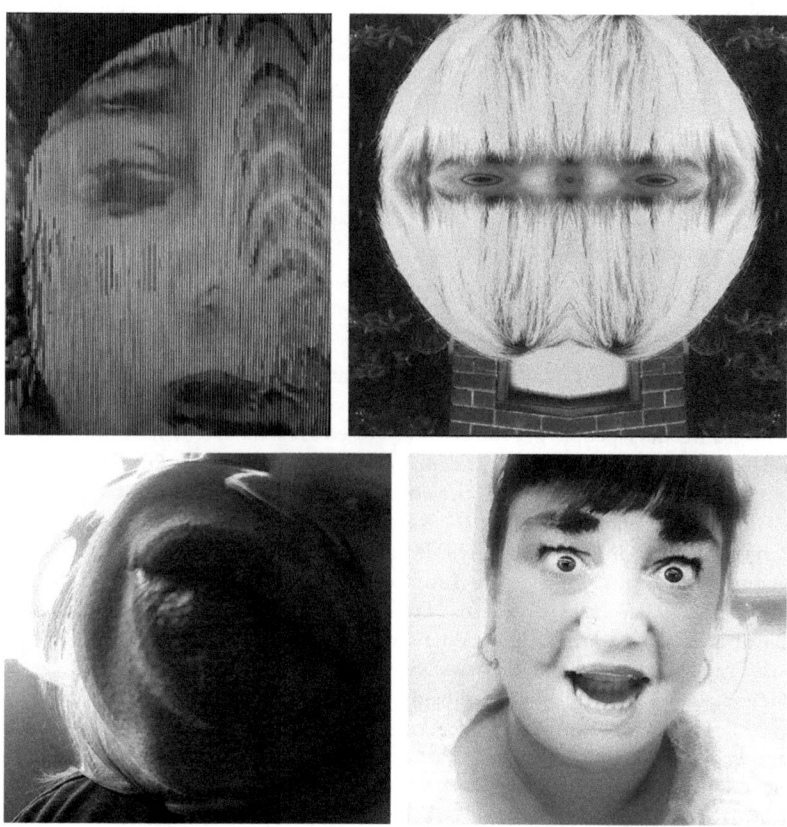

Figure 12.3 Selfie Portraits (Series). Asha Zappa, digital photographs and video stills, 2018.

As Asha's stories suggest, what is asked of therapists and of parents is symmetrical, albeit performed differently in the domains of parenting and Art Therapy, and can fold back into the nurturing we offer not only each other but ourselves.

Art Therapy itself is pregnant with transformative possibilities. Materially and discursively, it *matters*. If as Art Therapists we can remain open – *both* to practising an immanent critique of normative assumptions including their more subtly constraining inversions *and* to how our clients take up their lives within expanding repertoires of images and stories – we have at our fingertips the capacity to imagine and 'real-ise' a world of difference. Working together with our clients we can co-create a queer time and space to nurture rich, diverse and sustainable lives.

Acknowledgements

We acknowledge the Gadigal and Wangal Peoples of the Eora Nation, and the Burramattagal people of the Darug Nation, the traditional custodians of the lands on which we live and work. We offer our respects to the elders past and present.

Note

1 This chapter assumes a basic knowledge of queer-friendly, gender neutral and non-binary terminology. For a glossary of queer-friendly, gender neutral and non-binary terms, please see Hogan (2019).

References

Allen, S. 2019. It's Not Just Japan. Many US States Require Transgender People Get Sterilized. Available at: www.thedailybeast.com/its-not-just-japan-many-us-states-require-transgender-people-get-sterilized (accessed December 2019).

Barad, K. 2007. *Meeting the Universe Halfway: Quantum Physics and the Entanglement of Matter and Meaning*. Durham, NC: Duke University Press.

Bauer, G. R., Hammond, R., Travers, R., Kaay, M., Hohenadel, K. M., & Boyce, M. 2009. 'I Don't Think This Is Theoretical; This Is Our Lives': How Erasure Impacts Health Care for Transgender *People*. *Journal of the Association of Nurses in AIDS Care*, 20(5): 348–361.

Berlant, L. 2012. *Desire/Love*. Brooklyn, NY: Punctum Books.

Blanchard, S. K. 2019. Transgender Women Explain What It's Like When They Don't 'Look Trans'. *Vice*. Available at: www.vice.com/en_au/article/vb99dm/transgender-women-explain-what-its-like-when-they-dont-look-trans (accessed April 2020).

Blumer, M. L., Gavriel Ansara, Y., & Watson, C. M. 2013. Cisgenderism in Family Therapy: How Everyday Clinical Practices Can Delegitimize People's Gender Self-Designations. *Journal of Family Psychotherapy*, 24(4): 267–285.

Chadwick, R. 2018. *Bodies that Birth: Vitalizing Birth Politics*. Abingdon, Oxon: Routledge.

Dahl, U. 2018. Becoming Fertile in the Land of Organic Milk: Lesbian and Queer Reproductions of Femininity and Motherhood in Sweden. *Sexualities*, 2(7): 1021–1038.

Dempsey, S. 2013. *Same-Sex Parented Families in Australia*. Child Family Community Information Exchange Australia (CFCA) Paper no. 18. Accessed at: https://aifs.gov.au/cfca/publications/same-sex-parented-families-australia (accessed October 2019).

Durwood, L., McLaughlin, K. A., & Olson, K. R. 2017. Mental Health and Self-Worth in Socially Transitioned Transgender Youth. *Journal of the American Academy of Child & Adolescent Psychiatry*, 56(2): 116–123.

Ellis, M. L. 2007. Images of Sexualities: Language and Embodiment in Art Therapy. *International Journal of Art Therapy*, 12(2): 60–68.

Fenner, P. 2017. Art Therapy: Places, Forces, Flows, Matter and Becoming. *Art Therapy Online*, 8(1).

Finlay, J. 2019. *Seahorse*. A. Einsiedel (Producer), Grain Media, United Kingdom.

Halberstam, J. 2005. *In a Queer Time and Place: Transgender Bodies, Subcultural Lives*. New York and London: New York University Press.

Herthoni, L. 2015. *ARLA: The Land of Organic Milk*. Folke Film. Available at: https://vimeo.com/135063554 (accessed 6 December 2019).

Hochschild, A. R. 2012. *The Managed Heart: Commercialization of Human Feeling*. Berkeley, CA: University of California Press.

Hogan, S. 2001. *Healing Arts: The History of Art Therapy*. London: Jessica Kingsley Publishers.

Hogan, S., ed. 2002. *Gender Issues in Art Therapy*. London: Jessica Kingsley Publishers.

Hogan, S., ed. 2019. *Gender and Difference in Art Therapy: Inscribed on the Body*. London and New York: Routledge.

Holland, S. 2019. Pregnant with Possibility: The Importance of Visual Data in (Re)presenting Queer Women's Experiences of Reproduction. *Methodological Innovations*, January– April: 1–11.

Human Rights Campaign. 2019. Violence against the Transgender Community in 2019. Available at: www.hrc.org/resources/violence-against-the-transgender-community-in-2019 (accessed January 2020).

Lee, R. 2015. Forced Sterilization and Mandatory Divorce: How a Majority of Council of Europe Member States' Laws Regarding Gender Identity Violate the Internationally and Regionally Established Human Rights of Trans People. *Berkeley Journal of International Law*, 33: 114–152.

Lemay, M. 2019. *What We Will Become: A Mother, a Son, and a Journey of Transformation*. Boston, MA: Houghton Mifflin Harcourt.

Linnell, S. 2010. *Art Psychotherapy and Narrative Therapy: An Account of Practitioner Research*. Thousand Oaks, CA: Bentham Science Publishers.

Linnell, S 2019. Inter-Mission: An Enactment of How Art Psychotherapy and Narrative Therapy Shaped Teamwork and Therapeutic Practice in a Community-Based Counselling Service for Young People in Western Sydney. In A. Gilroy, S. Linnell, T. McKenna, & J. Westwood (eds.), *Art Therapy in Australia: Taking a Postcolonial, Aesthetic Turn*. Netherlands: Brill Sense, pp. 341–359.

McDowell, T., Emerick, P., & Garcia, M. 2014. Queering Couple and Family Therapy Education. *Journal of Feminist Family Therapy*, 26(2): 99–112.

McGregor, V. M. 2014. *Trans Temporality: Narrative, History, and Time*. Unpublished PhD thesis, University of Sydney, Sydney.

Moss, M. 2019. From Broken Circles to Different Identities: An Exploration of Identity for Children in Out-of-Home Care. In A. Gilroy, S. Linnell, T. McKenna, & J. Westwood (eds.), *Art Therapy in Australia: Taking a Postcolonial, Aesthetic Turn*. Leiden, Netherlands: Brill Sense, pp. 283–319.

Nahata, L., Curci, M. B., & Quinn, G. P. 2018. Exploring Fertility Preservation Intentions among Transgender Youth. *Journal of Adolescent Health*, 62(2): 123–125.

O'Connor, N. & Ryan, J. 1993. *Wild Desires and Mistaken Identities: Lesbianism and Psychoanalysis*. New York: Karner Books.

Padel, J. 1986, 'Ego in current thinking', In G Kohon (Ed) *The British School of psychoanalysis: the independent tradition*. Free Association Books, London, pp 154-172.

Peterson, C. 2013. The Lies that Bind: Heteronormative Constructions of 'Family' in Social Work Discourse. *Journal of Gay & Lesbian Social Services*, 25(4): 486–508.

Pyne, J. 2013. Complicating the Truth of Gender: Gender Literacy and the Possible Worlds of Trans Parenting. In F. Green & M. Friedman (eds.), *Chasing Rainbows: Exploring Gender Fluid Parenting Practices*. Toronto: New Demeter Press, pp. 127–144.

Pyne, J. 2014, Gender Independent Kids: A Paradigm Shift in Approaches to Gender Non-Conforming Children. *The Canadian Journal of Human Sexuality*, 23(1): 1–8.

Pyne, J., Bauer, G., & Bradley, K. 2015, Transphobia and Other Stressors Impacting Trans Parents. *Journal of GLBT Family Studies*, 11(2): 107–126.

Riggs, D. W., & Bartholomaeus, C. 2018. Fertility Preservation Decision Making amongst Australian Transgender and Non-Binary Adults. *Reproductive Health*, 15(1): article no. 181.

Talwar, S., ed. 2018. *Art Therapy for Social Justice: Radical Intersections*. New York: Routledge.

Vale, S. 2016. Forced and Coerced Sterilization: The Nightmare of Transgender and Intersex Individuals. *Impakter*. Available at: https://impakter.com/forced-and-coerced-sterilization-an-unnecessary-intervention-in-transgender-and-intersex-individuals/ (accessed December 2019).

Williams, C., & Linnell, S. 2006. 'When the Doctors Consulted the Narrative Therapist…' An Experiment in Questioning Dominant Stories of PhD Pedagogy. *The International Journal of Critical Psychology*, 18: 56–80.

Zappa, A. 2016. What's Blood Got to do with it? A Queer Exploration of the Genogram and its Application in Art Therapy. *ANZJAT: Australian and New Zealand Journal of Arts Therapy*, 11(1): 49–55.

Zappa, A. 2017. Beyond Erasure: The Ethics of Art Therapy Research with Trans and Gender-Independent *People. Art Therapy*, 34(3): 129–134.

13 Mothering mothers

An exploration of self-referred, self-funded, six-week Art Therapy groups for new mothers

Ros Taylor

Introduction

New motherhood can bring joy and positive expectations. It can also be a time of great struggle and turbulence. A shift in identity and relationships, hormonal changes, sleep deprivation, difficulties breastfeeding, experiences of traumatic births and a lack of community and social support creates a perfect storm for anxiety, depression and loneliness to set in. It has been reported that up to 20 per cent of women develop a mental illness during pregnancy or within the first year of their child's birth (Bauer et al. 2014, p. 3). Given this, and in spite of sound research findings that show long-term potential benefits to the mother and the child (Maselko et al. 2011; Oakley 1992; Oakley, Hickey & Rajan 1996, cited in Hogan, Sheffield & Woodward 2017, p. 171), there is currently very little in the way of routinely available support services for new mothers (Hogan 2008, 2012; Hogan et al. 2017). In the National Maternity Review (2016), many women said the care and support they received throughout their pregnancy had not continued into the postnatal period (Hogan et al. 2017). Eisenberg, Murkoff and Hathaway (1989, p. 546) describe the transition from pregnancy to motherhood as 'the reverse Cinderella', where 'the pregnant princess has become the postpartum peasant' with a 'wave of the obstetrician's wand'.

What is available in the way of provision for new mothers appears to be polarised, with a stark gap between inpatient mother and baby units for the very unwell and mother and baby drop-ins, which don't offer a suitable space to discuss difficult issues, emotional support or the opportunity for self-reflection, and where the focus is often only on the baby. This echoes what Sacks (2017) describes as the 'false-binary' that women are often left with after giving birth: 'They either have postpartum depression or they should breeze through the transition to motherhood' (Sacks 2017).

Having recently had my second child and familiar with the peaks and troughs of new motherhood, the importance of community and the extent to which art making can enable the expression of emotions, I imagined the potential powerfulness of Art Therapy groups for new mothers. I sought to set up groups with the aim of providing a safe space to support the wellbeing of new mothers, giving them the opportunity through art making and discussion to explore their feelings and personal experiences around pregnancy, birth and motherhood.

The literature

Hogan, Sheffield, and Woodward (2017) deliver a comprehensive review of the literature for perinatal art-based interventions and suggest that further research is needed to address the clinical efficacy and economic viability of such measures. They state:

> [T]here is a small evidence base emerging that points to the usefulness of art therapy during pregnancy and in the transition to motherhood. Social support is a crucial factor in women's ability to manage this transition and art therapy group based interventions, in particular, have been shown to improve women's self-confidence and self-esteem in ways that allow them to mediate the other stressors associated with new motherhood. The use of art making for self-reflection leading to greater self-knowledge is highlighted by several studies and linked to reductions in self-criticism. A small number of studies report on work with mother-infant dyads and report improved relationships and self-confidence in mothers.
>
> (Hogan et al. 2017, p. 175)

Within the literature there is very little that addresses the use of Art Therapy in post-natal care. An exception is Hogan (2003, 2008, 2012) who has documented a number of Art Therapy group-based interventions with new mothers that explore women's experiences of birth and the transition to motherhood. These groups were shown anecdotally to be of great value to the women who took part. These texts proved essential reading when setting up the groups and working with new mothers, and I found some of the ideas presented in the dyadic work to be helpful, most notably in Hosea (2006, 2017).

Setting up the groups

I put forward a proposal for the Art Therapy groups for new mothers to senior midwives at a large hospital in a south London National Health Service (NHS) trust, various London-based mental health charities and a number of children's centres within two south London boroughs. Everybody I approached and met with expressed huge enthusiasm for the groups and spoke of the pressing need for supportive spaces for new mothers, but in the current political climate of austerity, funding appeared unattainable. A paradox arose where it became evident that before funding could be made available, the groups would have to be tried and tested, and without funding, this couldn't happen. With personal financial assistance, I was eventually able to find funds to purchase art materials and hire a suitable space to hold the groups. These were self-referred and self-funded and mainly advertised via local forums in copy that I hoped would be encouraging and non-intimidating:

> Through art-making and discussion, in a safe, non-judgemental space, women will be given an opportunity to explore their feelings, birth stories

and changed senses of identity, boost their creativity and self-esteem and connect with a small group of other mothers who may be sharing similar experiences. Participants do not need to have any previous experience or expertise in art. Any woman who feels she may benefit from this small, creative group is welcome.

The groups were held in a room at the back of a ceramics café, popular with families, in a busy area of south-east London close to shops and a children's playground. The charge per person for each group covered my costs and gave me a modest fee. Five separate weekly six-week closed groups ran over a period of ten months. In total, 20 women accessed the therapy, with some of those choosing to participate in two consecutive groups. Each group consisted of no more than six women. Babies up to a year old were welcomed and present.

Women accessed the groups for a range of reasons and with different levels of need and were mixed in terms of first and second-time mothers. The majority of women were over 30, white, British, employed, in a relationship, and from middle-class backgrounds. I reserved one free place per group, in order to give someone unable to fund the group herself the opportunity to participate. It soon became clear that the demand for a subsidised place outstripped what I was able to offer and it felt unfair that there were no funds available to assist the mothers who contacted me without the means to pay. It was evident from the number of women who got in touch that there was a real need for and a desire to be part of this kind of supportive, creative group.

Some women didn't follow up their initial interest or cancelled their place at the last minute and I wondered why this might be and how I might have enabled them to come. Were they too depressed? Was the idea of attending too anxiety-provoking? Did their babies not conform to perceived ideals? Murray writes:

> Much of the information parents receive about infant development has tended to give the impression that there is a 'typical' or 'normal' infant – one, for example, who sleeps a lot between meals and is easily comforted. *If an infant does not match this image of the normal baby, a mother may easily feel that this is her fault.* In such cases mothers may be reluctant to avail themselves of support routes ... because they imagine that they will be met with disapproval or that they will be the only one with an infant who is crying.
>
> (1997, p. 335, emphasis in the original)

Running the groups

The sessions were 90 minutes long with the first half devoted to art making and the second to discussion. There were introductions at the start of the first session of each group and boundaries were discussed. A short period of talking between the mothers and 'checking in' with me followed. Participants were then able to choose from the wide range of art materials provided and work freely and without direction on their own pieces at separate tables. The art making process was generally done in silence.

I provided a large, soft play mat, which was placed in the middle of the room. To one side was a comfy sofa where mothers could feed their babies. Some babies sat on their mothers' laps while they made art, others slept close to their mothers in slings or in prams; high chairs were available for older babies who wanted to join in at the table with their mothers.

In the second half of the session, the group came together and artwork was laid out and shared with the group. This offered the opportunity for self-reflection and participants were able to share issues or concerns they might be experiencing and that may have been expressed through their art making; they were free to share as much or as little as they liked. It was important that everybody had the opportunity to speak and I regulated the time with that in mind.

Within the context of the group, it felt important to reveal that I was a mother and from time to time it felt appropriate to share with the group some of my experiences of being a new mother. Hogan (2003, p. 163) feels correspondingly and gives her reasons, with which I concur:

> I wished to make it clear to the group that I did not regard myself as 'sussed' and totally successful or model mother there to impart wisdom about how it should be done. Rather, I wanted to give permission for the expression of a range of feelings from euphoria to despair.

It was important that any disclosures I made weren't invasive and didn't divert me from my role as facilitator (Hogan 2003). The following excerpt from a group member emphasises the relevance of the facilitator imparting this information:

> I found being able to talk to you [the Art Therapist] and the other participants in a non-judgemental and open space really important. I really struggled in those first six months and felt really unsettled all the time, fretting about sleep and breastfeeding and what-ifs. I remember though in those sessions feeling much calmer. It helped so much just to be with other mothers and also importantly I feel, another mother who had been there before but who wasn't saying 'I've got it all right, learn from me', which you get a lot of!

When working therapeutically with new mothers, Stern (1995, p. 187) suggests that, 'the therapist can be more active, less abstinent emotionally ... more focused on assets, capacities and strengths than on pathology and conflicts'. Hosea (2017, p. 108) writes:

> Stern (1995) believes that the therapeutic setting in infant-parent psychotherapy is about the holding that allows mothers to develop their abilities. He believes that the transference from the therapist in this context works best as that of a benign mother/grandmother, who holds the new mother positively so she can find her innate repertoire of techniques.

This felt important for me to adhere to and be aware of when facilitating the groups.

Themes and issues

There were several themes and issues, all relevant to new motherhood, that cropped up in the sessions and I found many of these to be present in the literature discussing similar groups (Hogan 2003, 2008, 2012). Much that arose was complex and within this short chapter I can only touch on some aspects. All the women who participated in the groups spoke of the insurmountable exhaustion that accompanies new motherhood; the result of unrelenting nights of broken or very little sleep. This high level of fatigue, together with the continuous care that all babies need, can lead to feelings of anger and resentment, which, in turn, may produce feelings of guilt if mothers believe they shouldn't be having these negative emotions. Hogan (2012, p. 80) suggests that 'guilt, anger and depression are inexorably interlinked'. One participant admitted: 'I feel a huge sense of guilt if I'm not happy all the time; I should be feeling grateful, I have friends who have lost babies and others who are struggling to conceive'.

Guilt as a theme came up again and again in the groups and troubled all the mothers for a variety of reasons. Some felt guilty about their birth experiences and believed they were inadequate in some way if their births hadn't gone 'to plan' or how they had wished. Breastfeeding was a cause of major anxiety for a number of women and those who struggled felt they weren't 'good enough'. One group member said she had let herself and her baby down by not being able to breastfeed him.

Maternal ambivalence was discussed and thought about as a source of guilt within the groups; all the women identified with the feeling of wanting their baby close yet craving space for themselves. Ironically, when the women were given the opportunity to take time away from their baby, some of them admitted to either passing on the chance or not actually enjoying the freedom, worrying that the physical separation might cause the baby some form of emotional distress. Hogan (2012, 2016) suggests this anxiety and guilt felt by some mothers around leaving their baby for even a short amount of time with another caregiver might be due to these women internalising the 'negative aspect of object-relations theory' (Hogan 2012, p. 76). She writes that the theorist Bowlby helped to make the idea of 'maternal deprivation' popular by arguing 'that if women went out to work, their offspring could suffer irreparable psychological damage' (Rose 1990, cited in Hogan 2012, p. 77). Many women felt anxious and guilty about the prospect of going back to work and worried about the unrealistic expectations of unsympathetic bosses (both male and female) who lacked understanding. Some women felt guilt for perceiving they were asking too much from a partner.

Guilt was also prevalent among second-time mothers, who felt they might be neglecting the needs of their older child in favour of the baby. They feared that the relationship with and feelings towards their first-born had changed since the birth of their second child. Skaife (1997, p. 194) writes:

In my experience mothers pregnant with second children often fear that they cannot love two equally; there seems some impossibility about it. The special relationship with the first one before the birth that Rogers [1994] refers to is the shared awareness of an impending loss in that relationship. For a time after the birth, there is a period of adaptation which involves an inevitable change in the mother's feelings towards her first child.

One group member made a moving painting of her eldest waving goodbye to her on his first day of school. This was clearly a very emotional time for her and she described feeling 'grief'. The image metaphorically spoke of a departure from the former relationship they had together before the birth of his sister and simultaneously held sadness and joy; the loss of something cherished and the start of something new and wonderful.

Within the group, women spoke of changes to relationships and difficulties with their partners since the birth of their baby; some felt their partners didn't understand what they were going through and weren't supportive enough. Many women experienced a profound change and 'loss' of their former self. Stern (1995, 1998) maintains that the mother, with the birth of her child, gives birth to a new identity.

Several women in the group spoke about the humiliation they felt when members of the public passed comments or raised their eyebrows as they struggled to get their baby to stop crying in shops or on public transport. One described her experience on a bus as 'mortifying'. Women talked about feeling pressure from various people 'interfering'; these might be members of the public, family members, midwives and health visitors. They felt that such people had certain expectations of them and constantly made them feel as if they were doing something wrong. Hogan (2016, p. 2) writes: 'Women are policed, not just by the State, through health advice, pre-natal health-check regimes and hospital protocols, but also by relatives informed through and seeking to sustain a variety of community norms; this surveillance can feel oppressive'.

Highs and lows

There were many occasions during the sessions when new motherhood was celebrated as a joyful and rewarding time. The groups felt warm and there was often laughter during discussions. The more challenging parts of a new mother's experience could also be depicted, discussed and explored; these included feelings of self-doubt, claustrophobia, guilt, shock, resentment, loss, anger, sadness, anxiety and fear. One group member said: 'Being a mum for the first time is an unknown world ... I don't know how to cope and deal with my feelings'.

The poet Hollie McNish (2017, p. 123) eloquently captures the monotony, interminability and emotional highs and lows that come with caring for a very young baby:

'I feed her and she sleeps and I sleep and she wakes and I wake and I feed her and she wakes and he helps and he holds her so I sleep and she sleeps and I feed her and we go out and we come back and the tea's cold and I feel crap and I feel great and I feel calm and I wonder about my life this far and I cry and I weep and I breathe in and I breathe out…'

Almost all the participants reported that following the birth of their babies, they felt more lonely and isolated and craved having adult conversations and time for themselves. When reflecting on her time in the group, one member reported: 'It was really nice to get out and do something "grown up" that I could take my baby to and where I knew he was safe while I focused on me'.

Another wrote: 'I found the space doing something close to baby but not completely aimed at her really useful; it showed me that it was possible and in fact a good thing to not always be completely focused on her needs, but on my own as well'.

Having their babies present provided the mothers with a number of triggers and challenges; these provoked a range of strong feelings from joy, adoration and pride to less desirable emotions such as frustration, disappointment, shame and competition. That these emotions were palpable in the room allowed them to be explored. Mothers were able to see that other babies scream, fuss and struggle to be soothed, allowing myths perpetuated by some health professionals, family members and parenting books to be debunked. They witnessed first-hand that the group could tolerate and bear this 'difficult' behaviour from the babies. This alleviated feelings of shame and created a resilience that could be taken out of the group and into the outside community.

Several of the participants used the group to bring things that had happened to them between sessions into the open; others aired concerns and difficulties that were happening in the here and now. One group member painted an image of herself sitting on the pavement holding her baby in a sling. She told the group of how she had fallen the previous day. She was clearly still very shaken by the incident, but claimed that being able to 'paint it out and talk about it' had helped her immensely and allowed her to process the situation in a different way. Another reported: 'It really has been the highlight of my week to sit and paint and reflect on this time that's so very full of challenge and enormous feelings'.

A powerful image made from magazine cuttings that featured women in various roles was captioned 'You have got to be honest'. The participant claimed that making the image and discussing it with the others had given her a perspective on the situation and the strength to speak to her partner about things that had been worrying her. Several women said the groups had given them more confidence.

Sharing and shared experiences

Within a short period of time, the women in the groups felt safe enough to reveal and explore thoughts, feelings and experiences that they were unable to express elsewhere. One or two women sharing these allowed others to do the same. A participant wrote: 'Towards the end of the therapy I felt very comfortable with the group we had created and it became easier to open up and talk about fear, sadness and happiness in this new experience of being a mum.' Sharing thoughts and feelings with other mothers and realising that you are not alone is very comforting. Women spoke of how reassuring it was when they heard that others were going through what they were. One group member wrote: 'Sometimes what is difficult to say, is being said by someone else – helping and healing everyone.' And another: 'Listening to other people being in the same situation but with a different perspective really helped me to understand that I am not alone; it helps to relieve guilt, and the feeling you are always doing something wrong disappears'.

The confidential nature of the groups allowed for more taboo and difficult themes to be explored. A participant who had given birth to her daughter extremely prematurely wrote: 'My situation was particularly difficult and I was worried that I wouldn't be able to share it, but in the last session I let out a lot of emotion after two other mums shared their inner experiences and I felt a great sense of relief'.

Being part of a group enabled the women to make sense of and understand their birth and post-natal experiences and to build self-awareness. First-time mothers were able to learn and gather support from the experiences shared by second-time mothers. One participant reported: 'I found it really helpful to chat with people who had slightly older babies and second babies, getting a different perspective to what we manage in an NCT group of first-time mums with babies all the same age'.

Resonating images

Much of the art made in the groups resonated with the mothers and looking at each other's work acted as a catalyst and stirred up feelings in the women which were then able to be articulated through words. There were often echoes

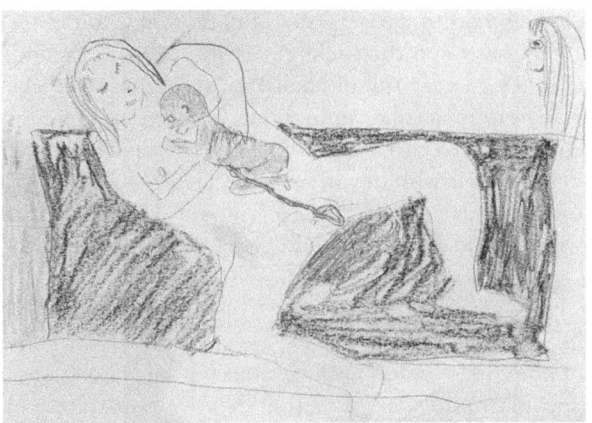

Figure 13.1 Post-Natal Bliss. Pencil and coloured pencil on paper, 2017.

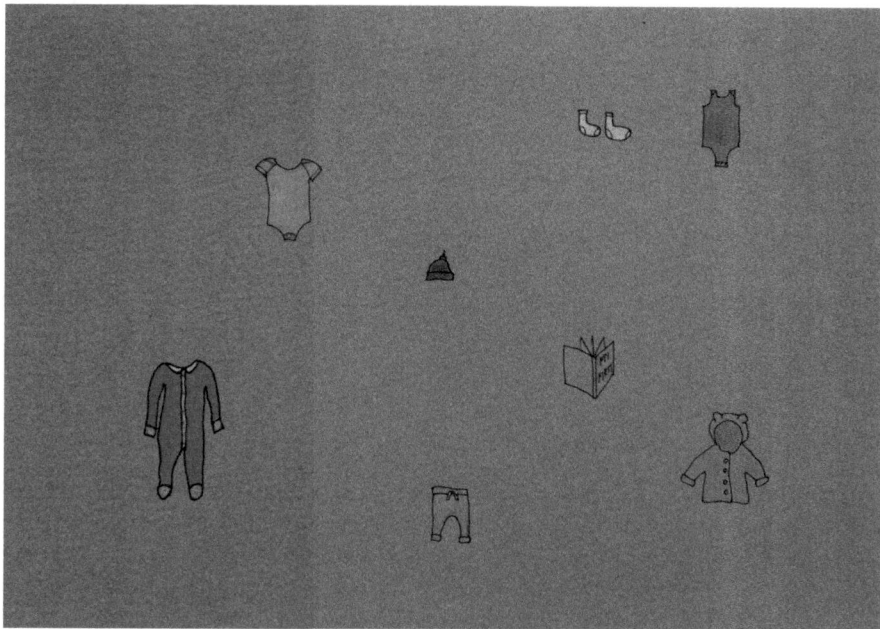

Figure 13.2 Outgrown Pen and coloured pencil on paper, 2017.

between group members' work. One participant drew a wave using chalk pastels. Her inspiration came from a mural depicting Hokusai's 'The Great Wave off Kanagawa' that she had walked past on her way to ante-natal appointments. The image spoke to the women of turbulence; in particular, the surge of un-dulating emotions. One woman said she felt 'as if she'd been hit by a wave' following the birth of her son. Several women said the picture reminded them of their contractions during labour. The tissues used to take off excess chalk and to blend the pastels were redeployed to create another artwork. All the women related the mopping up processes of art to bodily fluids – lochia, blood and tears and their babies' posset and excrement. Images and depictions of birth experi-ences were common within the groups; these gave women the opportunity to talk about their experiences and process them in a different way.

Several of the participants drew and painted images relating to nature. Mothers said that they were able to frequent parks and have more time to look around them; they appreciated this time and felt present in the moment in these open spaces. This seemed to be a happy time, when babies were most content and often slept, leaving mum to feel more at peace and to take in her surroundings.

With babies of varying ages present in the group, mothers could mourn stages lost and look forward to stages to come. All the mothers could relate to the sadness of leaving behind a stage in their babies' development; one group member likened the process to bereavement. Some of the women admitted that they would simultaneously find themselves wanting their babies to move on to the next thing and to be tiny again like other infants in the room with their mothers. A drawing by a participant of clothes that were now too small for her baby was understood and appreciated by the other mothers in the group for whom it brought up a sense of sadness and loss. A number of women chose to capture their baby at the time of the group and one drew her baby's current favourite toy. These fleeting moments could be preserved within the images.

Several women felt they had lost their sense of self since the birth of their baby and images were made in response to this. Hogan (2008, p. 209) suggests, 'the pictorial space provided by the use of the Art Therapy was very relevant to the women', it 'also afforded an opportunity for the reconstruction of a lost sense of self'.

The importance of the art making

Art making can be used to articulate feelings that cannot be described in words or might not be fully conscious, thus helping to promote self-understanding, ease emotional turmoil and bring comfort and relief. Jung understood the importance of art making in the context of psychotherapy and for his personal benefit. In the autobiography written at the end of his life in 1961, he wrote (Jung 1995, p. 201):

> To the extent that I managed to translate the emotions into images – that is to say to find the images which were concealed in the emotion – I was inwardly calmed and reassured. Had I left those images hidden in the emotions, I might have been torn to pieces by them.

Women in the group were able to express themselves and find a voice through the artwork. They found confidence in themselves and their artistic abilities and felt a sense of pride in what they created. It was as if the artwork gave them something that they could hold onto: something tangible. Hogan et al. (2017, p. 175) speak of emerging emotions that 'can be captured in art in ways that are fundamentally different and differently reachable to that of a language-based approach'.

All the women found the art making enjoyable and relieving and several began to continue with it at home. A number of women reported that they were amazed at what could be created in a relatively short amount of time. Second-time mothers said the sessions had inspired them to be creative with their older children and to make art together. It was interesting to hear that some participants had framed a picture made in the group. The frame seems symbolic, in that it holds an image of something meaningful that can then be protected. Simon (1996) writes: 'Sometimes the frame is used to draw attention to work as an object of value or reverence; such a frame may not necessarily enhance it in visual terms, but can contribute to its

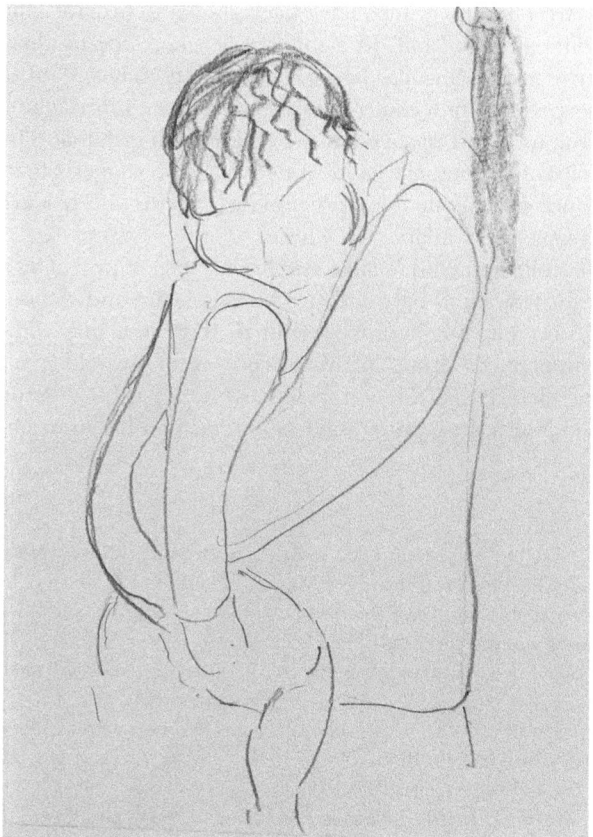

Figure 13.3 Mothering Mothers. Pencil on paper, 2017.

symbolic significance.' The following comment from a participant says much about the importance of the groups:

> I have framed the picture I drew of you holding Elsie and have it in my room. I look at it every day and think about 'mothering mothers' and community and Elsie and how much she's grown. It's one of my favourite things, so thank you.

Conclusion

Women struggle with the transition to motherhood. Post-natal depression, anxiety and loneliness are prevalent among new mothers in the UK and yet there is little support to hand. At a time of austerity with limited funding available, there is a risk that help might only be obtainable for those who can afford it. The focus of this chapter has been on a number of six-week Art Therapy groups for new mothers. Anecdotally, Art Therapy groups have been shown to provide valuable social support at this difficult transition. In a safe space where the mother feels supported, her confidence grows. She also has an opportunity to be creative. The art making allows the expression of feelings not easily articulated through words.

The feedback from the women I received at the end of each group and from a small number of participants I contacted almost two years on suggests that new mothers found the groups to be valuable and provided them with a level and quality of support that was not available elsewhere.

I hope this chapter has highlighted the value and importance of providing social and emotional support for women as part of their post-natal care and can serve as further anecdotal evidence that might prove useful to those working with new mothers. I share the sentiment of a group member, who wrote: 'I would love every new mother to have the chance and the opportunity to be a part of a group like this, where you can heal and feel supported and be understood by other mums'.

References

Bauer, A., Parsonage, M., Knapp, M., Lemmi, V., & Adelaja, B. 2014. *The Cost of Perinatal Mental Health Problems: Report Summary*. Central for Mental Health and London School of Economics, PSSRU. Available at: www.centreformentalhealth.org.uk/sites/default/files/2018-09/costsofperinatal.pdf (accessed November 2019).

Eisenberg, A., Murkoff, H. E., & Hathaway, S. E. 1989. *What to Expect the First Year*. New York: Workman.

Hogan, S. 2003. A Discussion of the Use of Art Therapy with Women who are Pregnant or who have Recently Given Birth. In S. Hogan (ed.), *Gender Issues in Art Therapy*. London: Jessica Kingsley Publishers, pp. 148–172.

Hogan, S. 2008. Angry Mothers. In M. Liebmann (ed.), *Art Therapy and Anger*. London: Jessica Kingsley Publishers, pp. 197–210.

Hogan, S. 2012. Post-Modernist but Not Post-Feminist! A Feminist Post-modernist Approach to Working with New Mothers. In H. Burt (ed.), *Creative Healing Through a Prism: Art Therapy and Postmodernism*. London: Jessica Kingsley Publishers, pp. 70–82.

Hogan, S. 2016. The Tyranny of Expectations of Post-Natal Delight: Gendered Happiness. *Journal of Gender Studies*, 26(1): 45–55.

Hogan, S., Sheffield, D., & Woodward, A. 2017. The Value of Art Therapy in Antenatal and Postnatal Care: A Brief Literature Review with Recommendations for Future Research. *International Journal of Art Therapy: Inscape*, 22(3–4): 169–179.

Hosea, H. 2006 The Brush's Footmark: Parents and Infants Paint Together in a Small Community Art Therapy Group. *The International Journal of Art Therapy: Inscape*, 11(2): 69–79.

Hosca, H. 2017. Amazing Mess: Mothers get in Touch with their Infants through the Vitality of Painting Together. In J. Meyerowitz-Katz & D. Reddick (eds), *Art Therapy in the Early Years*. London: Routledge, pp. 104–117.

Jung, C.G. 1995. *Memories, Dreams, Reflections*, 5th ed. London: Fontana Press.

McNish, H. 2017. *Nobody Told Me*. London: Blackfriars.

Maselko, J., Kubzansky, L., Lipsitt, L., & Buka, S. L. 2011. Mother's Affection at 8 Months Predicts Emotional Distress in Adulthood. *The Journal of Epidemiology Community Health*, 65(4): 621–625.

Murray, L. 1997. The Effect of Infants' Behaviour on Maternal Mental Health. *Health Visitor*, 70(9): 334–335.

National Maternity Review Report. 2016. *Better Births: Improving Outcomes of Maternity Services in England: A Five Year Forward View for Maternity Care.* England: NHS. Available at: www.england.nhs.uk/ourwork/futurenhs/mat-review (accessed November 2019).

Oakley, A. 1992. *Social Support and Motherhood.* Oxford: Basil Blackwell.

Oakley, A., Hickey, D., & Rajan, L. 1996. Social Support in Pregnancy: Does it have Long Term Effects? *Journal of Reproductive Psychology*, 14: 7–22.

Rogers, C. 1994. The Group and the Group Analyst's Pregnancies. *Group Analysis*, 27(1): 51–61.

Rose, N. 1990. *Governing the Souls. The Shaping of the Private Self.* London: Routledge.

Sacks, A. 2017. The Birth of a Mother. *The New York Times*, 8 May. Available at: www.nytimes.com/2017/05/08/well/family/the-birth-of-a-mother.amp.html (accessed November 2019).

Simon, J. 1996. *The Art of the Picture Frame.* London: National Portrait Gallery.

Skaife, S. 1997. The Pregnant Art Therapist. In S. Hogan (ed.), *Feminist Approaches to Art Therapy.* London: Routledge, pp. 177–196.

Stern, D. N. 1995 *The Motherhood Constellation: A Unified View of Parent–Infant Psychotherapy.* New York: Basic Books.

Stern, D. N. 1998. *The Birth of a Mother: How the Motherhood Experience Changes You Forever.* New York: Basic Books.

14 Mechanisms of change within a dyadic model of Art Therapy for parents and their infants

Victoria Gray Armstrong and Josephine Ross

Introduction

The practice of parent–infant art psychotherapy is an emerging field. The principle aim of this chapter is to bring the nascent research together and use it to develop a framework for understanding this practice area and its potential benefits. This will support practitioners and provide a solid basis for future research. This chapter builds upon an integrative literature review undertaken in October 2018 (Armstrong & Ross 2020) looking at those papers where Art Therapy was being used dyadically with parents and infants. Here we shall discuss what art psychotherapy with parent–infant dyads looks like, outlining the different models of practice, the difference between closed and open group formats, time limited and open durations, and directive and non-directive approaches. We shall then focus on the mechanisms of change in parent–infant work, based upon a thematic analysis of the literature which identified those aspects of art psychotherapy with this participant group which are consistent between different practitioners, formats and settings to build a model of change. A synthesis of key mechanisms for change can help to articulate what is unique about our practice and why it may be helpful for these vulnerable families. In this chapter we will outline each theme and its impact on the dyads and give a description of how this may look in practice, based on several years of developing parent–infant Art Therapy sessions (Armstrong, Dalinkeviciute & Ross 2019; Armstrong & Howatson 2015). We shall offer vignettes of specific groups or dyads from clinical practice in order to illustrate the concepts concretely. These vignettes are taken from Art Therapy groups running in the context of Art at the Start. This project began in 2018, based within the University of Dundee, in collaboration with Dundee Contemporary Arts Centre, to address the impact of early art experiences (https://sites.dundee.ac.uk/artatthestart/). One goal of Art at the Start has been to measure the outcomes of Art Therapy groups where the parent–infant relationship is considered to be vulnerable. All the parents involved agreed to their data being used for research and educational purposes but we have also changed names and identifying details.

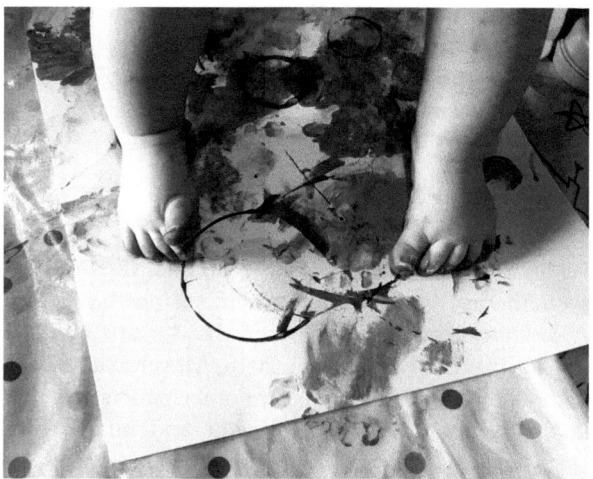

Figure 14.1 Infant engaged with painting.

Background

The central relationships in a child's first years of life have been demonstrated to build their capacity to regulate affect, to relate to others and to develop their sense of self (Bigelow et al. 2010; Schore 2001; Svanberg 1998) as well as affecting their future mental health and wellbeing (Belsky 2001; Sroufe 1996; Warren et al. 1997). The quality of early attachment relationships are shown to be impacted by the poor mental health of a parent (Cummings & Cicchetti 1990). An estimated 10–20 per cent of mothers develop mental health difficulties during pregnancy and in the year after birth (Bauer et al. 2014). Evidence of similar mental health difficulties for new fathers, and the impact of this on their children, is also growing (Khan 2017; Paulson & Bazemore 2010). It is therefore critical to both infant and parent wellbeing to offer post-partum psychological support where there are difficulties.

Dyadic approaches to addressing these difficulties have increasingly been championed (Baradon 2005) and within Art Therapy there has been growing interest in dyadic work (Taylor Buck, Dent-Brown & Parry 2013). Art psychotherapy with parents and infants together has the potential to address a number of concerns for families with very young children, such as the impact of traumatic birth experiences, concerns around attachment difficulties, post-natal depression, lack of confidence in parenting and social isolation (Armstrong et al. 2019; Arroyo & Fowler 2013; Hall 2008; Hogan, Sheffield & Woodward 2017; Hosea 2017). The All-Party Report on Arts in Health and Wellbeing (2017) highlighted the use of arts to improve health and wellbeing for parent–infant dyads in a participative arts context and a number of examples from this field (Black et al. 2015; Starcatchers 2014) demonstrate the practice. Art Therapy is similarly able to use the benefits of the art process and inherently engaging and sensory art materials. However, in addition there is the security created by a facilitator who, as a qualified Art Therapist, has an in-depth understanding of mental health and attachments and who is trained to create a safe space and to offer psychological support and containment.

What does art psychotherapy with parent–infant dyads look like?

Our review identified 11 published papers and two unpublished at the time which addressed art psychotherapy with parents and infants together (Armstrong et al. 2019; Armstrong & Howatson 2015; Arroyo & Fowler 2013; Hall 2008; Hosea 2006, 2011, 2017; Lavey-Khan & Reddick 2018; Meyerowitz-Katz 2017; Parashak 2008; Proulx 2000, 2002, 2003). There are other papers whose model works with either just the parent or with the parent and infant separately (Hamed-Agbariah & Rosenfeld 2015; Perry, Thurston & Osborn 2008; Ponteri 2001) but we focused on those where the work was entirely dyadic. All the models described in this literature took a group approach with various numbers of dyads brought together. In terms of the referral criteria for groups, some focused on specific populations, such as a diagnosis of post-natal depression, while others had broader criteria around improving relationships or increasing parental confidence. Most were for children under three, but some included children up to the age of five within their groups. All the groups were run by an art psychotherapist (in one case students with supervision, but qualified in all other cases) and at least one co-facilitator.

A variety of timeframes for work were described ranging from groups with no time limitations to blocks ranging from four to 20 weeks. The format for groups included open groups, closed groups and rolling groups. An open group is on-going and families can chose to join, when to come and when to end the work. In a closed groups the same set of parents and children are referred to the group for the duration of a fixed block of time, with the intention that all the dyads will complete the block. A rolling group sits somewhere in-between, where parents are invited to join, but they are able to join and leave an ongoing group as they please. There are benefits to each format, with open groups offering maximum flexibility and the potential to involve the greatest number of people, but with the risk of having too many or too few participants each week. A closed group offers the most consistency for the members and security about who will be there but the group duration offered may not suit the participants themselves and any drop-outs cannot be 'replaced'. A rolling group may offer a good compromise but difficulties may arise in knowing when a dyad has chosen to leave the group in order to have a recognition of endings and to offer those spaces to others.

A typical session may last from 60 to 90 minutes and involve between four and eight dyads with a focus on shared art making. The art psychotherapist in-troduces the art making and the materials and offers containment to the dyads, helping them to engage with art making and bringing everyone back together for some reflection time at the end. The papers reviewed reveal some geographical variation in the role of the Art Therapist. Art Therapists based in North America tended to be directive, with structured sessions and activities chosen as an intervention by the therapists, perhaps to support a particular difficulty. By contrast, Art Therapists in the UK tended to be more non-directive; although there was often structure around the use of time, the art making itself was left open to the dyads and the parents were encouraged to follow the infants' lead. The vignette below describes a typical Art Therapy session within the Art at the Start project to help visualise how a session may unfold in practice.

A group vignette

Our Art Therapy groups run in blocks of 12 weeks, taking referrals wherever there are concerns about the dyad's attachment relationship. This particular group has five mothers who come every week and another couple who dip in and out. The referrals came from health visitors and from a team working with young mothers. Several of the mothers have a diagnosis of post-natal depression and several have issues around anxiety. Some express feelings of isolation and a number of the mums have negative relationships with the children's fathers. The backgrounds of the mothers are socially and economically diverse but the art making and focus on the babies brings them together. The session lasts an hour and a half and starts with dyads arriving and settling themselves in, maybe making a cup of tea and getting little ones snacks or changed into messy clothes or just a nappy. One mum who has two children with her arrives quite late and a little flustered but the others welcome her in and we get her tea and give her time to settle while we play with the children. We introduce the art materials for the day. There are consistent materials every week and then additional things may be added following requests from the previous sessions or after consideration of materials which might benefit particular dyads. This week we have all our usual paints, papers, chalks, glues and collage materials but we have added in a collection of large boxes. The art making time is left open to the dyads and we emphasise to parents that they should follow their child's lead and see what materials interest them and take breaks when they lose attention. We have big plastic mats spread out on the floor so there are no worries about mess and we just need to keep mopping spills promptly so it doesn't get slippy. One of the youngest little ones in this group at six months is put in a box by mum so they can play peek with the flaps. We reflect to mum how much her little one is enjoying this game as this mum often seems nervous that she is not doing the right thing. Some of the older toddlers have ideas for building race cars and we help the mums to facilitate their ideas for them and to play together. A two-year-old girl is keen to use the paints, which we sense might be a little disappointing to her mum who had ideas of what she could build. We notice mum bring her back to the box activity several times and we gently reflect that she seems to be really interested in the paint this week. Mum takes this on board and is able to follow her lead and do some messy painting together. We allow dyads to find their own ending and there is a process of filling big buckets with water for baby baths, which for some is the favourite part. We have several buckets so a couple of little ones have a bath facing each other and splashing. After this, we regroup with some snacks to reflect on the work and think about next week. We sometimes find it hard to elicit suggestions from the mums who prefer us to give them some ideas but we are trying to move towards them feeling more ownership. We sing a few ending songs as a group. The co-facilitator for this group is also a music teacher and has introduced us to a goodbye song where each child is named in turn and all have responded to this with great delight.

Mechanisms of change

Through a process of thematic analysis of those papers in our review exercise we identified two encompassing themes in the literature on art psychotherapy groups for parents and infants, under which we were able to bring together detailed mechanisms of change. The first of these, which we called 'qualities of the group process', captured aspects of the therapeutic group experience that created change: namely, the kind of space created, the benefits of being a group member, the qualities the therapist brings, and the direct support for relationships. The second theme, which we called 'qualities specific to using art' captured those mechanisms of change that were unique to the art-making process: the materials, the process, the containment within the art and the final art works themselves. Detail of the mechanisms as described in the literature can be found in our review (Armstrong and Ross, 2020) and we do not seek to replicate this. Here we shall summarise each theme and then offer descriptions of how this looks within practice in our own project's sessions that we hope will feel useful to practitioners.

Qualities of the group process

The space created

The space of parent–infant Art Therapy groups conveys safety but also the potential for playfulness. Containment, or holding, is essential to creating safety and can be more about the physical containment through keeping boundaries or it can be psychological, about containing strong emotions for participants. Hall (2019) has given a useful visual description of the different levels of support that operate within her groups to keep them contained, both from the facilitators and from the systems around them. It matters how groups begin and end and how the facilitators keep consistency of space, time, participants and structure (Hall 2008; Hosea 2017).

Similarly it matters that everyone in the group feels the Art Therapist is able to contain difficult emotions and offer them support. Within Art Therapy sessions, there is an ethos of non-judgement and confidentiality that enables parents to feel safe. Within the safety created in the group there is the scope to be imaginative, to experiment, to be playful together and to view the relationship differently. It is a space outside of everyday life (Arroyo & Fowler 2013).

In the Art at the Start project, as the Art Therapist and co-facilitators, we find it useful during supervision to think about the different layers of containment operating. Sometimes, for example, we might be holding a parent, offering them support in order that they are in turn able to hold their infant. At other times we may be holding the group as a whole or perhaps an infant that their parent is unable to manage in that moment. Sometimes we might just be holding the space by not letting outside factors intrude into our room in a busy public gallery environment. We hold the boundaries of the space and the time through the Art Therapist starting off the group together in a circle and bringing it back together as an ending and through rituals such as bath time and the songs. In our groups the idea that the group is a space slightly outside of the everyday may be reflected by regular comments from parents that they are glad not to have to clear up the mess. Partly this allows us to show that we are looking after the parents as well as the infants but also emphasises that the normal rules may not apply here and that they can feel free to try a new activity but also a new way of behaving.

Group membership

Parent–infant Art Therapy groups offer a support network of other parents in similar circumstances acting as a community (Hosea 2017). Within this atmosphere of mutual support the parents can gain confidence, meet new people, form friendships, try new activities and learn from each other. The knowledge that there are shared experiences is important, allowing parents to share their own stories and the difficulties they are facing, both with practicalities and with mental health. In the groups, parents receive support from the other members and an understanding that others have similar struggles, lessening feelings of isolation and offering empowerment (Arroyo & Fowler 2013; Lavey-Khan & Reddick 2018).

In our sessions, we don't try to force any direct sharing of difficulties, and we reassure parents that this will not be expected of them as it is something they've been expecting and are nervous of. We only directly seek to reflect on how that day's session had been experienced for the group at the end. However, we find that parents gradually start to share with each other and move from only looking to the facilitators for support to looking to the group as a whole. We hear parents sharing difficulties and offering each other empathy. Other authors have acknowledged the need to balance some of the tensions within the group dynamics between one-to-one and group relationships; between interactions with the therapist rather than the group or between the engagement with the group and the need to keep the parents' focus on their infants (Lavey-Khan & Reddick 2018; Parashak 2008).

We have similarly found this to be true at times but overall we find that the benefits of the group far outweigh any challenges and that we are able to gently find a balance.

Vignette: Pria and Kye

Pria is feeling isolated at home with children and struggling with the loss of her previous work role which involved status as well as lots of interaction. We find that she comes to the group with a lot to share as if she has been keeping it in all week. We want to balance giving her the space and opportunity to vent this without losing the focus on the dyadic relationship. We also want to ensure all parents are given space without feeling overwhelmed by one member. Sometimes we may play with her baby (Kye, 13 months) for a little while after they first arrive to give her some time to chat with one of us or with other mums before directing her back towards Kye to start the art making. In this way we aim to keep the group as a positive experience for both of them. We noticed over the course of the sessions that Pria shifted her focus from only seeking to share and chat with us as facilitators to being much more happy to engage the whole group. She also gets positive validation now as other parents seek her out for advice and to share with.

Qualities of the therapist

The Art Therapists running parent–infant groups demonstrate sensitivity and empathy as well as the ability to scaffold experiences for the infant when the parent may not be managing to do this. Scaffolding describes the way the Art Therapist may step in temporarily to offer some support to an infant in lieu of their parent so that their experience is manageable and does not overwhelm them. The literature also include descriptions of therapists getting down on the floor and joining in (Hall 2008; Hosea 2006; Parashak 2008) and this may contribute to a less hierarchical feel compared with other services offered to parents as well as demonstrating a playful and engaged way of behaving with the infants. Many papers refer to the concept of modelling (Armstrong et al. 2019; Armstrong & Howatson 2015; Meyerowitz-Katz 2017; Proulx 2000), where the Art Therapist models a way of behaving and interacting with the infants. There is some caution too, with Parashak (2008) highlighting the need not to become 'the better mother' and Hosea describing the potential for 'grandmother' transference with the connotation of support and experience but also the risk of being seen as 'critical or withholding' (2006, 2017).

In our project we get down on the floor with the parents and the infants, although we do not tend to make paintings ourselves, and we engage playfully with the children. We try to give attention to the needs of both the parents and the infants and we aim to remain empathetic and non-judgemental. We know that sometimes one of us may need to play with a little one to give their parent time to process something difficult with the other facilitator. When we play we are modelling a way of following the lead of the infant and of valuing what they do. There is a balance to be struck when modelling positive behaviour as we do not want to take over or present ourselves as experts and therefore reinforce any feelings of inadequacy in the parents. Where possible we try to find ways to keep the parent themselves engaged with the play alongside or we may redirect the play to include them.

Vignette: Hannah and Blair

We notice in one session that Hannah and her daughter Blair (eight months) are slightly separate from the rest of the group. Hannah seems nervous to pick up Blair who is clearly seeking this and is tearful on the floor. Hannah seems overwhelmed and in fact moves further away from Blair towards the snacks, which Blair had not shown interest in. Blair is not yet able to crawl but, left on the floor, is attempting to move towards mum. It feels painful for both and we are wondering what it feels like for Hannah to be struggling to meet Blair's need for contact and what may have been happening for them that morning. We feel that we need to help scaffold this experience for Blair and so I move to sit with her on the floor and interest her in coloured scarves. I'm aware that I don't want to be seen as 'rescuing' Blair and replacing mum and so while we play gently I talk to Blair about how she is wondering where mum is and that mum is getting her some snacks and will be back soon. When mum returns with a snack I 'help' Blair to hide under the scarf for mum to discover and mum is able to engage with this game and start to play peek-a-boo under the scarf. Another slightly older little one also comes over to play with them and so we start a four-way game of peeking. Hannah seems to gain confidence and become more present and able to pick up Blair on her lap and to continue the game with the other child. We are also able to have time later in the group when Blair is tired from the art making to chat with Hannah and listen to her struggles that morning and her feeling that she never knows what Blair wants from her.

Support for the relationship

The relationship between parent and infant is of central importance in all the literature and is something worked on directly as well as through art materials. The techniques described are about increasing parental responsiveness and their emotional understanding of the infants. In practice this is done through helping parents to interpret infant's communications, building their attunement, their reflective capacity and skills at mentalising, and by reinforcing positive interactions when observed (Armstrong et al. 2019; Armstrong & Howatson 2015;

Arroyo & Fowler 2013; Hall 2008; Hosea 2006, 2017; Lavey-Khan & Reddick 2018; Parashak 2008).

In our sessions we often voice what we see the baby doing and what they might be looking for as a way of helping parents to see their infant's communications as meaningful. Really simple things like 'Katy you're picking up the brushes, are you trying to pass those to mummy?' help to draw a parent's attention to what their infant may be doing or communicating and the use of emotional language such as 'it looks like you're really excited about that paint' build on their capacities to be reflective about their infant's inner world. This is especially useful when it highlights a positive moment in the relationship, for example to say to a parent 'Charlie looked so happy when you were pouring the rice into his hands for him'.

Qualities specific to using art

Materials

Art Therapists' understanding of the qualities of art materials provides a unique benefit compared with parent–infant psychotherapies. The literature gives consideration to keeping the materials developmentally appropriate (Parashak 2008; Proulx 2000), to the qualities of colours (Hosea 2006) and to their somatic and symbolic qualities (Meyerowitz-Katz 2017; Proulx 2002). The specific qualities of certain materials may be used to address particular needs; for example, bubble paintings or puppets may promote eye contact, while collage may help parents to engage with their infants without the anxiety about mess or the need to be constantly putting in limits (Armstrong & Howatson 2015; Proulx 2000, 2002).

In our sessions we appreciate the physicality of the materials and how they may necessitate physical contact from parents to enable little ones to use them, helping to maximise the chances of positive interactions. We also find that presenting the materials to be inviting might encourage a parent to engage. The introduction of certain materials may also help to redirect interactions positively, for example by adding something more manageable for a particular dyad, or they may prolong a dyad's shared engagement, such as by adding a new texture or tool, like a sand shaker just at the point when the child loses interest in painting.

Vignette: Anna and Jamie

Jamie, 19 months, comes to the group with his mum Anna. He is very energetic and Anna is often frustrated at his behaviour when he gets boisterous. We suggest materials that allow him to be big and expansive. On a particularly bouncy day we tape rolls of paper to the floor and suggest to mum that they try to make the biggest footprints they can to engage her with his energy. They have fun together trying to balance each other while they do this and it later turns into a game of follow my leader with each making a funny walk that leaves painty footprints that the other tries to step in. We want mum to see the positives in his energy and we reflect back his sense of fun and how much he is enjoying this game with her. Jamie doesn't really like the brushes, maybe finding these fiddly, and so we offer them big paint rollers and he finds this much more engaging, rolling patterns across very big paper and mum joins in playfully by turning them into road ways for cars.

Art making process

The art process provides opportunity for playful engagement and the literature emphasises how the art making brought the parent and infant together. Hall (2008) describes how infants were always interested in being involved in painting with their parents and that the parents respond with interest. The sharing of the creative experience can give a dyad a point of contact around which to relate and may make their interaction feel easier by having this focus. The process is also fluid and can allow the dyads to engage at different levels depending on where they are in their relationship at that moment; they may be each making in parallel, a parent may be observing and supporting the art making of an infant, or the parent may be making themselves to encourage a little one to join in, or they may be mutually engaged in a shared art making.

In our groups we always start each session by encouraging parents to follow their child's lead and what is interesting them that day. As in the example of Jamie, this can lead to playful interaction and an enjoyment of each other. Activities that we found to be particularly engaging have been those which were new to both parent and child such as using shaving foam as a base for marbling, or using coloured salt dough clay. We find there is something extra special about trying a new experience together and sharing each other's reactions.

Vignette: Cassie and Nial

Cassie seems cautious in her interactions with Nial (12 months) as if anxious that she may make a mistake. When I observed them with toys on our initial home visit, she did not join in with him. The art making is engaging for both of them and so it draws them together. This usually happens quite naturally but sometimes it takes a little encouragement from us. We find that there are lots of the new sensations for Nial to try with the materials, such as the texture of cold wet paint or the soft feeling of feathers, and this gives lots of opportunity for us to encourage Cassie to observe and reflect back his responses. This seems to help her find a way that she is confident to join in with him. In later sessions we encourage her to notice and respond through the materials themselves, echoing the mirroring process of positive early relating. For example, when Nial was enjoying a very physical way of using paint by banging down the brushes, we suggested that Cassie might join in

> with him and she made lots of dots of paint, producing a sympathetic shared image. It felt very powerful to see this dyad engage in shared creation and Cassie took this work home to display.

Containment in the art

Containment has been discussed within the theme of safe spaces but containment can be provided within the art making itself. Some of the art materials have the potential to become very messy and there were descriptions in the literature of the therapist having to provide containment to stop the materials becoming overwhelming. This was true particularly where parents find the messy nature of some of the painting materials to be a challenge, and in these cases the Art Therapist may make adaptions to keep the art making fun rather than chaotic. Hosea (2006) explains that a role for the facilitators is to make the mess safe enough that the dyads can be playful. Proulx (2002) describes how the set-up of materials, for example with lots of small containers and trays to paint in, might build in some limits to provide containment and keep it pleasurable for the dyad. Although some materials have the potential for chaos, others may offer containment through their own qualities. Armstrong and Howatson (2015) give an example of using an activity with large cardboard boxes to offer playfully some contained spaces to very energetic twins who had been struggling to regulate, and Proulx (2003) describes an activity painting inside boxes to make aquariums where the use of the box rather than paper helps to contain the painting process and also becomes a literal container for cut-out fish.

In our sessions we notice parents who become anxious at the thought of the mess and make adaptions for them so as not to have this anxiety get in the way of their chance to be playful with their child. We want to maximise engagement and do not want a fear of mess to cause a parent to disengage. Simple steps like bringing in spare overalls to wear, or suggesting certain materials which parents may be more comfortable to start with before gradually introducing more mess. Where little ones are very keen on using a lot of paint and mums find this distressing we offer reassurance but also sometimes a practical suggestion such as painting into a box lid so that the paint can get very thick without pouring everywhere.

Final artwork

The final art works are a visible document of the relationship and in this way are powerfully symbolic. Many papers consider how final art works were invested with meaning, and described how they were displayed and carefully looked after by the facilitators (Armstrong et al. 2019; Armstrong & Howatson 2015; Hosea 2006, 2017). Proulx (2000) describes how the ritual of sticking a painting on a wall may allow for 'natural separation'. The artwork's impact can also extend beyond the session if they are reflected on the following week, or taken home and displayed.

In our sessions we do not stick with the convention of Art Therapy that all work is kept until the end of treatment and instead we tend to spread it out to reflect on at the end of the session and then we dry it carefully to return the week after. We think this reflects the different needs of work with very young children, where they need more immediacy and where art work may no longer be meaningful to them after long delay. If works are already dry they may even take them home that day. We find that the parents in our groups are keen to feed back to us that works have been appreciated and will share pictures on their phones of them decorating their fridges and doors. Sometimes we find that art works which are especially layered with paint and seem as if the paper may dissolve can be rescued by making a print of the image onto another page or by capturing the work with a photo. We try to carefully write names onto art works as often they are hard to pick out by the next week. Sometimes the parents do not seem as concerned about keeping track of their creations but by doing this for them we are modelling that they are important. When we value the art work we see ourselves as valuing the relationship that created them.

Conclusion

Art psychotherapy groups have been shown to benefit parent–infant relationships and to improve wellbeing for the dyad. Through a process of thematic analysis of the literature base we have brought out mechanisms of change that may be proving beneficial to the parents and infants that we work with. These included: change brought about by the group experience – from the space created by the Art Therapist; the chance to share with other parents; the therapist's way of behaving, and from the direct support to the dyadic relationship. Other benefits were specific to the use of art making: the materials themselves and the process of making art together; the symbolism of the final shared product, and the capacity to offer containment through the art materials themselves. In the *Art at the Start* project we have found this framework to be useful in our understanding of what is going on during our sessions and it is helpful in trying to break down the different elements of the process for reflection. Obviously, in reality, the different mechanisms are happening in parallel and complementary ways through the fluid process of the groups. When several different interactions are happening simultaneously it can be a challenge to pick apart what is happening for each dyad and what may be influencing the outcomes, so it is valuable to have a framework to come back to. It is our intention that this framework will be beneficial to those reflecting on their own parent–infant practice or those thinking of developing this way of working. We also find this framework useful as a starting point for further investigation as it offers a common way to think about parent–infant practice, even when the specific models have some variation between practitioners and contexts. Having a shared understanding of what is fundamental about the process will allow for comparisons and further research. It is important for this area of practice that there continues to be research and investigation in order to provide a solid evidence base that captures the benefits of art psychotherapy intervention that practitioners are observing.

References

All Party Parliamentary Group on Arts, Health and Wellbeing. 2017. *Creative Health Inquiry Report*, 2nd ed. London: AAPGAHW.

Armstrong, V. G., Dalinkeviciute, E., & Ross, J. 2019. A Dyadic Art Psychotherapy Group for Parents and Infants: Piloting Quantitative Methodologies for *Evaluation*. *International Journal of Art Therapy*, 24(3): 113–124.

Armstrong, V. G., & Howatson, R. 2015. Parent–Infant Art Psychotherapy: A Creative Dyadic Approach to Early Intervention. *Infant Mental Health Journal*, 36(2): 213–222.

Armstrong, V. G., & Ross, J. 2020. The Evidence Base for Art Therapy with Parent and Infant Dyads: An Integrative Literature Review. *International Journal of Art Therapy*, advance online publication. doi:10.1080/17454832.2020.1724165.

Arroyo, C., & Fowler, N. 2013. Before and After: A Mother and Infant Painting Group. *International Journal of Art Therapy*, 18(3): 98–112.

Baradon, T. 2005. *The Practice of Psychoanalytic Parent–Infant Psychotherapy: Claiming the Baby*. Abingdon, Oxon: Routledge.

Bauer, A., Parsonage, M., Knapp, M., Lemmi, V., & Adelaja, B. 2014. The Cost of Perinatal Mental Health Problems. Available at: www.nwcscnsenate.nhs.uk/files/3914/7030/1256/Costs_of_perinatal_mh.pdf (accessed April 2020).

Belsky, J. 2001. Developmental risks (Still) Associated With Early Child Care. *Journal of Child Psychology and Psychiatry*, 42(7): 845–859.

Bigelow, A. E., MacLean, K., Proctor, J., Myatt, T., Gillis, R., & Power, M. 2010. Maternal sensitivity throughout infancy: Continuity and relation to attachment security. *Infant Behavior and Development*, 33(1): 50–60.

Black, C., Ellis, M., Harris, L., Rooke, A., Slater, I., & Cuch, L. 2015. *Making it Together: An Evaluative Study of Creative Families an Arts and Mental Health Partnership between the South London Gallery and the Parental Mental Health Team*. London: South London Gallery.

Cummings, E. M., & Cicchetti, D. 1990. Toward a Transactional Model of Relations between Attachment and Depression. In M. T. Greenberg, D. Cicchetti, & E. M. Cummings (eds.), *Attachment in the Preschool Years*. Chicago: University of Chicago Press, pp. 339–372.

Hall, P. 2008. Painting Together: An Art Therapy Approach to Mother–Infant Relationships. In C. Case & T. Dalley (eds.), *Art Therapy with Children: From Infancy to Adolescence*. New York, NY: Routledge, pp. 20–35.

Hall, P. 2019. Can You Do Art Therapy with Mothers and Babies? Exploring a 40 Year Old Question. In *Holding and Being Held: BAAT Region 16 Conference*, Edinburgh.

Hamed-Agbariah, A., & Rosenfeld, Y. 2015. The Added Value of Art Therapy for Mothers with Post-Partum Depression in Arabic Society in Israel. *Harefuah*, 154(9): 568–572.

Hogan, S., Sheffield, D., & Woodward, A. 2017. The Value of Art Therapy in Antenatal and Postnatal Care: A Brief Literature Review with Recommendations for Future Research. *International Journal of Art Therapy: Inscape*, 22(4): 169–179.

Hosea, H. 2006. 'The Brush's Footmarks': Parents and Infants Paint Together in a Small Community Art Therapy Group. *International Journal of Art Therapy*, 11(2): 69–78.

Hosea, H. 2011. The Brush's Foot Marks: Researching a Small Community Art Therapy Group. In A. Gilroy (ed.), *Art Therapy Research in Practice*. Bern: Peter Lang, pp. 61–80.

Hosea, H. 2017. Amazing Mess: Mothers Get in Touch with their Infants through the Vitality of Painting Together. In J. Meyerowitz-Katz & D. Reddick (eds.), *Art Therapy in the Early Years: Therapeutic Interventions with Infants, Toddlers and their Families*. Abingdon, Oxon: Routledge, pp. 104–117.

Khan, L. 2017. *Briefing 50: Fatherhood: The Impact of Fatherhood on Children's Mental Health.* London: Centre for Mental Health.

Lavey-Khan, L., & Reddick, D. 2018. *Painting Together: A Dyadic Art Therapy Group.* Unpublished manuscript. Hertfordshire Partnership University NHS Foundation and Islington Council Early Years Education.

Meyerowitz-Katz, J. 2017. The Crisis of the Cream Cakes: An Infants Food Refusal as a Representation of Intergenerational Trauma. In J. Meyerowitz-Katz & D. Reddick (ed.), *Art Therapy in the Early Years: Therapeutic Interventions with Infants, Toddlers and their Families.* Abingdon, Oxon: Routledge, pp. 118–132.

Parashak, S. T. 2008. Object Relations and Attachment Theory: Creativity of Mother and Child in the Single Parent Family. In C. Kerr, Hoshino, J., Sutherland, J., Parashak, S. T., & McCarley, L. L. (ed.), *Family Art Therapy: Foundations of Theory and Practice.* Abingdon, Oxon: Routledge, pp. 65–93.

Paulson, J. F., & Bazemore, S. D. 2010. Prenatal and Postpartum Depression in Fathers and its Association with Maternal Depression: A Meta-Analysis. *The Journal of the American Medical Association,* 301(19): 1961–1969.

Perry, C., Thurston, M., & Osborn, T. 2008. Time for Me: the Arts as Therapy in Postnatal *Depression. Complementary Therapies in Clinical Practice,* 14(1): 38–45.

Ponteri, A. K. 2001. The Effect of Group Art Therapy on Depressed Mothers and Their Children. *Art Therapy,* 18(3): 148–157.

Proulx, L. 2000. Container, Contained, Containment: Group Art Therapy with Toddlers 18 to 30 Months and their Parent. *Canadian Art Therapy Association Journal,* 14: 3–6.

Proulx, L. 2002. Strengthening Ties, Parent–Child-Dyad: Group Art Therapy with Toddlers and Parents. *American Journal of Art Therapy,* 40(4): 238–258.

Proulx, L. 2003. *Strengthening Emotional Ties through Parent–Child Dyad Art Therapy: Interventions with Infants and Preschoolers.* London: Jessica Kingsley Publishers.

Schore, A. N. 2001. Effects of a Secure Attachment Relationship on Right Brain Development, Affect Regulation, and Infant Mental Health. *Infant Mental Health Journal,* 22: 7–66.

Starcatchers. 2014. *Expecting Something: A Public Health Initiative.* Edinburgh: NHS Lothian.

Svanberg, P. O. G. 1998. Attachment, Resilience and Prevention. *Journal of Mental Health,* 7(6): 543–578.

Taylor Buck, E., Dent-Brown, K., & Parry, G. (2013). Exploring a Dyadic Approach to Art Psychotherapy with Children and Young People: A Survey of British Art Psychotherapists. *International Journal of Art Therapy: Inscape,* 18(1): 20–28.

Warren, S. L., Huston, L., Egeland, B., & Sroufe, A. 1997. Child and Adolescent Anxiety Disorders and Early Attachment. *Journal of the American Academy of Child & Adolescent Psychiatry,* 36(5): 637–644.

15 And if the bough breaks

The use of individual Art Therapy within a perinatal mental health service

Bridget Grant

Introduction

In this chapter I will describe my work as an Art Therapist within a perinatal mental health service in the voluntary sector in central Scotland. The service works with both mothers and fathers but my focus here is on the women who use the service, offering a contribution to the under-reported area of individual Art Therapy with mothers experiencing perinatal distress. An exploration of themes and case material show how Art Therapy facilitates recovery and growth from perinatal distress such as post-natal depression (PND), anxiety and birth trauma.

Background

Idealisation and loss of authentic self

Loss of self and identify emerge as key themes in my work with women, in this time of massive change in their lives (Abrams & Curran 2011; Beck 2002a; Hogan 2012; Hogan, Sheffield & Woodward 2017; Mauthner 2010). Additionally, idealised notions of what or who a mother should be compound the symptoms of postnatal distress. Mauthner (2010) finds that women lose connection with their authentic selves when they strive to meet idealised expectations of motherhood (see Beck 2002b). This too resonates with observations from my own clinical work and I have come to wonder about what this means for the women it impacts so painfully.

In psychological terms, the act of idealisation may be a defence against the anxiety of knowing a part which is deemed not good enough or is unacceptable in some way; a fanciful imagining that allows temporary departure from the negatively perceived part within. In Kleinien object-relations theory, idealisation implies a splitting between 'good' and 'bad' (Klein 1986 [1946], p. 182). In order to preserve an acceptable version of the self, the unacceptable characteristic or part is suppressed and denied. The fear is that the two cannot co-exist as if the existence of the 'negative' extinguishes the good. The result is an idealised self, while a more realistic, 'warts and all' self is hoped to be avoided. However, seeking refuge in this idealised version leaves little or no space for experience that does not fit with the ideal criteria. In the process of disavowal, connection with the authentic self is lost. There may be many factors contributing to the psychological need to idealise in the face of becoming a mother, but for the purposes of this chapter I shall focus on one particular feature as an underlying theme drawn from my clinical work; the fear of 'maternal failure'.

Maternal failure

'Mother' may be one of the most powerful and evocative words in any language and culture. It alludes to the mystery of our origin, and our survival. 'Mother' evokes images rooted in archetypal psychology (Jung 1969 [1938]). We have powerful stories about both 'good' and 'bad' mothers which arise from the personal and the collective. They may be witches, queens, stepmothers or overwhelmed as in 'The Old Woman Who Lived in a Shoe'. While these stories bear little resemblance to real women, they express a psychological reality (Birkhauser-Oeri & Von Franz 1988, p. 13). Being labelled a failed or bad mother may be one of the most stigmatising and shaming attacks on a woman, for as Badinter (2010, p. 15) writes 'to admit you are not cut out to be a mother … would brand you a reckless monster'. Yet ideals regarding mothers are not fixed. While the biological facts of conceiving and giving birth remain static, societal attitudes regarding motherhood shift with time and culture (Gunderson 2019). Compare, for example, the view of the seventeenth-century French upper classes, who considered maternal mothering an impediment to fulfilling the duties of a distinguished wife and woman (Badinter 2010, p. 160), with 'attachment parenting' which is popular today (Attachment Parenting UK 2019).

To explore the fear of maternal failure, I shall first consider how societal and cultural constructs and expectations regarding mothers and babies impact on the woman's external and internal worlds (Rose 2018; Hogan 2012). Then, from a psychodynamic perspective, I shall reflect on how a woman's experience of being cared for as a baby herself might unconsciously play into the mix (Fraiberg, Adelson & Shapiro 1980).

In recent decades, a wide body of literature challenging and re-visioning dominant discourses on motherhood in Western society has come to the fore (Donath 2015). Examining motherhood in relation to identity, change and gender (Hogan 2012; Abrams & Curran 2011; Mauthner 2010; McMahon 1995) provides a deeper understanding of the impact cultural and psychological assumptions may have. Contextual cultural attitudes regarding gender and motherhood underpin how women experience PND (Abrams & Curran 2011) and impact mental health. Referring to aspects of object relations and attachment theory, Art Therapist Susan Hogan (2012, p. 81) argues that 'outdated, misogynistic theories continue to blight women's lives', warning such reductive theory can oppress our clients. As healthcare professionals, we have a responsibility to be aware of and to challenge the potentially harmful myths of motherhood (Beck 2002a). These myths and messages can be confusing and inconsistent. Women I work with describe a barrage of conflicting advice and opinions from health professionals, family, friends and even the stranger on the bus. In her study of the complex, paradoxical and often impossible projections mothers receive, Rose (2018) suggests that mothers are used as the scapegoats for the conflicts and failings which society does not wish to bear, assigning mothers the impossible task of 'repairing it all'. Badinter (2010) highlights the contradiction of promoting 'self-less' motherhood in an individualistic society while social media and online platforms operate as ubiquitous message delivery systems for society's often emotive and emphatic ideas about mothers and babies. It may not be surprising then that feelings of guilt and shame are prevalent in motherhood (Dunford and Granger 2017) and the mismatch between expectations and the actual experience of motherhood is linked to PND (Mauthner 2010; Beck 2002a).

Mothers have also once been a baby and have had the experience of 'mother' whether absent or present. How we make sense of, internalise and adapt to these early experiences are part of what forms our sense of who we are, to our self, to others and the world. Therefore, our thoughts around what constitutes 'mother' maybe powerful, unconscious and highly emotionally charged. Many of the women with whom I work express the desire to be different from their own mothers for fear of passing something 'bad' onto their baby. Sometimes, this deep anxiety creates an urge to fulfil an ideal based on the exact opposite and is unconsciously projected into the relationship with her baby, as an attempt to avoid any possibility of repeating her negative experience in childhood. For example, if her own mother's anger were an issue for her, she may not be able to tolerate *any* angry feelings in her relationship with her baby. However, as we have seen, idealisation leaves little space for authenticity. Suppressed feelings need to find a way out and like 'ghosts' from the past can haunt in the present (Fraiberg et al. 1980) and, with painful irony keep her more psychologically identified with her own mother or her internal image of mother than she realises, and perhaps vulnerable to enacting the very thing she fears most. Often a compassionate realisation of her own mother as a separate woman in her own right is part of the process of psychological separation.

Reflection

The institution of motherhood is held as an ultimately rewarding and fulfilling experience (Donath 2015), and for many women this is true. What happens then, if a mother's experience does not fit with, or reaches beyond the available discourse (Hollway 2011)? To use the metaphor from the nursery rhyme, what happens if the bough begins to break? Like the wind in the treetops, these factors may create a maelstrom of influences and pressures on a mother's psyche. Perhaps, in a painful attempt not to 'break' and let the 'baby fall' a rigidly held expectation of motherhood manifests. I suggest this idealisation, triggered as an anxious defence against the disturbing image of 'maternal failure', is a complicating factor lying at the heart of much perinatal distress. Allowing no space for states such as loss and grief (Hogan 2012; Beck 2002a), ambivalence

(Parker 1995) or post-traumatic stress from birth trauma (Birth Trauma Association 2019), it forces a disconnected self in which the symptoms of anxiety and depression can arise.

Context

Perinatal mental health

According to the Royal College of Obstetricians and Gynaecologists (RCOG), up to one in five women will experience mental health problems in the perinatal period (Russell et al. 2017). Of the 23,000 women surveyed by the RCOG, 81 per cent said they had experienced a maternal mental health problem and only 7 per cent of those were referred to specialist care (Russell et al. 2017, p. 9). The RCOG report found that mental health problems were attributed to a quarter of deaths of mothers in the time when the child was between six weeks to a year old (Russell et al. 2017, p. 9). In fact, suicide is the leading cause of death among women during the first year after pregnancy (MBRACE-UK 2018, p. 2). In Scotland there is recognition of the need to support perinatal mental health and the Scottish Government have recently allocated extensive funding for this area (Scottish Government 2019).

PND occurs across cultures and is not necessarily restricted to Western societies (Mauthner 2010). In addition, theories of PND vary, a biologically informed medical approach (Abdollahi, Lye & Zargami 2016; Mauthner 2010; Beck 2002b) contrasts with perspectives from the social sciences including psychosocial theories such as: interpersonal, feminist, attachment and self-labelling theory (Beck 2002b). Evolutionary theory views PND as an adaptive function to grieving loss and change (Abdollahi et al. 2016). It is also important to emphasise that men too experience PND and the research shows the statistics and risk factors are similar to those of women (Scarff 2019). Birth trauma is more widely understood in relation to perinatal mental health (Birth Trauma Association 2019). Distressing experiences during birth can result in post-traumatic stress disorder (Hogan et al. 2017) and the experience of maternity care staff in the hospital has a psychological impact on women in the post-partum period (Baker et al. 2005).

Art Therapy literature

Evidence indicating the efficacy of Art Therapy in perinatal mental healthcare is emerging (Hogan et al. 2017). Hogan and colleagues' (2017) literature review of arts-based interventions with pregnant women and new mothers found studies of group and parent–infant-dyadic Art Therapy, while individual Art Therapy with post-natal mothers was less evident. Art Therapy groups have been shown to improve mothers' self-esteem, self-confidence and self-awareness, while reducing self-criticism (Hogan et al. 2017) and enhance resilience in mothers at risk of developing PND (Kong 2019). A confidential arts-based group space in which socially unacceptable maternal anxieties can be depicted and explored was found to be of great value to new mothers (Hogan et al. 2017). Hogan developed multimedia arts groups for mothers to process experiences of birth trauma and iatrogenic hospital procedures (Jagminaite 2019). Sarid et al. (2017) integrate CBT and Art Therapy (CB-ART) helping to reframe and transform perinatal distress. In turn, mother–infant painting groups promote mentalisation and attuned interactions improving relationships (Hosea 2017; Armstrong & Howatson 2015). From a community perspective, Jagminaite (2017) proposes Art Therapy as a vehicle for women to explore, critique and analyse their experiences of birth and the conditions of motherhood, as a rite of passage in preparation for the realities to come.

The perinatal service and Art Therapy

The service

The service offers counselling and support to families experiencing perinatal distress. Referrals are taken for parents who have a child under the age of two, either as a self-referral, or from a health and/or social care professional. Referrals for fathers are encouraged, but the majority are for mothers. In 2019 only 6.5 per cent of referrals were for fathers. Increasingly there are some referrals from same sex and transgender parents. The onsite crèche is pivotal, allowing an element of connection alongside separation as a parent takes therapeutic space for themselves (Rayment 2017).

Art Therapy

Historically, Art Therapy has formed a key support offered within the service. A dedicated, fully equipped Art Therapy room has existed in the service since the late 1990s, providing space for both individual and group work. The value an organisation places on Art Therapy has a significant impact on the quality of the clinical work (Meyerowitz-Katz & Reddick 2017). The Art Therapy room in the service frequently evokes a positive response when people first enter, whether to make art or not. It has been described as the 'heart' of the building and we often gather in its light airy space to hold our team meetings.

Viewing motherhood as a developmental life stage and event (Abrams & Curran 2011; Birksted-Breen 1986) or a rite of passage (Jagminaite 2019), offers the opportunity to redefine self and identity and learn new ways of being (Abrams & Curran 2011). Integrating these experiences and working through internal conflicts of the psyche (Birksted-Breen 1986) may require a deeper engagement with life, self and external relationships, challenging both internal and external norms and letting go of systems that are no longer relevant. The multiplicity of meaning in images is particularly well suited to working with women making this transition. The special properties of art materials and images offer a container in which to hold and process the irreducible, shifting states, and images have capacity to hold the archetypes and symbols that may arise from the unconscious at this time. Haywood (2019) observes how art materials can help to ground the uncertainty inherent within transition; the art materials help us to play in the limbo while also providing a physical container.

Art Therapy is a brain-mind-body process. The tactile, sensory and physical properties of art materials, combined with the movement in art making, offer a way to the unconscious and neurological processes required to effect psychological change (Hass-Cohen & Findlay 2015; Elbrecht & Antcliff 2015). The somatic nature of Art Therapy corresponds with the bodily events of pregnancy and birth and caring for a new baby (another body) when the physiology of a mother's ecosystem may be distressed and deregulated.

Working as an Art Therapist in this service stirs deep and primal layers within my psyche. Powerful mother archetypes (Birkhauser-Oeri & Von Franz 1988) are activated alongside less resolved younger parts of self. Loss and grief are ever-present (Beck 2002a) and birth connects us with death. My countertransference can feel painfully intense and raw and at times form into powerful projective

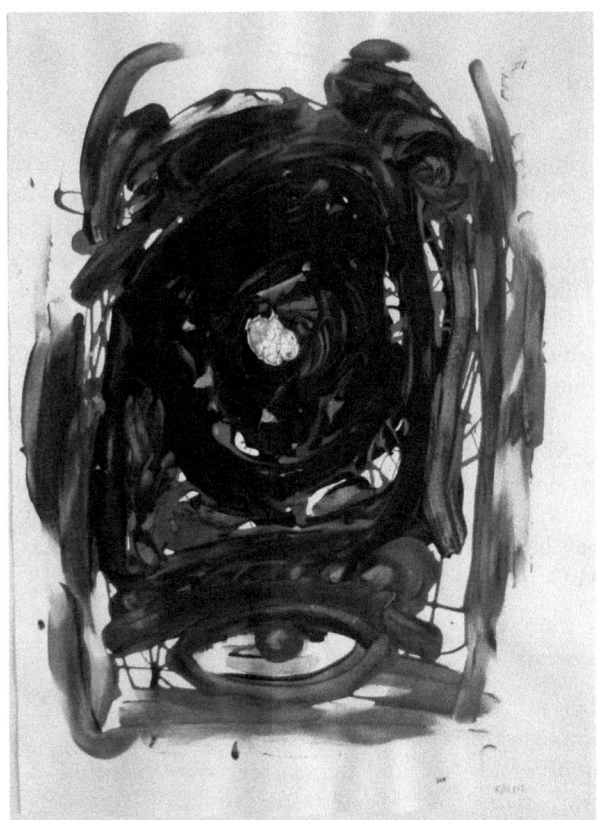

Figure 15.1 Untitled. Bridget Grant.

identifications (Ogden 1982). Clinical supervision is essential and post-session response art is a way to begin to process and reveal unconscious aspects within the therapeutic relationship (Brown, Meyerowitz-Katz & Ryde 2007). The physicality of the art materials helps metabolise and release the processes, expanding my capacity for reflection with the client (Rowe 2017). Figure 15.1 is a painting I made when I first began at the service, before I had 'acclimatised' so to speak. Eight years on, it remains for me an embodied and symbolic expression of how my internal world met the worlds of the clients and the perinatal service at that time.

My work includes group and parent–child-dyadic Art Therapy in addition to individual Art Therapy. Alongside broad-ranging psychodynamic and Art Therapy theory, my practice is informed by somatic and body-work approaches arising from converging findings within the fields of developmental and inter-personal neuroscience and the physiology of trauma (Rothschild 2000, 2017; Schore & Sieff 2015; van der Kolk 2015;). In mediating inner states via art materials, I am also influenced by Focusing Orientated Art Therapy (Rappaport 2009) which uses Gendlin's (2003) concept of 'felt sense' and his work on focusing, designed to enquire within the body as a way of accessing the unconscious.

Case study: Nicola

This case study provides an account of the making of and reflecting on four images made in individual Art Therapy with Nicola, a new mother, who attended for 16 sessions following a traumatising hospital experience. Working with a somatic, felt sense approach to trauma (Rappaport 2009; Rothschild 2000), the study shows how the images were pivotal in unlocking Nicola's sub-conscious feelings of failure as a mother and revealing how she had become caught in a projective identification whereby her traumatic experience of the hospital environment was internalised as her own maternal failure. Art Therapy allowed suppressed thoughts and feelings to become available for integration, therapeutically holding the potentially breaking 'bough'. The images helped Nicola to hear her own voice and begin the process of psychological separation from her mother. Thus, she was able to release her defences, reconnect with her sense of self and continue her journey into motherhood in more creative and growthful ways. Names have been changed and the the material has been published with the client's consent.

Referral and assessment

Nicola, a woman in her twenties was referred to the perinatal service by her health visitor, for symptoms of post-natal depression and anxiety, when Marie, her baby, was four months old. She and her partner were first-time parents. They had just moved in together and he had begun a new job.

Marie's birth was prolonged and difficult, involving epidural and forceps delivery, culminating in emergency life-saving surgery. Nicola powerfully recalled the brief sensation of holding her baby just after birth followed by the abrupt separation and the sickening thought she might never see her again if she did not survive the operation. Nicola underwent 90 minutes of surgery, requiring multiple blood transfusions. She had a local anaesthetic and was conscious throughout. Listening, I felt something of this horror, like a silent scream within me. Nicola said she could not control catastrophic thoughts and replayed the experience over and over. She was consumed with anxiety and emotions that were hard to make sense of. The fear and panic she felt in her body bore the hallmarks of a flashback, associated with the effects of post-traumatic stress (Rothschild 2017; Ogden 2017; van der Kolk 2015). This affected her relationship with Marie, and she seemed angry and critical of herself.

Nicola often felt unheard, particularly by her mother. While speaking warmly of her, she felt controlled by her mother's anxiety and did not want to 'pass this on' to her daughter. I wondered how her mother's anxiety had shaped Nicola's emotional security in childhood (Schore & Sieff 2015). Nicola's need to be heard and reformulate the relationship with her mother, alongside the need to process the hospital trauma seemed clear. Her internal world and identity appeared in a state of flux. Combined with the non-verbal aspects of trauma (Ogden 2017; Schore & Sieff 2015; van der Kolk 2015), this indicated there might be much that could not be put in words. I suggested Art Therapy could help express what needed to be both heard and seen in Nicola (Case and Dalley 2014) and introduced Rothschild's (2000, 2017) approach in 'organising and outlining a trauma memory' as a way to structure and contain the work. This procedure can be tailored to individual processes and may be interwoven with other aspects of the client's process as they arise. Such a focus required individual work and Nicola was curious and open about using Art Therapy.

Making a container

Laying the foundations for working with the traumatic memory involved organising the sequence of events into manageable pieces, including an overall title and a beginning and end (Rothschild 2000 2017). Rothschild (2000, 2017) also emphasises the importance of pacing the process through tracking and regulating the autonomic nervous system and identifying an 'anchor', as an internal safe space. Using a piece of cartridge paper, folded in two Nicola wrote a title and a series of simple sentences, like chapter headings for each part of the experience. This book-image became an important object in the Art Therapy, to be referred and returned to, providing a holding container for the trauma work (Rothschild 2000, 2017).

Voicing the fear of maternal failure

Nicola's first drawing unlocked her unspoken fear that she was a bad mother. Listening to Nicola describing how Marie cried when she could not sleep at night, I sensed that Nicola's distress was linked to something deeply disturbing.

This felt not verbal, but somatically based in a primal anxiety. I suggested she use art materials to make an image of the felt sense (Gendlin 2003) of this (Rappaport 2009).

Nicola chose a box of soft coloured pastels and a sheet of white cartridge paper and spent 20 minutes making a drawing. We looked at what she had made (Figure 15.2). At the centre Nicola identified a dark 'unbearable' part, encircled with black, purple then red and yellow which she said represented the anger she felt. She associated the radiating red rings with the piercing sensation of Marie's cries and the clock her longing for the sun and daylight to appear again. I was struck by the grid-like marks, in the centre evoking in me a sense of tightness in my chest, which felt meaningful in a way I did not understand. Reflecting on this, Nicola disclosed a strict routine she had devised for Marie's sleep-time. The rules were that she must not let in any light or leave the room until Marie had stopped crying and gone back to sleep, no matter how long it took. The 'unbearable' began to make sense in terms of the isolation and loneliness she felt as her partner slept in the other room. Nicola expressed shame at feeling imprisoned by Marie as if it was wrong to feel this way in relation to her baby. Reflecting on the quality of 'imprisonment' at the centre of her drawing, we made the connection with the imprisoning routine she had imposed upon herself. Wondering what purpose this might serve in keeping something in, or out, revealed a fear in Nicola that she was, underneath it all, a 'bad mother'. This admission felt like a painful release, almost too dangerous to voice, as if saying it would make it true. Nicola allowed this hidden thought to rise to the surface. She began to cry and I was deeply moved to hear her. We did not yet know the root of Nicola's sense of maternal failure, but we saw that the rigidity of the sleep routine, demanding a kind of 'perfection', was like a structure she had erected around and within herself to protect against the anxiety and shame of this. Yet, the idealised expectation had, in itself become a prison, generating and trapping her in anxiety and depression.

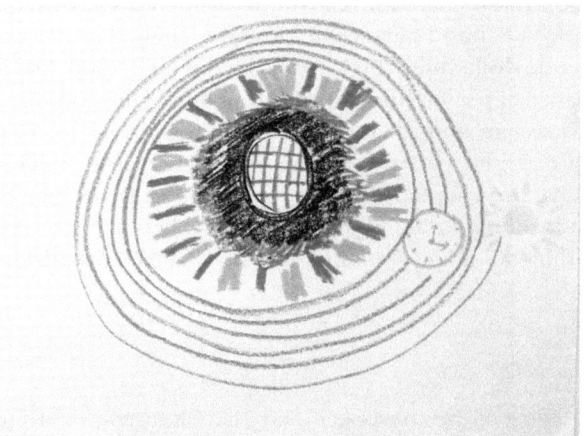

Figure 15.2 A Dark 'Unbearable' Part. Nicola.

Before it had appeared in the image it had not been possible to see this and make these connections. Once it was voiced, and heard, Nicola cried and expressed relief. We were then able to start safely dismantling it, and begin to 'play' (Winnicott 1971, p. 54) with more creative ideas about how she could manage the long nights, such as going downstairs with Marie to make a cup of tea and seeking support from her partner.

Reflection

Nicola's image was complex and embodied providing a symbolic container in which multiple emotions could be held in one place and reflected back, becoming available for psychological integration (Schaverien 1987, 1999). Picking up on the 'aesthetic-counter-transferential fragment' (Leclerc 2006, p. 132) at the centre of her drawing had helped to unlock the anxiety it both hid and hid from.

The following week Nicola said she had relaxed her routine and that she and Marie had slept much better. It seemed that a significant shift had taken place. Nicola was starting to get in touch with and trust her own needs and instincts and to let these guide her.

'Euphoric Moment'

Alongside processing difficult and painful feelings, identifying and taking in 'the good' (Hanson 2011) offers a way to cultivate necessary resources (Wilson 2017). The next image Nicola made (Figure 15.3) represented the time she first held Marie in the hospital, just *before* she was rushed into emergency theatre. She named it the 'Euphoric Moment'. It was important to remember and reconnect with this event, knowing that it was also still there inside her. The gold in the image both holds and accentuates the precious pink centre while radiating a

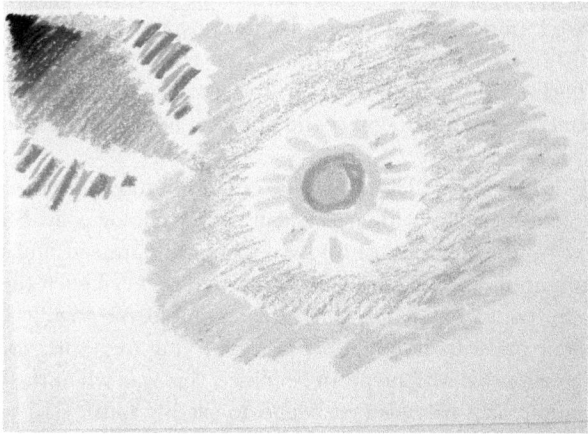

Figure 15.3 Euphoric Moment. Nicola.

sense of goodness. The imminent trauma is depicted as the threatening blue and black tornado-like shape in the top left hand. I saw a breast-like quality in this image and recognised its similarity to the preceding picture, but with a very different feel. In that session I had felt I was working with a younger Nicola, who needed me as a containing mother (Bion 2004) to help her with frightening unprocessed thoughts and feelings.

In contrast, the aesthetic countertransference (Schaverien 2011) of this image evoked a sense of safety and stability inviting me as a guiding grandmother. On reflection, in relation to the first image, I am also reminded of Nicola's painful struggle with breastfeeding.

My sense of Nicola's resourceful and emerging self was reinforced as she spoke about finding time to undertake her own creative activities. She had begun to set boundaries with her own mother, not reacting immediately to anxious texts or voice messages. The sense of her confidence and knowledge as a mother was growing as she imagined the kind of life she wanted for herself and new family.

There was also sadness as she remembered the pain of 'not knowing' but feeling she *ought* to know, when Marie was first born. She remembered people saying that her mothering instinct would just kick in, and the expectation was, if she only allowed it, she would know how to feed and respond to Marie. When, amid the effects of post-traumatic stress, this 'knowing' did not come, and in fact she felt increasingly lost within herself, she began to think she must be an un-natural or bad mother.

Hospital

In our eleventh meeting Nicola said she had felt anxious about coming today, knowing she wanted to move onto the next 'part' of the trauma. Our conversation turned to her experience of the hospital environment and she chose, rather than follow the linear outline of the trauma narrative to use art materials, to explore her sense of the hospital environment. Nicola said the drawing expressed feeling overlooked, unheard and unseen by the hospital staff both before and following the birth and surgery (Figure 15.4). She felt that overstretched, under-resourced staff had not listened to her warning about having a condition that made her vulnerable to haemorrhaging, and she was angry that this might happen to someone else.

Nicola had nearly died. Following the surgery she could not move. Her wounds meant she could barely hold her baby either physically or psychologically. She felt this was not understood by the nurses and midwives, whose harassed and pragmatic attitudes felt lacking in the gentle kindness she needed then. She felt the staff were impatient when she could not reach the toilet and told me vividly about feeling violated as an older midwife, handled her breasts trying to get her to feed. She remembered feeling ashamed and inept and realised this was when the belief that she must be inadequate as a mother first began to silently form.

In this drawing, Nicola depicts her sense of being surrounded by countless, faceless, indistinguishable healthcare professionals. They do not appear as

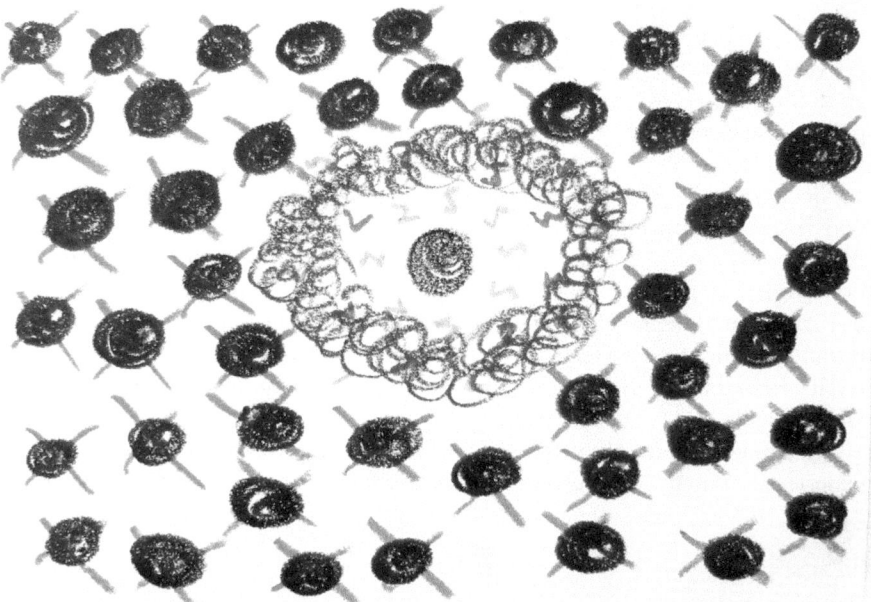

Figure 15.4 Overlooked, Unheard and Unseen. Nicola.

people, becoming a non-human 'system'. It is as if Nicola too has lost her humanity, reduced to a black spot indistinguishable from the others. The purple scribbles represent her feelings of bewilderment at not being seen and heard. We recognised how this resonated with the familiar experience of finding it hard to find her voice and express her needs.

We think of hospitals as caregiving places in which we are looked after. Reflecting on the image and Nicola's experiences we began to see the short-comings of the hospital environment as repeating a kind of 'maternal failure' for Nicola, perhaps echoing past experiences with her mother. Menzies' (1960) study of nurses in a hospital shows how organisational structures and culture can form as a defence against anxiety evoked by the primary task; dealing with life and death. In Nicola's drawing, the apparent loss of herself as an individual, and her forming belief that she was already failing as a mother, suggested she had in-ternalised the hospital environment's disowned anxiety and inadequacy as her own. Seeing this in her drawing helped her know it was not *her* failure. This insight was an important turning point.

Surgery

The conscious and unconscious symbolic representations within the preceding images and the deepening trust within our therapeutic relationship paved the way for Nicola to move into the work of processing the most terrifying part of the hospital experience, undergoing surgery. She was visibly fearful and reported a racing heart, light head and churning stomach. The very thought of the memory activated her threat system preparing for a fight, flight, freeze or submit response as if the danger was present *now*. This indicated a need to help ground her physiological self in the physical and psychological safety of the present (van der Kolk 2015).

Nicola said she preferred to make an image rather than talk. The brain-mind-body processes of using art materials held within the therapeutic relationship of Art Therapy can offer containment and grounding. The memory of trauma may be encoded as dissociated, unprocessed fragments of experience (van der Kolk 2015). Art making's sub-cortical processing could account for its capacity to facilitate without overwhelming the emergence of unprocessed disturbing material or content, in preparation for psychological integration through cognition and words.

This image (Figure 15.5) allowed Nicola to finally put words to her frightening experience. The drawing is reminiscent of a torture scene, and this is how it had

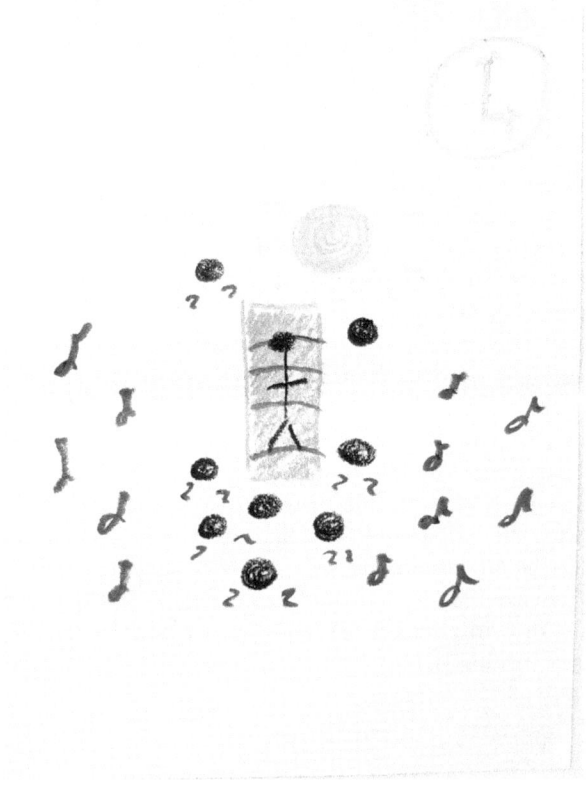

Figure 15.5 Trapped. Nicola.

felt to her. It seemed there were countless people in the room. She was given a local anaesthetic and was awake and conscious. There was a light above her with a large metal shade which, to her horror, she realised reflected the whole scene below. She could not bear to watch but was unable to move her head. When she tried to close her eyes, she was told to keep them open so her responses could be tracked. Nicola asked the nurse beside her if she was going to die, and she replied that they were doing all they could. At this moment in the session, I was the witnessing Art Therapist (Learmonth 1994) alongside Nicola, sharing with her the combination of overwhelming sadness and terror, trapped in this scene of horror.

Lack of mirroring is a feature of trauma (van der Kolk 2015). Here, 'mirroring' refers to receiving the attuned recognition of another. Nicola's unrecognised distress at being trapped beneath the harsh reflection of the 'mirror' in the operating theatre compounded the trauma increasing her experience of powerlessness. The aerial perspective in her drawing, as if we are looking down on the scene, accentuates this and is reminiscent of out-of-body experiences associated with shock and dissociation. Making this image helped to reflect her experience in a way she could control, assimilate and safely share with me.

Ending

The following week, Nicola said she was amazed that the intrusive images and thoughts about the surgery and hospital had gone. She felt sadness but this was different and felt an important step towards cultivating self-compassion. She reflected that she and her mother were also forming a better relationship, which could now tolerate disagreement. She decided she was ready to end Art Therapy.

It seemed fitting when Nicola spontaneously brought Marie into our last session. Laying a blanket between us I welcomed her into the space. It was a privileged hour as I followed the natural flow back-and-forth between the three of us. Nicola said that Art Therapy had played an important part in helping her recover. She decided to leave her artwork with me, in the service, saying she felt this part was 'closed'.

Reflection

Nicola's traumatic experience had ruptured her internal containment (Loban 2014). This, combined with the immense changes and responsibility of motherhood, was overwhelming. Art Therapy within the one-to-one therapeutic relationship provided the necessary container when the outer containers of her mother and hospital failed to hold.

Conclusion

Experiences of motherhood may differ greatly from societal and personal expectations. In this pressured and tumultuous time, an ideal of mother can manifest as a defence against the anxiety of maternal failure. Connections are made linking idealisation, loss of authentic self, depression and anxiety. Art Therapy's non-verbal processes offer a way to bridge disconnected feelings and fears of shaming 'maternal failure' which may feel too disturbing to voice.

Art Therapy groups with mothers and mother–infant dyads are effective in addressing perinatal mental health problems but little is written about individual Art Therapy with new mothers. The focused work with Nicola necessitated individual sessions and the space without her baby allowed her to re-find herself as a woman *and* as mother. Alongside group and dyadic work, opportunities for individual Art Therapy are crucial in providing space to process separately, away from the baby, and group work is not appropriate for every client's process. This chapter has shown how when the bough began to break, individual Art Therapy helped a woman, becoming a mother, to *catch* herself: cradle and all.

References

Abdollahi, F., Lye, M. S., & Zargami, M. 2016. Perspective of Postpartum Depression Theories: A Narrative Literature Review. *North American Journal of Medical Sciences*, 8(6): 232–236.

Abrams, L., & Curran, L. 2011. Maternal Identity Negotiations among Low-Income Women with Symptoms of Postpartum Depression. *Qualitative Health Research*, 21(3): 373–385.

Attachment Parenting UK. 2019. Available at: https://attachmentparenting.co.uk/ (accessed 16 November 2019).

Armstrong, V. G., & Howatson, R. 2015. Parent Infant Art Psychotherapy: A Creative Dyadic Approach to Early Intervention. *Infant Mental Health Journal*, 36(2): 213–222.

Badinter, E. 2010. *The Conflict: How Modern Motherhood Undermines the Status of Women*. New York: Metropolitan Books.

Baker, R. S., Choi, P. Y. L., Henshaw, C. A., & Tree, J. 2005. I Felt as though I'd Been in Jail: Women's Experiences of Maternity Care during Labour, Delivery and the Immediate Postpartum. *Feminism & Psychology*, 15(3): 315–342.

Beck, C. 2002a. Postpartum Depression: A Metasynthesis. *Qualitative Health Research*, 12(4): 453–472.

Beck, C. 2002b. Theoretical Perspectives of Postpartum Depression and their Treatment Implications. *The American Journal of Maternal Child Nursing*, 27(5): 282–287.

Bion, W. 2004. *Learning from Experience*, 4th ed. Lanham, MD: Rowman & Littlefield Publishers.

Birkhauser-Oeri, S., & Von Franz, M. L., eds. 1988. *The Mother: Archetypal Image in Fairy Tales*. Toronto: Inner City Books.

Birksted-Breen, D. 1986. The Experience of Having a Baby: A Developmental View. *Free Associations*, 4: 22–35.

Birth Trauma Association. 2019. Available at: https://birthtraumaassociation.org.uk. (accessed June 2019).

Brown, C., Meyerowitz-Katz, J., & Ryde, J. 2007. Thinking with Image Making: Supervising Student Art Therapists. In J. Schaverien & C. Case (eds.), *Supervision of Art Psychotherapy: A Theoretical and Practical Handbook*. Abingdon, Oxon: Routledge, pp. 168–181.

Case, C., & Dalley, T. 2014. *The Handbook of Art Therapy*, 3rd ed. Abingdon, Oxon: Routledge.

Donath, O. 2015. Regretting Motherhood: A Sociopolitical Analysis. *Signs: Journal of Women in Culture and Society*, 40(2): 343–367.

Dunford, E., & Granger, C. 2017. Maternal Guilt and Shame: Relationship to Postnatal Depression and Attitudes Towards Help-Seeking. *Journal of Child and Family Studies*, 26: 1692–1701.

Elbrecht, C., & Antcliff, L. R. 2014. Being Touched through Touch: Trauma treatment through Haptic Perception at the Clay Field: A Sensorimotor Art Therapy. *International Journal of Art Therapy: Inscape*, 19(1): 19–30.

Fraiberg, S., Adelson, E., & Shapiro, V. 1980. Ghosts in the Nursery: A Psychoanalytic Approach to the Problems of Impaired Infant–Mother Relationships. In S. Fraiberg (ed.), *Clinical Studies in Infant Mental Health*. New York: Basic Books, pp. 164–192.

Gendlin, E. T. 2003. *Focussing*, 3rd ed. London: Rider.

Gunderson, J. 2019. The Historical Rise of Intensive Mothering and its Implications for Women. *Academia.edu*. Available at: www.academia.edu/1370587/ (accessed November 2019).

Hanson, R. 2011. *Just One Thing: Developing a Buddha Brain One Simple Practice at a Time*. Oakland, CA: New Harbinger Publications.

Hass-Cohen, N., & Findlay, J. 2015. *Art Therapy and the Neuroscience of Relationships, Creativity and Resiliency*. New York and London: W. W. Norton and Company.

Haywood, S. 2019. Holding and Being Held at Times of Transition and Change. Conference paper presented at *Holding and Being Held: BAAT region 16 Conference 2019*, 28 September, City of Edinburgh Methodist Church, Edinburgh.

Hogan, S. 2012. Postmodernist but Not Post-Feminist. In H. Burt (ed.), *Art Therapy and Postmodernism Creative Healing Through a Prism*. London: Jessica Kingsley Publishers, pp. 70–82.

Hogan, S., Sheffield, D., & Woodward, A. 2017. The Value of Art Therapy in Antenatal and Postnatal Care: A Brief Literature Review with Recommendations for Future Research. *International Journal of Art Therapy: Inscape*, 22(4): 169–179.

Hollway, W. 2011. Rereading Winnicott's 'Primary Maternal Preoccupation'. *Feminism & Psychology*, 22(1): 20–40.

Hosea, H. 2017. Amazing Mess: Mothers Get in Touch with their Infants through the Vitality of Painting Together. In J. Meyerowitz-Katz & D. Reddick (eds.), *Art Therapy in the Early Years: Therapeutic Interventions with Infants, Toddlers and their Families*. London and New York: Routledge, pp. 104–117.

Jagminaite, E. 2019. Art Therapy and Motherhood as a Rite of Passage. In S. Hogan (ed.), *Gender and Difference in the Arts Therapies: Inscribed on the Body*. London and New York: Routledge, pp. 163–180.

Jung, C. W. 1969 [1938]. Psychological Aspects of the Mother Archetype. *In Archetypes and the Collective Unconscious*. Princeton, NJ: Princeton University Press.

Klein, M. 1986 [1946]. Notes on Some Schizoid Mechanisms. In J. Mitchel (ed.), *The Selected Melanie Klein*. London: Penguin Books Ltd., pp. 176–200.

Kong, M. 2019. Development of a Group-Based Art Therapy Program to Enhance the Resilience of Mothers at Risk for Postpartum *Depression. Korean Journal of Art Therapy*, 26(1): 111–136.

Learmonth, M. 1994. Witness and Witnessing in Art Therapy. *Inscape*, 1: 19–22.

Leclerc, J. 2006. The Unconscious as Paradox: Impact of the Epistemological Stance of the Art Psychotherapist. *The Arts in Psychotherapy*, 33: 130–134.

Loban, J. 2014. The Invisible Wound: Veterans' Art Therapy. *International Journal of Art Therapy: Inscape*, 19(1): 3–18.

Mauthner, N. 2010. 'I Wasn't Being True to Myself': Women's Narratives of Postpartum Depression. In D. Jack & A. Ali (eds.), *Depression and Gender in the Social World*. Oxford: Oxford University Press.

MBRACE-UK. 2018. Saving Lives, Improving Mothers' Care 2018: Lay Summary. Available at: www.npeu.ox.ac.uk/downloads/files/mbrrace-uk/reports/MBRRACE-UK %20Maternal%20Report%202018%20-%20Lay%20Summary%20v1.0.pdf (accessed November 2019).

McMahon, M. 1995. *Engendering Motherhood: Identity and Self Transformation in Women's Lives*. New York: Guilford.

Menzies, I. E. P. 1960. A Case-Study in the Functioning of Social Systems as a Defence against Anxiety: A Report on a Study of the Nursing Service of a General Hospital. *Human Relations*, 13(2): 95–121.

Meyerowitz-Katz. J., & Reddick, D. 2017. Art Therapy: A Transformational Object. In J. Meyerowitz-Katz & D. Reddick (eds.), *Art Therapy in the Early Years: Therapeutic Interventions with Infants, Toddlers and their Families*. London and New York: Routledge, pp. 178–193.

Ogden, P. 2017. Beyond Words: A Sensorimotor Psychotherapy Perspective. In M. Solomon & D. Siegel (eds.), *How People Change: Relationships and Neuroplasticity in Psychotherapy*. New York: W. W. Norton and Company, pp. 97–125.

Ogden, T. H. 1982. *Projective Identification and Psychotherapeutic Technique*. London: Karnac.

Parker, R. 1995. *Torn In Two: The Experience of Maternal Ambivalence*. London: Virago Press.

Rappaport, L. 2009. *Focussing-Orientated Art Therapy, Accessing the Body's Wisdom and Creative Intelligence*. London: Jessica Kingsley Publishers.

Rayment, A. 2017. Side by Side: An Early Years Art Therapy Group with a Parallel Therapeutic Parent Support Group. In J. Meyerowitz-Katz & D. Reddick (eds.), *Art Therapy in the Early Years: Therapeutic Interventions with Infants, Toddlers and their Families*. London and New York: Routledge, pp. 165–177.

Rose, J. 2018. *Mothers: An Essay on Love and Cruelty*. London: Faber & Faber.

Rothschild, B. 2000. *The Body Remembers: The Psychophysiology of Trauma and Trauma Treatment*. New York and London: W. W. Norton and Company.

Rothschild, B. 2017. *The Body Remembers, Volume 2: Revolutionizing Trauma Treatment*. New York and London: W. W. Norton and Company.

Rowe, P. 2017. On Mark Making and Leaving a Mark: Processing the Experience of Art Therapy with a Preschool Child. In J. Meyerowitz-Katz & D. Reddick (eds.), *Art Therapy in the Early Years: Therapeutic Interventions with Infants, Toddlers and their Families*. London and New York: Routledge, pp. 32–45.

Russell, K., Ashley, A., Chan, G., Gibson, S., & Jones, R. (2017). *Maternal Health – Women's Voices*. Royal College of Obstetricians and Gynaecologists. Available at: www.rcog.org.uk/ globalassets/documents/patients/information/maternalmental-healthwomens-voices.pdf (accessed August 2019).

Sarid, O., Cwikel, J., Czamanski-Cohen, J., & Huss, E. 2017. Treating Women with Perinatal Mood and Anxiety Disorders (PMADs) with a Hybrid Cognitive Behavioural and Art Therapy Treatment (CB-ART). *Archives of Women's Mental Health*, 20: 229–231.

Scarff, J. R. 2019. Postpartum Depression in Men. *Innovations in Clinical Neuroscience*, 16(5–6): 11–14.

Schaverien, J. 1987. The Scapegoat and the Talisman: Transference in Art Therapy. In T. Dalley, C. Case, J. Schaverien, F. Weir, D. Halliday, P. Hall, & D. Waller (eds.), *Images of Art Therapy: New Developments in Theory and Practice*. London and New York: Routledge.

Schaverien, J. 1999. *The Revealing Image: Analytical Art Psychotherapy in Theory and Practice*. London: Jessica Kingsley Publishers.

Schaverien, J. 2011. Aesthetic Counter-Transference. In C. Wood (ed.), *Navigating Art Therapy: A Therapist's Companion*. London and New York: Routledge.

Schore, A., & Sieff, D. 2015. On the Same Wave Length, How Our Emotional Brain is Shaped by Human Relationships. In D. Sieff (ed.), *Understanding and Healing Emotional Trauma: Conversations with Pioneering Clinicians and Researchers*. London and New York: Routledge, pp. 111–136.

Scottish Government. 2019. Mental Health Care for New Mums. Available at: www.gov. scot/news/mental-health-care-for-new-mums/ (accessed June 2019).

van der Kolk, B. 2015. *The Body Keeps the Score: Mind, Brain and Body in the Transformation of Trauma*. London: Penguin Books.

Wilson, M. 2017. *Resource Focused Counselling and Psychotherapy: An Introduction*. London and New York: Routledge.

Winnicott, D. 1971. *Playing and Reality*. London and New York: Routledge.

16 Cases on the border

Perinatal parent–infant work involving migrants, video analysis and art psychotherapy

Diane Bruce

Cases on the border

This chapter discusses how the arts fit into a perinatal parent–infant frame to form a creative space for migrant mothers and their developing infants suffering from interrelational and emotional trauma. It draws from my experience of working as an art psychotherapist in perinatal parent–infant mental health within a large UK NHS Trust. Policy and service constraints have challenged art psychotherapy in this field, given its limited evidence-base (Hogan, Sheffield & Woodward 2017; Bruce & Hackett 2020). This in part led me to train as a Video Intervention Positive Parenting (VIPP) intervener[1] to benefit from its strong research trajectory (Juffer, Bakermans-Kranenburg & Ijzendoorn 2008, 2015). My service has been tailored to combine VIPP with the tactile qualities of art psychotherapy to address the needs of parents and infants who come from an area where second- and third-generation ethnic minorities make up a large proportion of the community's population. More than half of residents are Asian, black, black British and northern European. They retain complex cultural histories and have been raised in a range of faiths. Muslims make up a quarter of the population. Other prominent faiths include Christianity. One in four do not speak English as their main language. Interpreters are available to those who are referred, but this facility is often abandoned because words are lost in translation or cannot convey the layers of emotional feelings that have led parents and their infants to the service. The families I talk about are high-functioning, educated and intelligent. They are challenged by political uncertainty, socio-economic deprivation, physical and emotional violations, sexual abuse, coercive abuse and transnational exploitation. Each case brings relational foibles and personal traits that mix historic parenting traditions with UK social values. Nuances from these influences fade, dilute or combine with personal, educational, religious, societal and social media influences to form rich and cultural hybridity. A pie chart showing the demographics of my recent caseload provided a visual representation of this spectacular kaleidoscope of identities.

Parent–infant cases cited here are drawn from two clinically overlapping secondary care departments. Fiscal pressure and indistinct service borders with hard-to-define mental health criteria mean that *at risk* families can easily be neglected. A recent audit found that at least 17 per cent of cases are returned to general practitioners because it was thought that the parent–infant problem could be managed by visiting community health teams, other agencies or pharmaceuticals. A similar incongruity concerns the infant's age and at what point the parent–infant pair are considered as separate mental health entities. This can result in the maternal (less commonly paternal) *problem* being referred to adult services while the infant is deemed non-clinical. The *patient* in this work is the 'relationship between' (Bruce 2018). Although obvious, this fact often seems to be overlooked. It can mean that 'illnesses of transgenerational relational origin' (Jones 2019 p. 53) can sometimes slip under the radar, or certainly be at risk of doing so. By this I mean that relational trauma is stored as an unseen ghost within the body/developing personality of the infant and outward behaviour fuses (or confuses) with normal Oedipal struggles (Britton 1989). Only in acute situations, if the child is removed and fostered within the care system for instance, is the trauma noticed in the young infant (here referred to as developmental trauma). It otherwise remains unseen until interrelations are expected to develop in school environments and where the impartiality of the teacher now provides the objective lens.

Over 60 per cent of perinatal stress, anxiety and depression caused by relational trauma reportedly remains untreated in the UK. Parents are often reluctant to seek help for fear of their child being removed. Perinatal illnesses that *are* recognised are estimated to carry a long-term cost to society of £8.1 billion per annum. This is said to equate to £10,000 per new birth. Allocation of these costs suggests that 28 per cent relates to *the mother* and 72 per cent relates to *the child* (Marmot Review 2017). This quantitative allocation is confusing, not least because the father is excluded from these statistics. While co-parenting and the value of the father is increasingly recognised and written about (e.g., Baradon 2019), meta-studies on transgenerational attachment transmissions (Verhage et al. 2016) remain gender-biased in that the father is cited far less than the mother. There are various reasons why it is not always possible to work therapeutically with the father. Nevertheless, his or the mother's absence can elucidate the *aliveness* of the internalised parent. I am speaking here of an infant's maternal grandparents: the values, cultures, traditions and beliefs that come to mould parental minds. A mother's pre-verbal experiences and the environment in which she was conceived and raised impact her mindset and her relational choices, not least in the attraction she has to her baby's father. These subtle but perplexing influences all come to affect the parent–infant relationship and the developing personality of the infant: what seeps through skin borders (Anzieu 1989) is now ever-more complex than Winnicott's 1960 understanding of a *total environment* (Winnicott 1960, p. 43).

Let me be clear, the women spoken of here may not (now) be ill enough to be psychiatrically diagnosed with a 'serious mental illness' (ICD-10 1990). For some their problems are noted as *moderate*. For others any diagnosis may have always bordered on what might be termed *delusional*, making the location of the illness difficult to fathom, though seemingly still *her* problem. What proves even harder to untangle is how complex ecological circumstances combine with unconscious defence patterns to form a transgenerational relational infrastructure – the force of which can easily infect vulnerable minds. This not only leaves perinatal mothers at high risk, but it risks them unknowingly distorting the developing personalities of their infants. Fear fertilises the infection and impoverished surroundings subsequently propagate it.

Touch, video and trauma

Touch was first brought to my attention by John Berger (1977) when he spoke of how we always look at an object in relation to ourselves or to another. He points out that our vision is constantly active: changing and adjusting from microscopic to telescopic views. In contrast, the proximity of touch is limited, only reachable by arm's-length or body proportion. Touch as a form of containment is grounding. This in particular was extremely useful for one mother I speak of later. First, I would like us to consider Merleau-Ponty's philosophical description of touch as it helps us consider the challenges of self-observation in parent–infant video work. His words emphasise the relational qualities of self-touching similar to the touching of art media in art psychotherapy:

> I touch myself touching; my body accomplishes 'a sort of reflection.' In it, through it, there is not just the unidirectional relationship of the one who perceives to what he perceives. The relationship is reversed, the touched hand becomes the touching hand, and I am obliged to say that the sense of touch here is defused into the body – that the body is a 'perceiving thing,' a 'subject-object.'
>
> (Merleau-Ponty 1964, p. 166)

At the beginning of a pre-arranged video feedback session a mother I have named Mina[2] arrived late, agitated and very stressed. She was restless and unable to concentrate or think clearly. I encouraged her to turn one palm upwards and using the index finger on her other hand, lightly run the tip of her finger over her hand and fingers before repeating this on the other. My intention was to calm her troubling emotions and help her to feel her body in that present moment.

Skin-to-skin touch is encouraged between parent and infant during the first moments of life to help re-orientate the baby to an outside-in connection and to ground the baby's new existence (Merleau-Ponty 1968). Mina seemed to need reminding of this orientation too. This short exercise enabled her to relax and think about what we could both see happening in the videos I had previously filmed of her with baby Sep as they played together with some bricks. I come back to Mina and Sep later in the chapter.

In preparation for this session, as in other similar cases, I analysed video footage to find knots of a visual story that depicted sensitive moments highlighting the mother's good parenting. I scripted these into words to describe the child's non-verbal expressions. Each of these was matched to a carefully chosen video still to accentuate tender moments of touching, eye-to-eye contact and gentle embrace. The idea being that video feedback enables parents to grow to recognise these moments and adjust their style of parenting to the pace and rhythm of their infant (Raphael-Leff 1983). Keeping the infant in mind in this way reinforces the potential for reflective capacity or the ability to mentalise, i.e., to think about the infant, reflect on what he or she might be thinking while also thinking of their own intentions within the situation.

Self-observation and looking together at videos conjures a dialogue known to improve parent–infant attachment, but I believe it does not altogether address what sometimes feels like an elephant in the room. On many occasions I found myself offering mothers like Mina crayons to hold, clay to prod or wool to knit or crochet a tactile story: one that maximised the physicality of touch as a narrative choice. In some cases this activity settled mothers sufficiently for them to watch and listen. It helped others to speak of the harrowing truth about what brought them to the service. Either way, this tangible approach seemed to provide a sensual gateway to non-verbal, primitive feelings that made direct links to relational experiences, not least those arising from difficult childhoods. Being propelled to such depths during the short perinatal window requires bravery and tenacity, since what is remembered can be painful – yet the sense of urgency that comes with working with a new baby can push generational connections (Faimberg 2005) and provide the answer to why a mother finds it hard to be in the moment with her infant.

I am speaking here about touch and its sensual link to the unpredictable and unwelcome presence of trauma. That is to say the residue left from horrific afflictions that creep into the body then outwardly present as an awkward gait, a rounded posture or a gripped jaw seen as a mother struggles with physical pain when reaching to take her baby into her arms from the floor, for instance. This anguish, hardship and hurt echoed loudly in the slow-motion of the videos I analysed. Clips sometimes revealed uncomfortable moments: a baby's fearful hesitation or prolonged stare as he or she raises her or his face to meet the sorrow, sometimes terror of a mother's worried look. Artwork made by the mothers captured something different: raw and expressionistic in understanding, but equally as potent. I am reminded of Elkins' poetic words:

> Paint records the most delicate gesture and the most tense. It tells whether the painter sat, stood or crouched in front of the canvas. Paint is a cast made of the painter's movements, a portrait of the painter's body and thoughts.
>
> (Elkins 2000, p. 5)

Dollery and Briggs (2002, p. 177) differently exemplify the shame that comes with the spilling from the inside-out into the public domain when they write of a woman's caesarean scar breaking open. I witnessed mothers describe the weight of their birth experiences as they spilt – sometimes flooded their stories *out* onto torn jagged paper, or as they scratched them into paintings. I saw how they glued clay or tightly stitched cloth to hold together worn defences. All to prove they were coping; that they were sane; that they were humanly doing their best for their babies. There were of course times when the elephant shrank and where attuned moments were marked and impactful progress of a positive nature was made. Notwithstanding this, it feels irresponsible to ignore the deep impression of emotional trauma and the countertransference strongly felt in the room and the artwork.

Maternal preoccupation is known to restrict reflective functioning (Slade et al. 2005). In randomised control trials of parent–infant psychotherapy, Fonagy, Sleed and Baradon (2016) suggest integrating video to facilitate triangular thinking, not least because it exercises a mother's mentalising muscle. We do, of course, know that art psychotherapy works in the same way (Verfaille 2011, for instance). There is good evidence that proves positive video feedback increases reflective functioning (e.g., Juffer et al. 2008; Jones 2006; Kennedy 2011), but not all mothers commit to this activity. A third of recent cases were offered VIPP alongside art psychotherapy. Most were sceptical about being filmed. It is the therapist's responsibility to sensitively hold these feelings, filter what is seen, pace the feedback and praise the steps being bravely embarked upon. This includes acknowledging trauma when it unexpectedly arises, as it did in the example of Mina.

Bessel van der Kolk tells us, 'trauma is not the story of something that happened back then … it's the current imprint of that pain, horror, and fear living inside people' (2014). This dynamic aliveness is augmented by video and a moving image seen in slow-motion can be provocative. Mulvey (1989) refers to the positioning of the male gaze in the context of narrative cinema and from a feminist perspective she speaks of the cultural other as the male in third person. He is the active one looking at the vulnerable, *wanted* woman. The woman becomes desexualised, undesirable and something to flee from once copulation has occurred (Mulvey 1989; Tuffery 2011). When an infant has been conceived this way, it is highly comprehensible that a mother will feel judged, embarrassment and shamed at being watched by a camera.

The lens here shines a light on what Freud referred to as the mind's superego (Freud 1923). The internalised critical parent may cause a mother to look at her baby and see the face of her perpetrator. One mother admitted that as we watched a video-clip all she could see was *her mother's bitter mannerisms staring back at her*. Another said she could not bear to look at the way she unknowingly but *harshly shoved her baby to one side* to enable her to enjoy the pleasure of fitting together a wooden jigsaw puzzle. A third commented on the forceful way she saw herself *push a spoon of food into her baby's mouth*. Watching her baby retch caused her to retch as it reminded her of her perpetrator forcing himself on her when she was a teenager. As the person holding the camera, I did at times also feel like the violator, positioned away from the scene, viewing the mother–infant as objects within a metaphorically negative space: leaving them to carry society's guilt and shame. In much the same way Copjec speaks of the splitting of the ego where the woman becomes the object of the man's fetish: '[when] the Chinese man mutilates the woman's foot … it is the foot that wears the mark, not the Chinese man' (Copjec 1994, p. 111). This leaves not he, but she curtailed. Conflicting religions or cultural pressures compress the isolation felt by a woman with such experiences. Poverty further exasperates situations. This irritant can cause coldness, intrusiveness and resentment in a mother's attachment to her infant. In one case it led a mother to say 'my baby had stolen the person I was'. In another, 'I couldn't kill myself now even if I wanted to'.

Turning this negativity around can be hard, especially in the presence of the baby. The process requires sensitivity, flexibility, alliance and vigilant safeguarding. This includes in-depth discussions with multidisciplinary teams and strong relationships with community agencies familiar with the family. Service restraints squeeze therapy ideals, making intense integrative interventions the only choice. With these points in mind, I next share two case vignettes before returning to Mina and Sep's story. Here I hope to further illustrate how the combination of self-touching, self-observation and looking together provided a contained space for migrant mothers to confront residues of trauma while rekindling helpful childhood memories to fertilise positive and meaningful relationships with their infants.

Abi and Abla

Mother Abi and baby Abla were referred because Abi was finding it hard to speak to Abla with comprehensible words. English was not her mother tongue. They came from a mother and baby unit (MBU) where they had been admitted following a mental illness exasperated by the shock of Abi's mother's recent death. Abi literally *lost her words*, triggered by being unable to say goodbye to her mother who was 4,000 miles away. Figure 16.1 shows a pencil drawing of Abi in her Asian homeland where she grew up. The image illustrates how she and her family are separated by the frame divisions of a bedroom window. None have mouths or lips and one has no facial features at all. Abi was raised by her aunt and uncle who could not have children. Her birth mother apparently died at her birth. She believed her aunt and uncle were her biological parents until her late teens, when a family member with learning disabilities *blurted out* that she was adopted. Abi said this confirmed the *hollow aloneness* she had sensed from an early age. She felt vulnerable and confused by this realisation and arrived in the UK disorientated and perplexed. She fell pregnant with Abla following a chance meeting with a stranger who sexually assaulted her before fleeing the scene. She felt afraid and ashamed to talk about this and feared the consequences of termination. She felt obliged to continue with the pregnancy while homeless and destitute. Figure 16.2 shows a fragile clay baby with limbs glued onto its torso. It rests on tissue paper and is placed carefully in a box. The text beneath speaks of a nostalgic plea for the happy and guiltless times to which Abi longed to escape. During a reflective session, she shared her thoughts about images made. Abi related a photographic image of some body-bags to the death

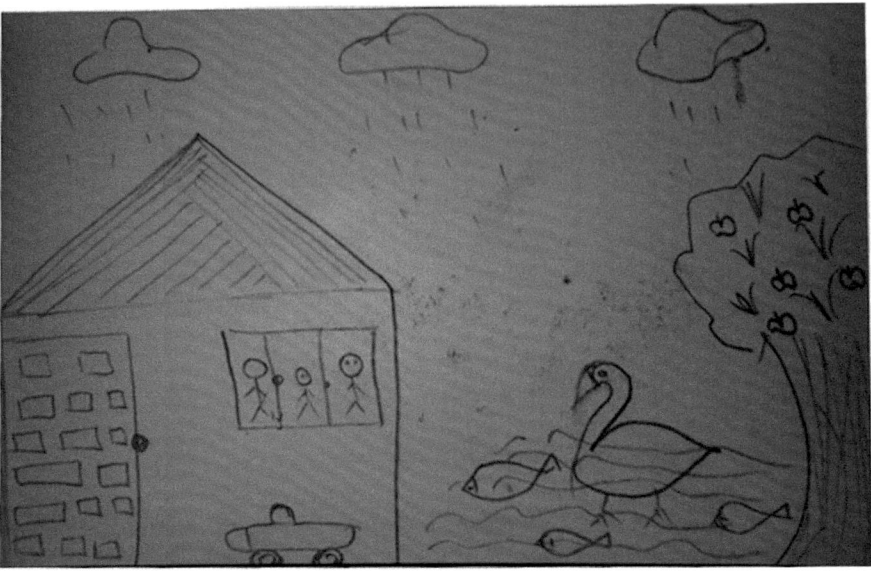

Figure 16.1 Homeland. Abi, pencil on card, 2019.

of her biological and adoptive parents. While this chosen image relates to the clay baby in Figure 16.2, its fragility may also depict her own sexually assaulted body. The promising feature in Figure 16.1 is a fruiting tree which is grounded. This enabled Abi to remember she had a happy childhood surrounded by plants and greenery and with parents who provided warmth, comfort and reassurance. She related a photographic image of a grandmother with a young child enfolded in her arms. Abi said she saw them looking far ahead and this helped her to feel hope for her and her son's future.

My analytical observations of the pair's video-clips showed a succession of shots that revealed Abi encroaching on Abla's space as he tried to enjoy the task of playing together with his mother. Abla could be seen pushing his mother out of the way to find the space he yearned to develop independent play. The MORS[3] attachment questionnaire (Oates & Gervai 2003) depicted a good level of warmth but a high level of intrusiveness. This matched what was seen in the clips. It also illustrates how the traumatic intrusiveness that Abi had previously experienced was repeating itself in her and Abla's interactions. Subsequent sessions addressed this worrying transmission. Abi was encouraged to create space for Abla to freely explore his environment. Abi's mind remained clear enough to see and think about her son's requests because the intrusive trauma was being held in the artwork. This integration of video feedback and art psychotherapy also saw the return of Abi's vocabulary. Shifts made helped regulate their interactions and attunement.

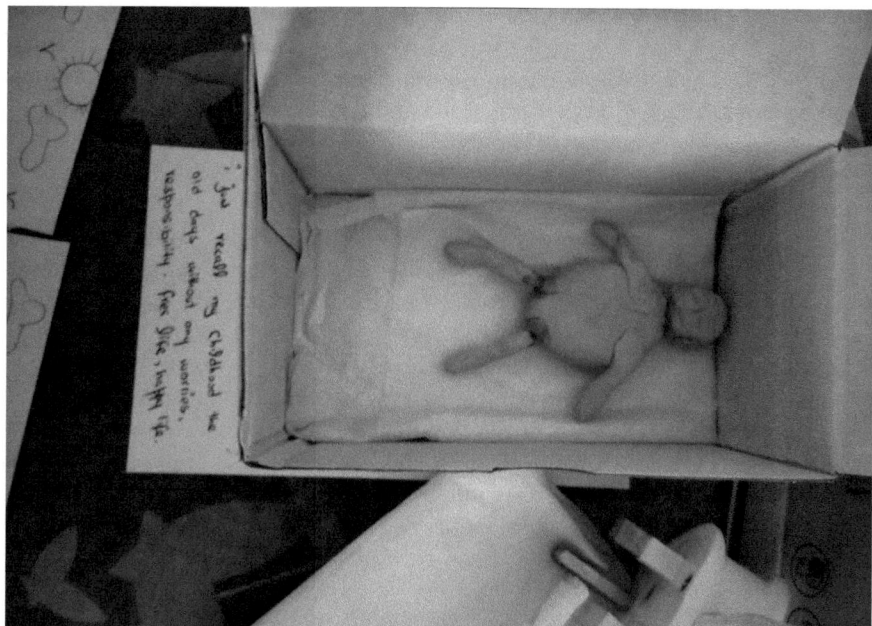

Figure 16.2 Clay Baby. Abi, clay, tissue, glue and cardboard, 2019.

Khadija and Sabine

This parent–infant pair were cautiously referred by my supervisor who showed me a video-clip of a mother quietly encouraging her 13-month-old to play with a toy spinning wheel. It was hard to decipher what mother Khadija was saying because her voice was so faint. What was apparent was her animated hand movements set against the black of her full hijab. Khadija was apparently artistic and had tried to rekindle her love of crochet but never felt able to 'get going' on anything. When the harsh voices she was prone to hearing overpowered her mind, she would repeatedly bang her head on a hard surface in an attempt to make them stop. As they were no longer at a MBU, most sessions took place in their home, where I observed Sabine draw and play happily with her sibling. Their father and wider family members were on hand in different rooms. Khadija struggled to cast a stitch onto her crochet hook. The wool kept un-knotting and it then became difficult to find the right loop to try again. She said she felt 'out of rhythm'. With encouragement she kept trying. Each stich brought a feeling of achievement. As she became more confident, she began speaking about the chronic social anxiety she suffered as a child and why this was. She told me how she did not attend much school but would instead 'curl up and lose herself in a book'. Books were her saviour. During a later session, Khadija made a book from clay saying it was a symbol of her courage and of her strengthening relationship with Sabine. She wrote: 'Sabine has started to enjoy reading books and turning the pages. She likes it when I am sat with her and we read the book together.' She chose two photographs from a selection. They enabled us to talk about the importance of prayer in her life and the importance to her of bringing her palms together. [This bringing together of hands in prayer relates to Mina's touching hands and to Merleau-Ponty's (1964) many references to the meaning of touch]. Khadija said she wanted to crochet a doll for Sabine. By the end of the final session she had completed the 3D head of a doll wearing a mauve coloured hat. At this stage the facial features were absent, although this *whole object* symbolised Khadija's own wholeness and how far she had come as a woman and as a parent to Sabine.

Khadija did not want to be filmed at first because she was so hateful of her self-image. During the first session, I suggested she hold the camera and film me with Sabine while we were drawing. She then handed the camera to me to film her hands interact and entwine with Sabine's as they passed pens and crayons back and forth to each other. Gradually Khadija felt more relaxed about letting me film her face. The footage encouraged her to see how her coiled torso released each time she lifted her head to meet Sabine's wanting eyes. As she allowed her spine to straighten, the animation I had first seen in Khadija's expressive hands spread to her arms, neck and shoulders. She integrated this bodily awareness into her daily prayer practice. With each feedback session, we both observed positive changes in her and Sabine's interactions. Sabine liked how much her mother was opening up. In her home I was privileged to see Khadija without her hijab. While her voice remained discreet, by the final session I noticed how colourful her clothing was becoming and how this positively reflected her changing mood.

Mina and Sep

Mother Mina and baby Sep are second-generation migrants. They were referred by a worried health visitor who had had ongoing concerns since Sep's birth 16 months earlier. Sep was delayed in walking and mother–infant bonding was ambiguous due to Mina's previous acts of self-harm and suicidal idealisations. This was augmented by a complex family system. Sep's father was 17 years older than mother Mina. They were from different countries, practised different religions and their cultures expressed different attitudes towards males and females. While Mina was intelligent and held down a good job, she was in love and naïvely believed Sep's father felt the same way. She was led to believe they would marry before discovering he was already married with grown up children. Mina fell pregnant with her daughter Sep within three months of her male baby dying very late into gestation. Sep's father was apparently insensitive to the meaning of this loss. He was unpredictable and highly strung. He managed his failings by projecting derogatory verbal abuse at Mina. Mina's own family controlled her money and Sep's father amplified this control by limiting her income and threatening to leave her and Sep destitute. Mina lived in constant fear and anxiety. The birth of each of Mina's babies required caesarean surgery. This was complicated by ongoing vaginal bleeding and crippling spinal pain that at times caused her legs to become numb. Mina made a trunk shape with clay. She bent it into a curve and said it was a foetus. The stretching of the clay tubular shape caused the clay spine to rip open. Other marks also punctured the clay skin. Mina wrote about making this form: 'I'm not sure what I felt. I made a foetus. Not sure I engaged with baby growing inside me.' Mina told me about her own infancy and how she was separated from her mother for the first few months of her life because her mother was ill in hospital. She related that she and her mother were never close. Her mother was ambiguous in her feelings towards Mina. Mina grew up thinking her mother preferred her younger siblings to her. She saw herself as an outcast. In a different session she chose two photographic images. One was of a mother and baby. Other children are hiding their faces from the camera. Mina said the photograph (taken by Dorothea Lange in 1936) showed a woman who looked like a woman who had 'experienced a hard life and had a lot on her mind'. Lange's work shines a light on American migrants from the 1930s. Lange titled this particular image 'Migrant Mother'. Mina was unaware of this fact, although coincidentally it did reflect the hardship she had experienced. Mina also chose an image of some elephants. She said the adult elephant must be 'old and wise'. The baby elephant in the foreground is being nourished from a distance source – with water (that looks like milk). This may relate to the positioning of Mina's own mother who was distant during her early infancy.

Analysis of early video-clips revealed a mother who hit her head with her hand while expressing how stupid she was (this was far from the truth). Baby Sep was heard imitating her mother's self-deprecating words. This scenario echoed what happened in the family home on a regular basis. The slow-motion of video stills revealed Sep reaching for her teddy, perhaps for comfort, before she felt confident enough to lift her head to meet her mother's worried look. When Mina realised how this might feel for Sep, she cried. In a different clip Mina saw herself take over Sep's exploring. She recognised how much she herself wanted to play. She could not recall playing with her own mother or father. The clips helped Mina see how intrusive and forceful she was in response to Sep's desire to explore. Like Abi, Mina's painful realisation saw her step back and allow space for Sep to unfold the book flaps herself while enjoying the pleasure of naming the animals beneath. The understanding Mina gained about her own relationship with her parents freed her to think about how she interacted with Sep. It helped her to think about the relationship she had with Sep's father. The process of making the foetus gave Mina time to mourn and begin to grieve over significant losses. Subsequent videos showed Mina's increased closeness to Sep and the positive adjustments made. It was a joy to see their attuned *moo* sounds. Their facial profiles mirrored attunement like twin bookends. Sep eventually began walking, not least because of Mina's tenacity and determination to offer her daughter an infancy that was loving, equal in gender opportunity and free from infirmity.

Discussion

I would like to begin this section by further paraphrasing Descartes then Fonagy, from *my mother thinks, I think, therefore I am* to *my mother feels, I feel, therefore I think*. This implies that to think properly one needs to be able to feel: touch in the context of the work I have spoken of here relates to the psychic function of the skin – first vested in the infant's whole body surface, now in the touching hand (Anzieu 1990, pp. 72–73). As an infant's independence increases, touch and feel become a place where thoughts and words begin to form. The infant's hand soon becomes the containing function. This directly relates to the tactile qualities of art psychotherapy. In their writing about trauma healing and the importance of touch, Elbrecht and Meyerowitz-Katz each speak of the reflective nature of clay (Elbrecht 2013; Meyerowitz-Katz 2003). Like Merleau-Ponty they suggest that in touching malleable art materials, they *touch the body back*. The mothers here thus came face-to-face with their separateness. They were able to feel themselves and their infants as separate humans no longer fused in reverie. The phenomenology of touch is, as Merleau-Ponty (1964) says, always relational and poignant to a mother feeling herself in the present moment for her developing infant. If the mother is able to feel her skin as a boundary and as a surface that represents the border between her inside self and the outside world, this will in turn help her infant to feel that difference too, thus encouraging him, to securely and confidently develop a healthy relationship with his caregiver while adjusting his understanding and proximity to the subject-objects in his new world.

The baby's point of view

Hope for the new generation is always at the forefront of perinatal parent–infant work. Development of the baby's personality is paramount. The perinatal period provides a window of time to propel creative changes for parents. The work described here sets out to encourage mothers to consider what it might be like to understand the world from their infant's viewpoint. The objectivity of video work provided a triangular forum for this to be reviewed and thought about. This media enables special moments to be shared that may reveal an infant's beaming eyes when they hear the sound of their mother return to the room, or a loving smile missed in real time. Looking together enabled mothers to think objectively, like co-psychoanalytical observers. Seeing themselves as expert parents enabled them to feel liberated. It enabled them to establish a *female gaze* that strengthened their confidence. The slow-motion video clips enabled them to understand how their infant might reads their face as a series of still shots or as a chain of fine body movements. Sharing moments where the reach was too sharp or too hesitant or where their infant wanted more encouragement, helped them to see for themselves – without judgement – how they could adjust and do it differently next time. Sights, sounds, smells, touches and tastes combine like instantaneous *slices* of feelings in an infant's mind. These *feelings* create a permanency with repetition. We know from Stern (1985, p. 122) that singularly these slices have no coherent meaning: a mother's face might be viewed by the infant as a misaligned image, perhaps similar to a Picasso portrait. This gradually comes into focus the more the same expression is repeated. Uncoordinated misalignments happen not only in facial but in bodily expressions too. They may stick if repeatedly marked and mirrored back to the infant in a negative way. This may leave a baby confused about how to read genuine smiles or a funny laugh. An infant may feel perplexed by a hand that reaches out too slowly or too quickly. Guided self-observation using video helps explain what happens when an infant repeatedly experiences smiling eyes, a welcoming beam or a gentle embrace. A mother is then more empowered to comprehend the positive impact this can have on her infant's forming personality.

Concluding thoughts

In this chapter I have attempted to reflect on the use of video as a means of creating space where migrant mothers can view their interactions in line with their infant's developing self. I wanted to emphasise the proximity of touch that is prevalent in art psychotherapy and its importance when addressing issues involving interrelational trauma. Perinatal parent–infant work requires a long and broad view from which to absorb not only the depth of what is passed from generation to generation (Faimberg 2005), but also to include the breadth of what flows through political and religious discourses and practices prevalent in multi-cultural communities. This milieu is representational of the community where I work. Self-looking through video work provides a dynamic space to observe the self and the superego as defined by Freud (1923). This cannot altogether reach parameters associated with very primitive feelings and what is often at the root of the perinatal problem. Words can rarely be found to describe the invasive and potent nature of pre-verbal feelings associated with transgenerational trauma, making it difficult to define. It is difficult to express the immediacy of their existence. Yet as van der Kolk (2014) emphasises, their presence is strongly felt. If accessed through the touching hand in the containment of perinatal parent–infant art psychotherapy, there is a chance that the intrusion on new life can be halted or changed. I have focused here on selected cases affected by the intrusiveness of trauma seen in the slow-motion of mother–infant interactions and the touch of art materials. Trauma does not recognise race, gender or status in its victim choice. Instead it engulfs feelings collated worldwide and like an alchemist it mixes horrific experiences of war, natural disaster and relational abuse with internalised discourse. This toxic mix can plague vulnerable perinatal parent–infants and the continuum that follows when intervention is not possible or unable to be sought. The perinatal period provides a window of time large enough for women that are brave enough, to halt the transgenerational transmission of trauma while simultaneously promoting a more positive style of parenting for the trajectory of the next generation.

   Touch and the creative activity of art making provide an important link between a parent's *alive past* and the interactions between the parent–infant in the *present* moment. Sensitive video feedback using the pre-verbal voice of the infant keeps the parent's mind buoyant with her infant's needs and developmental states while art psychotherapy safely contains what might also be active in the parent's mind and alive in the room. In summary, video promotes a mother's visual thinking and reflective capacity whilst the tactility of art making helps her to feel herself enough to form space for bi-directional creativity, thus promoting positive change for both.

Notes

1 I am a registered Video Intervention Positive Parenting (VIPP) intervener (www. leidenattachmentresearchprogramme.eu/vipp/en). The programme is based on attachment theory. There are other recognised ways of using video to help improve parent–infant relationships. Kennedy (2011) and Jones (2006) offer two further adaptions. Each has similar and overlapping principles in that they include videoing the parent–infant and the intervener who then join as co-observers (Kennedy, Landor & Todd 2015). Practice is regulated by registered supervisors. The continuum of these reflective experiences is based on the intersubjective principles first pioneered by Colwyn Trevarthen's infant development work during the latter part of the last century (Trevarthen & Aitkin 2001).
2 All names in this chapter have been changed to protect anonymity.
3 MORS (Oates & Gervai 2003) is a carefully designed attachment questionnaire that measures the warmth-coldness, intrusive-nonintrusive bi-directional polarities of parent–infant relationships. This measure was used with all VIPP cases mentioned here. Clarity and change can sometimes be seen in pre- and post-treatment scoring, although, in my experience, should be viewed within the broader context of case formulation.

References

Anzieu, D. 1989. *The Skin Ego.* New Haven and London: Yale University Press.
Anzieu, D. 1990. *A Skin for Thought.* London and New York: Karnac.
Baradon, T. 2019. *Working with Fathers in Psychoanalytic Parent–Infant Psychotherapy.* London and New York: Routledge.
Berger, J. 1977. *Ways of Seeing.* London: Penguin.
Britton, R. 1989. The Missing Link: Parental Sexuality in the Oedipus Complex. In R. Britton, M. Feldman, and E. O'Shaughnessy (eds.), *The Oedipus Complex*, ed. J. Steiner. London: Karnac.
Bruce, D. 2018. The Long View: Attachment, Trauma and Intergenerational Approach to Art Therapies in Perinatal Parent–Infant Mental Health. *News-Briefing: British Association of Art Therapists (BAAT), winter.* 18.
Bruce, D., & Hackett, S. S. 2020. Developing Art Therapy Practice Within Perinatal Parent–Infant Mental Health. *International Journal of Art Therapy: Inscape.* (This paper is at the peer review stage and editorial discretion).
Copjec, J. 1994. *Read My Desire: Lacan against the Historicists.* Cambridge, MA: MIT Press.
Dollery, J., & Briggs, A. 2002. Secondary Skin and Culture: Reflections on Teaching Traveller Children. In A. Briggs (ed.), *Surviving Space, Papers on Infant Observation.* London: Karnac, pp. 172–187.
Elbrecht, C. 2013. *Trauma Healing at the Clay Field: A Sensorimotor Art Therapy Approach.* London: Jessica Kingsley Publishers.

Elkins, J. 2000. *What Painting Is.* London: Routledge.

Faimberg, H. 2005. *The Telescoping of Generations: Listening to the Narcissistic Links between Generations.* London and New York: Routledge.

Fonagy, P., Sleed, M., & Baradon, T. 2016. Randomized Controlled Trial of Parent–Infant Psychotherapy and Treatment as Usual for Parents with Mental Health Problems and Young Infants. *Infant Mental Health Journal*, 37(2): 97–114.

Freud, S. 1923. *The Ego and the Id.* London: Hogarth Press.

Hogan, S., Sheffield, D., & Woodward, A. 2017. The Value of Art Therapy in Antenatal and Postnatal Care: A Brief Literature Review with Recommendations for Further Research. *International Journal of Art Therapy*, 22(4): 169–179.

ICD-10. 1990. *The International Classification of Diseases, Version 10.* Hyattsville, MD: National Centre for Health Statistics.

Jones, A. 2006. How Video Can Bring to View Pathological Defensive Processes and Facilitate the Creation of Triangular Space in Perinatal Parent–Infant Psychotherapy. *Infant Observation*, 9(2): 109–123.

Jones, A. 2019. When Working Therapeutically with a Baby's Father is Not Possible. In, T. Baradon (ed.), *Working with Fathers in Psychoanalytic Parent-Infant Psychotherapy.* London and New York: Routledge, pp. 50–63.

Juffer, F., Bakermans-Kranenburg, M. J., & van Ijzendoorn, M. H. 2008. *Promoting Positive Parenting: An Attachment-Based Intervention.* London and New York: Routledge.

Juffer, F., Bakermans-Kranenburg, M. J., & van Ijzendoorn M. H. 2015. *Manual VIPP-SD Video-Feedback Intervention to Positive Parenting and Sensitive Discipline*, version 3.0. Netherlands: Leiden University.

Kennedy, H. 2011. What is Video Interaction Guidance (VIG)? In H. Kennedy, M. Landor, & L. Todd (eds.), *Video Interaction Guidance: A Relationship Based Intervention to Promote Attunement, Empathy and Wellbeing.* London: Jessica Kingsley Publishers, pp. 20–43.

Kennedy, H., Landor, M., & Todd, L. 2015. *Video Enhanced Reflective Practice: Professional Development through Attuned Interactions.* London: Jessica Kingsley Publishers.

Marmot Review. 2017. *Creative Health: The Arts for Health and Wellbeing.* Available at: www.artshealthandwellbeing.org.uk/appg-inquiry/Publications/Creative_Health_Inquiry_Report_2017.pdf (accessed September 2019).

Merleau-Ponty, M. 1964. The Philosopher and His Shadow. In *Signs*, trans. R. C. McCleary. Evanston, IL: Northwestern University Press, pp. 159–181.

Merleau-Ponty, M. 1968. *The Visible and the Invisible.* Evanston, IL: Northwestern University Press.

Meyerowitz-Katz, J. 2003. Art Materials and Processes – a Place of Meeting: Art Psychotherapy with a Four-Year-Old Boy. *Inscape*, 8(2): 60–69.

Mulvey, L. 1989. *Visual and Other Pleasures.* New York: Palgrave Macmillan.

Oates, J. M., & Gervai, J. 2003. *Mothers' Object Relations Scales.* Paper presented at the 11th European Conference on Developmental Psychology, Milan, Italy.

Raphael-Leff, J. 1983. Facilitators and Regulators: Two Approaches to Mothering. *British Journal of Medical Psychology*, 56: 379–390.

Slade, A., Grienenberger, J., Bernbach, E., Levy, D., & Locker, A. 2005. Maternal Reflective Functioning, Attachment, and the Transmission Gap: A Preliminary Study. *Attachment and Human Development*, 7(3): 283–298.

Stern, D. N. 1985. *The Interpersonal World of the Infant.* New York: Basic Books.

Trevarthen, C., & Aitken, J. 2001. Infant Intersubjectivity: Research, Theory and Clinical Applications. *Journal of Child Psychology, Psychiatry*, 2(1): 3–48.

Tuffery, H. 2011. Are You Looking at Me? The Reciprocal Gaze and Art Psychotherapy. *Art Therapy Online: ATOL*, 1(3).

van der Kolk, B. 2014. *The Body Keeps the Score: Mind Brain and Body in the Transformation of Trauma*. USA: Viking Penguin.

Verhage, M. L., Schuengel, C., Fearson, R. M. P., Cassibba, R., Madigan, S., Oosterman, M., Bakermans-Kranenburg, M. J., & van Ijzendoorn, M. H. 2016. Narrowing the Transmission Gap: Synthesis of Three Decades of Research on Intergenerational Transmission of Attachment. *Psychological Bulletin* 142(4): 337–366.

Verfaille, M. 2011. *Mentalizing in Arts Therapies*. London: Karnac.

Winnicott, D. W. 1960. Parent–Infant Relationship. In *The Maturational Processes and the Facilitating Environment*. Madison, CT: International Universities Press, Inc., pp. 37–55.

17 Art Therapy for motherhood and families as a way to support positive parenting

Lucia Hervás Hermida

Introduction

> We have reflected on parenthood. And well, I see it, we see it, as our life is always a green tree, and then paternity/maternity arrives and everything changes. As autumn comes, everything falls, it is not a relative change, it is a radical change, and until you begin to roll and settle, you do not return to life...".[1]

As these parents said, parenting is about change (see Figure 17.1). New parents need to face a completely new situation, while society is transforming as well. We are witnessing very important changes in the situation of the family and with respect to reproduction. There is plenty of literature advocating the significance of the parental role for children's development, and there is a new conceptualisation of family, as a

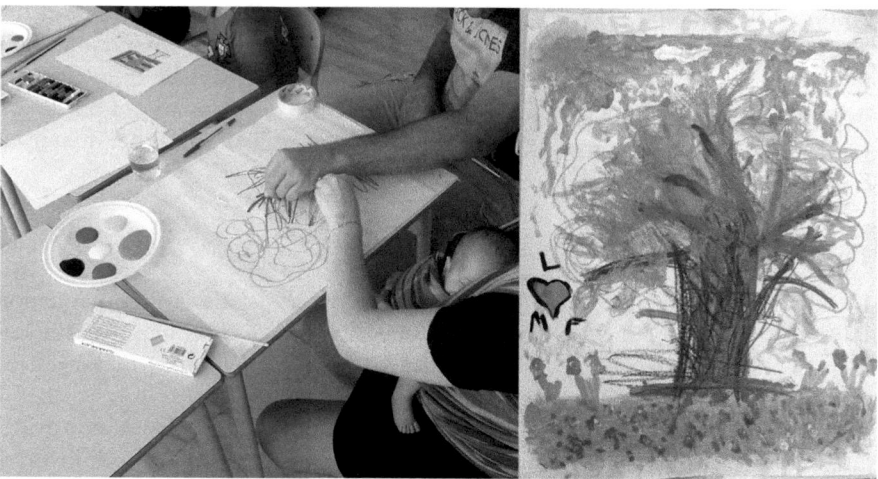

Figure 17.1 The Tree of Life. Art Therapy in the perinatal period, pregnant women or recent mothers with their partners. Image and text by the participants of the Art Therapy workshop developed in Calpe, Spain, 2017.

learning space for the development of each of its members. In addition, nowadays, we can observe a broader diversity of family models. We can evidence a greater recognition of women's rights and participation in public life that has unavoidable consequences for family dynamics. However, from a feminist perspective, motherhood is still one of the main conflicts with respect to women's identity. Self-identity is also a key factor for resilience through all this social change, new family patterns, assisted reproduction and the new roles in parenting.

The awareness of the public dimension of the family and its socialising and educational function has contributed to the emergence of the positive parenting model, on both policies and research, regarding the implementation of measures for family support. The European Social Charter (Council of Europe 1996) recognises these family needs in Article 16: 'the family, as the fundamental basic unit of society, has the right to receive social, legal and economic support and protection to ensure all its development potential' (p. 2).

This positive approach implies a change in family intervention, emphasising the development of educational and preventive measures that focus on the potentials and abilities of parental roles, rather than their difficulties or problems (Rodrigo López 2015). For that purpose, Art Therapy has shown its suitability, as research suggests. A feminist perspective is also included, regarding women's experiences in the transition to motherhood.

This chapter will develop the theoretical and methodological basis for this positive parenting feminist Art Therapy model, and will show its possibilities and scope (Hervás Hermida 2018). Three kinds of settings have been explored, the format of Art Therapy with families through a dyadic approach (in this dyadic approach the emphasis is on parent–child interaction and bonding); the format of Art Therapy with mothers, fathers and relatives (in group work aimed at giving social support with no children present); and the format of Art Therapy in the perinatal period (with pregnant women and their partners, and new mothers and their partners). Through several case vignettes it will be illustrated how Art Therapy can foster the development of parenting skills, resilience and good family interactions as well as promote maternal wellbeing.

Positive parenting

In 2006 the Council of Ministers of Europe, published the recommendation REC (2006) 19 on Policy to Support Positive Parenting. This important document sets guidelines among the states for the implementation of measures for family support. Positive parenting there refers to:

'parental behaviour based on the best interests of the child that is nurturing, empowering, non-violent and provides recognition and guidance which involves setting of boundaries to enable the full development of the child' (p. 1).

The main principles that characterise positive parenting are the following: respect for the needs of children, strengthening of secure affective bonds and resolution of conflicts in a non-violent manner (González Sánchez, Martin

Morales & Roig Tomas, 2013). According to Rodrigo Lopez, Máiquez Chaves & Martín Quintana (2010) there are three fundamental assumptions on which the positive parenting model is based:

1   The importance of the family, as the basic nucleus of society, considering the diversity of family forms and the respect for their privacy and autonomy.
2   The ecological-systemic family conception, as a complex system of relationships in a social and historical context in a process of constant change.
3   The acceptance of all fathers' and mothers' needs, not only for therapeutic or rehabilitative support, but from a preventive and developmental perspective as well.

For this preventative purpose, parental education programmes develop care, education and guidance strategies. The aim of this type of educational intervention is to improve parents' educational and interpersonal skills with their children and within the family; and parental competences, attachment, resilience and non-violent attitudes (see Table 17.1). The most recent programmes aim to improve family functioning as a system, through multi-context interventions. They foster relationships and co-parenting, and the development of parental skills and resilience, focusing on each family's needs and resources, and not looking at any ideal parenting model (Martín-Quintana et al. 2009). As Rodrigo López et al. (2015) explain, this new type of experiential methodology is based on parents' own experiences; and promotes reflection and analysis of their own ideas and behaviour. The group process favours the shared construction of knowledge, so parents are encouraged to actively participate and to take responsibility of their process, developing empowerment.

Motherhood from the feminist and gender perspective

As mentioned above, despite the advances in co-parenting and the incorporation of women to work and public life, literature states that parental responsibility still belongs mostly to women, so reproduction is a factor in inequality. Moreover, according to Bernal Martínez de Soria and Sandoval Estupiñan (2013), there is a certain uncritical discourse within the positive parenting model, an absence of

Table 17.1 Principles of positive parenting (Rodrigo Lopez et al. 2010 p. 12)

- Warm, protective and stable affective bonds.
- A structured environment, which provides a model in which children can learn the rules and values.
- Stimulation and support for daily learning, promotion of motivation and its capabilities.
- Recognition of the value of children as persons.
- Training of daughters and sons, as competent and active agents.
- Education without violence.

true debate around the cultural meanings around family life and its implications for women's lives. This is not surprising, as maternal experiences have been historically overlooked (Hogan et al. 2015; Hogan 2017; Miller 1980).

As I observed through my research, and according to the literature, there are several issues arising regarding the changes and difficulties that mothers usually experience in their transition to parenthood (see Table 17.2). There are basic personal needs that are usually not being satisfied, like the need for proper rest and having time for their own issues, but also other important needs related to the couple and their social support as well as for their children. Women usually complain about the difficulties in achieving a healthy work–life balance.

I also found an overwhelming perception of responsibility, added to the social pressure and lack of support, that provokes a situation of chronic stress and crisis. The inclination to define parenting in terms of responsibility drives parents, and especially mothers, to focus on children's wellbeing, forgetting about their own self-care. This is a source of maternal ambivalence, as Badinter argues (2011). Although most women perceive motherhood as a valuable part of their lives and identities, it is also the core of significant distress. This refers to the paradox that Nussbaum (2000) explained about the domestic space as contradictory. For women, motherhood and family life still can be a space for both love and oppression.

So, in this chapter I focus on motherhood within family intervention, looking at the specific conditions experienced by women in their maternal role, from a feminist perspective. I propose a broader look at the phenomena, as I explained previously:

> Motherhood is not only the state reached by women when giving birth, but as described by Stern, Bruschweiler-Stern, and Freeland (1999), it is a complex psychological process that begins sometime before the birth, culminates after the birth of the child, and lasts throughout life, even when the children have become independent or after their loss. Téllez Infantes and Heras González (2004) emphasise this issue by noting the expectation of permanent availability, which is extended in an unlimited way through the symbolic union of woman with her children during life. Beyond that, motherhood is a social construction that derives from the symbolic attributions and discourses maintained throughout history, and

Table 17.2 Mothers' issues, difficulties and needs (Hervás Hermida 2018)

- Life changes and feeling of loss.
- Couple and family changes.
- Lack of social support.
- Feeling of loneliness and isolation.
- Stress, exhaustion, overwhelm.
- Fears, doubts, insecurity.
- Children concerns.

affects the identity of women who are mothers as well as those who are not, having very strong implications for the bodies and lives of all women.

> For this reason, I propose a broader definition of it, understanding motherhood as a process, in contrast to the notion of state. Motherhood is a psychological, social and cultural process, which alludes to the experience and identity of the mother as well as to her role with her children and society (Rich 1978), including the cultural and symbolic aspects of it (Lozano Estivalis 2006). At the intersection of these, I introduce the creative dimension, placing the focus on the potential of creation that involves motherhood, at both physical, emotional, psychical, social and cultural levels.
>
> (Hervás Hermida 2018, pp. 824–825)

The inclusion of a feminist perspective implies a special look at the cultural issues and images created by women, focusing on the improvement of women's lives and the deconstruction of inequalities (Alonso Garrido 2012; Lopez Fernandez Cao 2000). Feminist Art Therapy then focuses on the generation of a space for mutual support where there can be a process of re-elaboration of experiences, beliefs and representations regarding gender (Hogan 1997, 2003). This provides multiple benefits for mothers: emotional support, the elaboration of experiences of transition to motherhood, the deconstruction and reflection on the beliefs and discourses that preserve inequalities, and the reconstruction of the maternal identity, strengthening self-esteem, increasing autonomy and empowerment (Hauser Dacer 2016; Hogan 2012). As Swan-Foster (2012) observes, motherhood can be understood as a creative process, an initiation process, which develops at all physical, emotional, social and spiritual levels. Through the exploration of this creative dimension of motherhood and family life it is intended to facilitate the elaboration of the experience in all its complexity.

Art Therapy for motherhood and families as a way to support positive parenting

Learning from the literature of both the positive parenting model, the parental education programmes and feminist and gender theories, I have developed a 'preventive' Art Therapy model for motherhood and family care. This proposal stems from family Art Therapy literature, especially the systemic approach (Kerr et al. 2011) and the development of the dyad modality (Armstrong & Howatson 2015; Proulx 2003; Regev & Snir 2015; Taylor Buck 2015; Taylor Buck et al. 2014). The benefits of Art Therapy in this context have to do with the art language, which provides an alternative to verbal communication, and allows exploration of the dynamics of the family system through art creation (Riley & Malchiodi 2003).

It offers a space where parents and especially mothers can articulate their concerns and find social support. As Hogan, Sheffield and Woodward (2017) conclude in their literature review about Art Therapy and motherhood, Art

Therapy fosters an improvement in self-esteem, self-confidence, self-reflection and self-knowledge of women in their transition to motherhood, as well as an improvement in their relationships with children, as assessed through both forms of work, with mothers and in mother–child dyads.

In my experience, the three kinds of settings explored have been useful in this regard, in various ways, as we will see:

- **In the family setting (dyadic format)**, the focus was on parent–child interaction and bonding. Within this setting, findings showed the need to pay special attention to the balance of the needs of each member of the dyad, and the conflicts of autonomy. It has also been important to note the presence of children and their effect on the process, enhancing its positive effects: play, spontaneity, affectivity, etc., as well as the possibility to invite other members of the family: brothers and sisters, grandparents, etc. (see Figure 17.2).

Susan, a woman who participated in the family group, came during one session with her daughter (aged two) and her mother-in-law (Sally), and they made this painting together. She commented about the image: 'I am the blue circle in the middle. My children appear there, entering and leaving the circle. She (her daughter) is joining us.' Then she explained how she felt upset when Sally started to spread along the painting. 'I felt a little invaded, and somewhat uncomfortable. Then I solved it by painting my circle more intense blue, as if I said "Here I am".' Then she explained how she could look at her contribution to the painting in a different way. 'I really like what

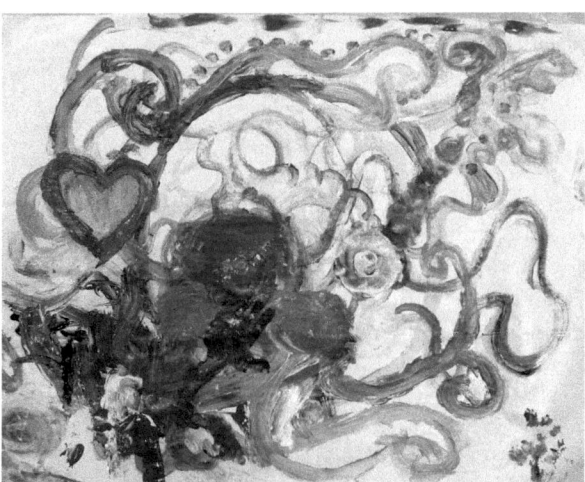

Figure 17.2 Glow of Hope. Family Art Therapy with other members of the family. Image and text by the participants of the Art Therapy workshop developed in Aranjuez, Spain, 2015.

she has painted because it gives us a lot of light, and it is true she brings us joy [...] I liked it a lot, and it even surprised me [...] I have had a very nice experience.'

Sally then said about the painting: 'I enter and leave her world, and also paint abroad, because I need to interact with more people, and then I come back in, but not wanting to invade [laughs when saying this] but wanting to contribute, because I also consider that I belong to this world.'

- **In the mothers, parents and relatives setting** (with no children participating), the focus was on the creation of a space for social support, personal growth and empowerment, with special emphasis on group interaction and shared reflection as a mean of mutual learning.

For Leonard, a father of three participating in the parents group who was not very satisfied with his work–life balance, a very significant moment happened when he modelled a boat with clay. He realised that putting the oars on was an act of self-care and empowerment, as an insight of the need to take responsibility. After this session he thought he could start his own business, feeling more confident about his abilities and possibilities for growth.

- **The perinatal setting** included both groups with pregnant women and during the post-partum period (with their partners), focusing on the transition to motherhood. The emphasis there was on the creation of a space for emotional support, as well as attachment and bonding issues. In these groups, findings showed the importance of containment and holding the special emotional sensitivity of this stage as well as the attention to the specific physiological needs of pregnancy and body issues.

Laura, a late pregnant woman said about her drawing, 'At the beginning the circle was my life, I had everything within the circle, I had a planned life, and being a mother wasn't part of my plans. And when it happened, I was very afraid, and denied it, because I couldn't believe I was pregnant. It took me a few months to assume it and step out from what I had always been used to, to make it possible. I think that unconsciously I had always run away from babies, rarely I have held a baby in my arms. Now I have a friend who has recently given birth, and then I started to break up with everything, and held the baby. For me this is a therapy, and the fear is gone, and everything is new, I really don't know … It's a very long road, being a mother, there are many things that I don't know, and I want to do it well, and I believe that love is what will lead me to become a good mother … is all very new for me … and my family are not here they are far away. So it's going to be myself, my pregnancy, the baby … but I prefer that way, so I have no opinions, only my partner's … He is afraid, because he knows much more than me, he has many nephews. As I now know that it is possible, now I am sorry, I know that it is possible, and it is all out of my control, my life changes completely. Something new that no longer scares me, for now on I am very calm, and I hope it continues like this.'

Beyond the differences of each type of intervention, the guiding principles are very similar, and they stand from the recognition of each family and each participant's needs. As the outcomes of the research showed, and according to the literature, the fundamental principle that should guide the intervention is respect as well as the attention to their needs, seeking to promote the development of each of its members as well as the family as a whole.

In that sense, the main aim of the intervention (see Table 17.3) is to involve parents in their personal development, as a way to foster children's development, through the improvement of interaction. A relevant outcome in this regard has been the amelioration of parents' identity and self-esteem through the development of creativity, raising self-connection, wellbeing, empowerment and resilience. Most of the parents did not have so many previous experiences of art creation, so it was an invitation for them to explore this facet of their lives, and an opportunity to share this new way of communication with their children. The inclusion of art works, images and metaphors has many benefits. In the first place we can affirm that it fosters awareness processes and communication. According to Demecs, Fenwick and Gamble (2011) and Hogan (1997, 2003, 2015, 2016, 2017), the realisation of creative group activities facilitates a space for mutual support, where the sharing of information among mothers and parents can occur, and so emotional expression and personal reflection. In the second place, images can be useful not only as a means of expression and elaboration, but can also help to understand the subjective experiences of the mother and her bond with her child, and serve to prevent possible problems and pathologies (Swan-Foster 1989, 2012; Swan-Foster, Foster & Dorsey 2003). Third, we have observed that the active, experiential and artistic methodology facilitates the development of parental competences related to positive parenting, good interaction and

Table 17.3 Objectives of the intervention (Hervás Hermida 2018, p. 849)

- To promote wellbeing, relaxation from stress, disconnection from routine and foster internal connection.
- To offer a space of emotional support and an opportunity for emotional expression, reflection and elaboration on the experience of parenting and family life.
- To encourage personal development, better self-esteem, autonomy and empowerment, through a better awareness of one's own needs and skills.
- To raise the development of healthy bonding, both with the children, as well as with the couple, the family, and the group, as a network of mutual support.
- To foster the development of parental skills, especially those based on resilience and good interaction.
- To boost a rich, creative and healthy perception of the experience of motherhood and upbringing.

resilience. The exploration of family patterns through the creative process and artworks allows the visualisation of the family as a system and the creation of new ways of interaction that include positive discipline and the setting of limits. This is very important as it fosters the transformation of insecure attachment styles and violent interaction patterns, developing greater confidence and strengthening bonds. Finally, as Grosser Villar (2007) emphasises, Art Therapy can boost resilience as a protective factor for mothers having difficulties, aiding them to connect with their motherhood in a positive way and have a better future perspective. Parenting then becomes a source of strength, motivation and empowerment.

Art Therapy methods for motherhood and family care: Guidelines for practice

The evaluation and comparative analysis of the different aspects of the Art Therapy intervention developed in my research and the analysis of literature allowed me to draw some conclusions and findings in terms of guidelines and recommendations for practice. In general terms, as explained above, I propose an active, experiential and creative methodology, where group creation works as a learning environment. This is based on the interactive group Art Therapy modality developed by Waller (1993), emphasising the role of the Art Therapist as mediator of the process.

Findings showed that participants valued especially the quality of the therapeutic relationship as a key element for the creation of a space for deepening of their awareness of personal issues and thus having an impact on their lives. The fact that I am a mother as well was appreciated, as empathy and resonances naturally emerged. Nevertheless, it also made me face my struggles with my own maternity experience, so in this kind of intervention where deep personal and family contents are revealed, it is especially important for the therapist to attend personal therapy and supervision.

The intervention followed a semi-directive approach, with open theme-centred directives. These were proposed attending to participants' needs, taking into account the symbolical potential of art materials and metaphors. Findings revealed participants valued the environment of respect, confidence and freedom created, as well as the importance of art materials and the creative process, as it provided moments of connection, joy and acknowledged significant family experiences. The sharing of information and collective reflection appeared as well as a key aspect, attending to resonances between the group members, with no expectancies, judgement or ideal parenting models. Parental competences and self-knowledge emerged from their own experience.

Other characteristics of the methodology are:

- The use of varied materials: drawing, painting, clay modelling, sculpture, play, puppets, etc. Specially the use of home-related materials: food, flour, cloth, recycled items, etc. which inspired them to talk about daily issues like feeding, sleeping, conflicts, limits, etc.

- The use of projective, creative and integrative techniques in order to enhance awareness and articulation of their issues.
- Other techniques such as relaxation and visualisation techniques, meditation, breathing exercises, massage, movement, dance, music, storytelling, etc.

Another important issue to take to account, especially within the dyadic setting, is the impact of children and parents participating together. On the one hand, children assist in the creation of an environment of spontaneity, joy and play necessary for the development of the Art Therapy process. But, on the other hand, it is important to highlight how this boosts the appearance of conflicts of autonomy and limits, and the need to manage this issue in order to avoid chaotic discharge and promote awareness, empowerment and non-violent solutions (see Figure 17.3).

> Ramona had a revealing experience related to the conflicts of autonomy and limits in the family group. When modelling with her son (aged three), she said about the choice of colour that she wanted to take the dark blue but her son wanted yellow, and so it all became green. She explained that she wanted to create something related to the sea, and then she was not able, and this made her feel upset. This experience aided her to articulate her fear to confront her son, and her doubts about whether she was letting him take more decisions than he should, and consider the need to clarify and set limits.

Looking at the duration of the intervention, the different timeframes experienced, from two to 20 sessions long, and the good results obtained in the evaluation of each

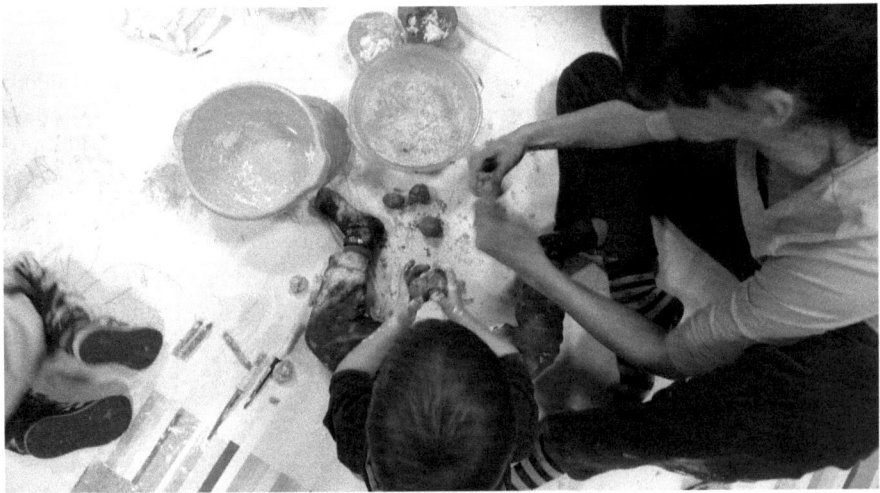

Figure 17.3 Green Bowl. Family Art Therapy with a dyadic approach, mothers and infants participating together. Image and text by the participants of the Art Therapy workshop developed in Aranjuez, Spain, 2015.

of them, make me conclude that it can be pretty flexible. Even short interventions can foster a process of awareness and change. The difficulties expressed by women for work–life balance imply that the possibility to participate in a short but effective intervention is highly valued. This is consistent with Ponteri (2001), Demecs et al. (2011), as well as Proulx (2003), who maintain that an eight-session format is suitable and cost-effective. Nevertheless, a longer duration would allow a deeper process.

Conclusions

As we have observed, there are many ways in which Art Therapy can be useful to support positive parenting. In each kind of setting, the presence of the art language within the group learning environment shows the possibilities for the exploration of maternal and family issues, and the development of parental competences. This is very relevant, as it affords a unique way of preventive intervention that incorporates the creative dimension of motherhood and family life, while seeking to develop more egalitarian and respectful family dynamics. The main principle that guides the intervention is then respect, a deep and sensitive respect given to all members of the family, their situation, feelings and needs, in order to promote the development of each person as an individual, as well as the family as a system. It is able to look at the conflicts of autonomy within the multiple levels of the family system, as well as to embrace diverse conceptions of parenting and family models. In that sense, I would like to emphasise the importance of the participants' involvement in the process, including the assessment and the evaluation stages.

Finally, I would like to reflect on the value of this proposal for social transformation. An intervention like this could play a highly powerful role for the co-construction of new symbolic representations of parenting and motherhood, through the active exploration and broadening of the collective imagination. This has a very important impact, as Muraro (1991), Sau (1995) and other feminist authors argued, about the need to create new models of maternal experience that could help women to overcome the maternal crisis. As Friedan (1963) said, the breaking of the invisible chains that constitute beliefs is imperative, for which Art Therapy can be an ally.

Note

1 Figures and quotations in this chapter are images created by parents in the Art Therapy interventions undertaken for my PhD research in Aranjuez and Calpe during the years 2015–2017.

References

Alonso Garrido, M. Á. 2012. *Mujeres y arteterapia*. PhD, Universidad Complutense of Madrid.

Armstrong, V. G., & Howatson, R. 2015. Parent–Infant Art Psychotherapy: A Creative Dyadic Approach to Early Intervention. *Infant Mental Health Journal*, 36: 213–222.

Badinter, E. 2011. *The Conflict: Women and Mother.* Melbourne: Text Publishing Company.

Bernal Martínez de Soria, A., & Sandoval Estupiñan, L.Y. 2013. Positive Parenting or Being Parents in the Family Education. *Estudios sobre Educación*, 25: 133–149.

Council of Europe. 1996. European Social Charter (revised). European Treaty Series, No. 163.

Council of Europe. 2006. Recommendation Rec 19.

Council of Europe, 1996. European Social Charter (revised). European Treaty Series – No. 163.

Demecs, I. P., Fenwick, J., & Gamble, J. 2011. Women's Experiences of Attending a Creative Arts Program during their Pregnancy. *Women and Birth*, 24: 112–121.

Friedan, B. 1963. *The Feminine Mystique.* New York: Norton and Co. Publishers.

González Sánchez, R., Martin Morales, S., & Roig Tomas, S. 2013. *Queriendo se entiende la familia. Guía de intervención sobre parentalidad positiva para profesionales.* Madrid: Save the Children.

Grosser Villar, H., 2007. El embarazo como un renacer. Una intervención de Arte Terapia en una mujer embarazada víctima de violencia intrafamiliar. Master's Thesis. Universidad de Chile, Santiago de Chile.

Hauser Dacer, J. 2016. Embarazo y Maternidad, las Desigualdades de Género y los Aportes del Arteterapia. Papeles Arteterapia Educ. *Artística Para Inclusión Soc*, 11: 151–161.

Hervás Hermida, L. 2018. *Arteterapia para la maternidad y la familia. Una vía de apoyo a la parentalidad positiva.* PhD, Universidad Autonoma of Madrid.

Hogan, S., 2012. Revisiting feminist approaches to art therapy. Berghahn Books, New York.

Hogan, S., 2003. Gender issues in art therapy. Jessica Kingsley Publishers, London.

Hogan, S. 1997. *Feminist Approaches in Art Therapy.* London: Routledge.

Hogan, S. 2003. *Gender Issues in Art Therapy.* London: Jessica Kingsley Publishers.

Hogan, S. 2012. Revisiting Feminist Approaches to Art Therapy. New York: Berghahn Books.

Hogan, S. 2015. Mothers Make Art: Using Participatory Art to Explore the Transition to Motherhood. *Journal of Applied Arts & Health*, 6(1): 23–32.

Hogan, S. 2016. *The Birth Project: Using the Arts to Explore Birth.* Interim report. University of Derby.

Hogan, S. 2017. The Tyranny of Expectations of Post-Natal Delight: Gendered Happiness. *Journal of Gender Studies*, 26: 45–55.

Hogan, S., Baker, C., Cornish, S., McCloskey, P., & Watts, L. 2015. Birth Shock: Exploring Pregnancy, Birth and the Transition to Motherhood Using Participatory Arts. In N. Burton (ed.), *Natal Signs Cultural Representations of Pregnancy, Birth and Parenting. Ontario: Demeter Press*, pp. 272–298.

Hogan, S., Sheffield, D., & Woodward, A. 2017. The Value of Art Therapy in Antenatal and Postnatal Care: A Brief Literature Review with Recommendations for Future Research. *International Journal of Art Therapy*, 22(4): 169–179.

Kerr, C., Hoshino, J., Sutherland, J., Parashak, S. T., & McCarley, L. L. 2011. *Family Art Therapy: Foundations of Theory and Practice.* New York: Routledge.

Lopez Fernandez Cao, M. 2000. *Creación artística y mujeres: recuperar la memoria.* Madrid: Narcea.

Lozano Estivalis, M. 2006. *La maternidad en escena. Mujeres, reproducción y representación cultural.* Zaragoza: Prensas Universitarias de Zaragoza.

Martín-Quintana, J. C., Máiquez Chaves, M., Rodrigo López, M., Byme, S., Rodríguez Ruiz, B., & Rodríguez Suárez, G. 2009. Programas de educación parental. *Interv Psicosoc*, 18: 121–133.

Miller, A. 1980. *For Your Own Good.* New York: Noonday Press.

Muraro, L. 1991. The Symbolic Order of the Mother. New York: SUNY Press.

Nussbaum, M. C. 2000. *Women and Human Development: The Capabilities Approach.* Cambridge: Cambridge University Press.

Ponteri, A. K. 2001. The Effect of Group Art Therapy on Depressed Mothers and their Children. *Art Therapy*, 18: 148–157.

Proulx, L. 2003. Strengthening Emotional Ties through Parent–Child-Dyad Art Therapy: Interventions with Infants and Preschoolers. London: Jessica Kingsley Publishers.

Regev, D., & Snir, S. 2015. Objectives, Interventions and Challenges in Parent–Child Art Psychotherapy. *The Arts in Psychotherapy*, 42: 50–56.

Rich, A. 1978. *Of Woman Born: Motherhood as Experience and Institution.* New York: Norton and Co. Publishers.

Riley, S., & Malchiodi, C. A. 2003. Family Art Therapy. In C. A. Malchuidi (ed.), *Handbook of Art Therapy.* New York: Guilford Press, pp. 387–398.

Rodrigo López, M. J. 2015. *Manual práctico de parentalidad positiva.* Madrid: De sintesis.

Rodrigo López, M. J., Amorós Martí, P., Arranz Freijo, E., Hidalgo García, M. V., Máiquez Chaves, M. L., Martín Quintana, J. C., Martínez González, R. A., & Ochaita Alderete, E. 2015. *Guía de buenas prácticas de parentalidad positiva. Un recurso para apoyar la práctica profesional con familias.* Ministerio de Sanidad, Servicios Sociales e Igualdad. Federación Española de Municipios y Provincias.

Rodrigo Lopez, M. J., Máiquez Chaves, M. L., & Martín Quintana, J. C. 2010. *Parentalidad positiva y politicas locales de apoyo.* Madrid: FEMP Federación Española de Municipios y Provincias.

Sau, V. 1995. *El vacío de la maternidad. Madre no hay más que ninguna.* Barcelona: Icaria Editorial.

Stern, D. N., Bruschweiler-Stern, N., & Freeland, A. 1999. *The Birth of a Mother: How the Motherhood Experience Changes You Forever.* New York: Basic Books.

Swan-Foster, N. 1989. Images of Pregnant Women: Art Therapy as a Tool for Transformation. *The Arts in Psychotherapy*, 16: 283–292.

Swan-Foster, N. 2012. Pregnancy as a Feminine Initiation. *Journal of Prenatal & Perinatal Psychology & Health*, 26(4): 207–235.

Swan-Foster, N., Foster, S., & Dorsey, A. 2003. The Use of the Human Figure Drawing with Pregnant Women. *Journal of Reproductive and Infant Psychology*, 21: 293–307.

Taylor Buck, E. 2015. *Development of a Manual for Dyadic Parent–Child Art Therapy*, PhD, University of Sheffield.

Taylor Buck, E., Dent-Brown, K., Parry, G., & Boote, J. 2014. Dyadic Art Psychotherapy: Key Principles, Practices and Competences. *The Arts in Psychotherapy*, 41: 163–173.

Téllez Infantes, A., & Heras González, P. 2004. Representaciones de género y ma- tenridad: una aproximación desde la antropología sociocultural. In S. Capporale Bizzini (ed.), *Discursos Teóricos En Torno a La(s) Maternidad(Es). Una Visión Integradora.* Madrid: Entinema, pp. 63–101.

Waller, D. 1993. *Group Interactive Art Therapy: Its Use in Training and Treatment.* London: Routledge.

Index

abortion 20, 23–24, 27–29, 33, 41, 99, 101–102, 132, 164
abuse 124–125, 136–167, 146–147, 154, 163, 236, 239; abuse of power 4–6, 8, 162, 236; sexual abuse 42, 44, 228
abnormality (foetal) 24
ageing 86
ambivalence 1, 5, 72, 74–76, 80, 107, 110–113, 121, 127, 131, 140, 144, 151, 187, 212, 226, 246
anaesthetic 217, 223
analytical (Jungian) 85, 211, 223, 227
anger 9, 14, 19, 28–29, 72, 75–76, 80, 85; socialised not to express anger 28
antenatal 8, 51, 194, 208, 225, 241, 254 (all same reference)
asexual 99

baby blues 77
beauty 84, 88, 98
birthplan 45, 49, 51; guilt at not going to plan 187
blackness 124; disproportionately high death rate 5; binary 72; see also multi-cultural 142, 136, 228, 233
bleeding 66, 237
blood transfusion 217
body image (release of toxic feelings) 34, 43, 44–48, 52, 79; (failure of), 54, 63, 66–67; cultural 71–73, 84, 86, 91, 98, 100, 104, 110–111, 159; of colour, 157; in relation to violence 163, 222, 227, 234; trans 178; PTS 217
breast feeding 2, 7, 71, 73, 76, 86, 93, 183, 186–187, 220

caesarean section 4, 43, 72, 101
capitalism 103

conception 66, 85, 161, 168
contractions 2, 26, 191

deaths 4, 8, 13, 15, 21, 23, 25–27, 31, 35, 38, 40–42, 57, 59, 85, 91, 96, 98, 111, 133–134, 144–145, 152, 156, 174, 213, 215, 221, 233
danger 90–91, 222; in relation to abortion 99; trans 178; bad mother 218
depression xviii, 7, 9, 42–43, 52, 72–77, 85–87, 107; challenge to term post-natal depression 6; in relation to miscarriage 27–28, 34; infertility 33
domestic abuse 124; see also violence against women

ectopic pregnancy 23, 53, 66–67
embryos 24, 36, 66, 139
empowering 17, 19, 23, 78, 84–85, 115, 117, 138, 141, 201, 239; for positive parenting 244–247, 249–252
epidural 216
episiotomy 4; lack of informed consent 4
equality 3, 7; onset of inequality 3, 98–99, 245
expressionistic 231

fallopian tubes 66
fear 24, 31–32, 34, 80, 115–116, 113, 117, 206, 210–212, 217–218, 222, 224, 230–233, 237, 246, 249, 252; fear of death 26, 42–52; fear of child's removal 2, 229; of commitment 5; loving two children 187–190; women feared 89–90
feminism 87, 106, 112, 171, 174, 224–225
fertility 10–11, 51, 88–89, 174; trans 168–169, 182. See also infertility
flourishing 142

foetal 24, 57, 135–136, 139, 169, 237; remains 27; maternal-foetal attachment 126, 128, 132
forceps 216

gender 84–87, 102, 104, 111, 124, 136, 154, 157, 165–182, 194, 211, 214, 225–226, 229, 237, 239, 245, 247, 254
gestation 8, 56, 102, 236
group art therapy 251; see also social support
gynaecologist 84, 213, 226

haemorrhaging 220; see also bleeding
hope; words of hope 2; hopes and fears 24–26, 31–34, 37, 39, 45, 52–59, 61, 66, 115, 118, 135, 139, 142–148, 210, 234, 238, 248, 250

iatrogenic 7, 214
in-utero 124–125, 129, 132, 134
induction 3–4
infertility 1, 9, 13–14, 18–22, 24–25, 27–28, 31–35, 38–41, 53–56, 58–61, 88
IVF 13, 23, 63–64, 67, 169

labour 73–74, 138, 169–170, 191, 224; length 3–4; risks and benefits discussed 4
liminality 1, 171
loss 26; fear of 44, 51; ill-treatment during labour 154; division of labour 77, 99
love 5, 25, 34, 72, 84, 86, 88, 108, 113–114, 117–122, 145–148, 160, 172, 180, 188, 194, 226, 235–236, 246, 249; unconditionally 6, 75, 140

matrescence 71–80, 82–87
metaphor 1, 6, 9, 16, 18–19, 21, 53–54, 63, 69, 77, 82, 94, 138, 141–143, 149, 188, 212, 232, 250–251
midwife 43–44, 49, 72, 84, 122–123, 154, 157, 220
motherhood; foreword; changed identity 1–8
mutual support 2, 118, 201, 247, 249–250

natural conception 67; mothering as natural (and essentialism) 75, 103–104,

150, 161, 220; time of labour 3; research process 11, 15; birth 101; trans 165, 168; art making 205–206, 223, 251
newborn 91

obstetrician 84, 183, 213, 226; obstetric abuse and violence 4, 7, 152–155, 157–164
oppression; foreword 103, 165, 170, 246

patriarchy 95
postnatal distress 138, 210; care into 183; value of 194, 208, 241
postnatal depression 87, 183, 208, 209–210, 225; non identification with term 7
prematurity 190

queering 165–175, 177–181

racism 5, 93

social support, importance of 1, 6, 72–79, 84, 118, 149, 155, 164, 176, 183–184, 194–195, 197, 199, 213–214, 226, 244–249, 253, 255; supporting families 22; 247–253, 255; support in getting to the group 134
surrogacy 103–105; in trans context 168
stillbirth 4, 8, 22–23, 27, 28, 33–35, 39, 40–41, 53

termination of pregnancy 24, 53, 57, 68, 233, 237; see also abortion
trauma, traumatic birth 1, 5, 20, 42, 44, 48; loss 26–27, 31–37

ultrasound 27, 29, 63
uterus 23, 37, 66

violence against women; during pregnancy 6–7, 155, 163–164; in relationships 6–8; obstetric violence 4, 152–164; societal 98, 136; against trans women of colour 169, 181

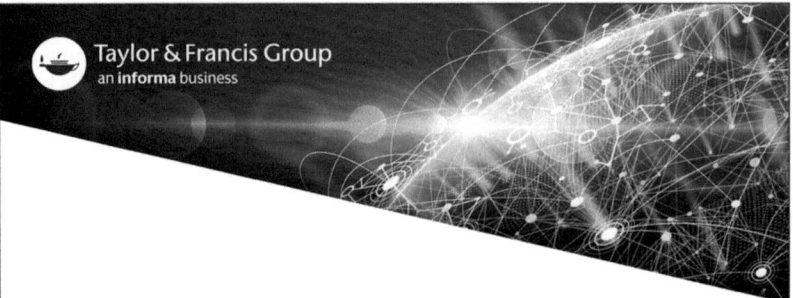
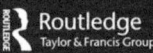
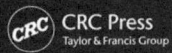